Oxford Handbook of
Clinical Skills for Children's and Young People's Nursing

Paula Dawson MSc in Advanced
Nursing Practice, RGN, RSCN, PGCHE

Lecturer, Child Health
School of Nursing, Midwifery and Physiotherapy, University of Nottingham, UK

Louise Cook BSc, RN Child, PGCHE

Lecturer, Child Health
School of Nursing, Midwifery and Physiotherapy,
University of Nottingham, UK

Laura-Jane Holliday Master of
Nursing Science, RN Child

Practitioner Health Lecturer, Child Health
School of Nursing, Midwifery and Physiotherapy,
University of Nottingham, UK;
Preceptorship Development Nurse, Medicine and
Respiratory Staff Nurse
Nottingham Children's Hospital, Nottingham
University Hospitals NHS Trust, Nottingham, UK

Helen Reddy MA with Education,
BSc (Hons) in Neurological Care, Diploma of
Higher Education in Nursing, RN Child

Practitioner Health Lecturer, Child Health
School of Nursing, Midwifery and Physiotherapy,
University of Nottingham, UK;
Junior Sister, Paediatric Neurosciences
Nottingham Children's Hospital, Nottingham University Hospitals
NHS Trust, Nottingham, UK

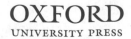

OXFORD
UNIVERSITY PRESS

OXFORD
UNIVERSITY PRESS

Great Clarendon Street, Oxford OX2 6DP
United Kingdom

Oxford University Press is a department of the University of Oxford.
It furthers the University's objective of excellence in research, scholarship,
and education by publishing worldwide. Oxford is a registered trade mark of
Oxford University Press in the UK and in certain other countries

First Edition published in 2012
Impression: 1

British Library Cataloguing in Publication Data
Data available

Library of Congress Cataloguing in Publication Data
Data available

ISBN 978–0–19–959346–0

Printed in China
on acid-free paper by
C&C Offset Printing

Oxford University Press makes no representation, express or implied, that the
drug dosages in this book are correct. Readers must therefore always check
the product information and clinical procedures with the most up-to-date
published product information and data sheets provided by the manufacturers
and the most recent codes of conduct and safety regulations. The authors and
the publishers do not accept responsibility or legal liability for any errors in the
text or for the misuse or misapplication of material in this work. Except where
otherwise stated, drug dosages and recommendations are for the non-pregnant
adult who is not breast-feeding

Links to third party websites are provided by Oxford in good faith and
for information only. Oxford disclaims any responsibility for the materials
contained in any third party website referenced in this work.

Foreword

Healthcare is under considerable pressure to continuously improve and respond to the changing needs of populations with safe, high quality care. For children and young people's services this is particularly intense for a range of reasons, not least because they are a highly vulnerable care group, often unable to speak for themselves. However, two key reasons stand out in particular. First, children are surviving longer because treatments and technologies are advancing at an extraordinary pace. As a result there is an increasing number of children who need highly effective nursing interventions because of their complex conditions. Secondly, the focus of attention is now on the whole child. This means nurses increasingly have not only to ensure they consider the prevention of ill health, but also to encourage the maintenance of good health. Both are core, but often forgotten components of all care delivery.

In addition nurses need to be confident to work across a range of different agencies, ensuring children are treated as individuals and that their families are fully involved. Collaboration is crucial to ensure working together in a planned way, not only making professional sense, but also leading to children and young people receiving the services they deserve. The focus should always be on the things that matter to them and the best possible outcome of their health care.

Nurses therefore need practical concise reference tools that provide them with both clinical guidance and importantly, the best evidence available on which to confidently base their decisions. This book adds to the rich body of evidence already available and will be a valuable resource to assist nurses in not only providing the very best clinical care possible, but also enabling them to speak up for children and young people about their health needs.

Professor Dame Elizabeth Fradd DBE
Independent Health Services Adviser
Fellow of the Royal College of Nursing
Fellow of the Queens Nursing Institute
Honorary Fellow of the Royal College of Paediatrics and Child Health
Honorary Member of the faculty of Public Health
Honorary Dsc Wolverhampton University
Honorary D University Central England. Hon LLD Nottingham
Ambassador for Children's Hospices UK
Vice President of Rainbows Hospice for Children and Young People
Honorary Professor Nottingham University
Visiting Professor Birmingham City University
Member of Nottingham University Council
Chair National HV Taskforce
June 2011

Preface

The assessment, planning, and delivery of evidence-based and skilled nursing care forms the very bedrock of an excellent care experience for children, young people and their families.

This book aims to provide a concise, current, and evidence-based guide to clinical skills relating to the care of children and young people.

All content has been thoroughly researched and reviewed to ensure that it is current and reliable. Theory underpinning the principles and procedures has been kept to a minimum within the text, with the emphasis being to provide information that will be directly relevant to the skill being undertaken in the care setting. Key references to seminal papers, guidelines, and websites are included at the end of each topic.

Members of the University of Nottingham's Division of Nursing Child Health Team are delighted to have worked on this text, in collaboration with children and young people's nurses from all around the UK.

Practising nursing professionals have contributed their knowledge and expertise by developing the evidence-based guidelines, and adding their own personal tips for good practice, gained through experience, consultation, and collaboration with children, young people, families, and colleagues.

We hope that this will become a well-thumbed volume, which takes its place in your bag or pocket as a reliable companion, as you work to develop and enhance your clinical skills to the very highest standard for the children and young people in your care.

Paula Dawson
Louise Cook
Laura Holliday
Helen Reddy

Contents

Contributors

Krystina Alex
Advanced Neonatal Nurse
Practitioner
Diana, Princess of Wales Hospital
Grimsby, UK

Carol Arme
Named Nurse for Safeguarding
Children
Nottingham Children's Hospital
Nottingham University Hospitals
NHS Trust, UK

Katie Bagstaff
Senior Sister, Paediatric Recovery
Cambridge University Hospitals
NHS Foundation Trust, UK

Michelle Bennett
Clinical Nurse Specialist,
Children's Pain Management
Nottingham Children's Hospital
Nottingham University Hospitals
NHS Trust, UK

Karen Blair
PGCLT Honorary Lecturer,
Canterbury Christchurch
University
Paediatric Constipation Nurse
Specialist
Norfolk and Norwich University
Hospital and Looked After
Children Specialist Nurse
Great Yarmouth and Waveney
Community Services, UK

Diane Blyton
Paediatric Renal Nurse
Educator, Children's Renal and
Urology Unit
Nottingham Children's Hospital
Nottingham University Hospitals
NHS Trust, UK

Rachel Bower
Retrieval Coordinator, PICU
Nottingham Children's Hospital
Nottingham University Hospitals
NHS Trust, UK

Lorna Bramwells
Matron, Acute Paediatrics
Queen Mary's Hospital for
Children
Epsom & St Helier NHS Trust, UK

Mary Brown
University Teacher
School of Nursing, Midwifery and
Physiotherapy
Nottingham University, UK

Gozia Brykcynska
Senior Lecturer in Child Health
University of West London, UK

Claire Burville
Senior Staff Nurse, Paediatric
Surgery
Children's Hospital
Oxford Radcliffe NHS Trust, UK

Carol Chamley
Senior Lecturer, Children and
Young People's Nursing
Coventry University, UK

Dave Clarke
Lecturer and Programme Manager
Children and Young People's
Nursing
School of Nursing and Midwifery
Studies
Cardiff University, UK

Mitch Clarke
Infection Prevention and Control
Nurse Specialist
Nottingham University Hospitals
NHS Trust, UK

David Coan
Senior Matron for Children
Services
New Cross Hospital
Wolverhampton, UK

Jacqueline Collin
Lecturer
Keele University, UK

Steven Collis
Clinical Nurse Specialist, Home
Oxygen Assessment
Chesterfield Royal Hospital NHS
Foundation Trust, UK

Roy Connell
Independent Nurse Prescriber
Nottingham Children's Hospital
Nottingham University Hospitals
NHS Trust, UK

Rebecca Cooke
Transition Nurse Coordinator,
Paediatric Haemoglobinopathy
Birmingham Children's Hospital,
UK

Marianne Craig
Eye Clinic Liaison Nurse
Great Ormond Street Hospital for
Children
London, UK

Jane Davies
Senior Lecturer and Professional
Head, Children and Young
People's Nursing
School of Nursing and Midwifery
Studies
Cardiff University, UK

Patric Devitt
Senior Lecturer in Child Health
School of Nursing, Midwifery &
Social Work
The University of Salford, UK

Sue Doherty
Paediatric Diabetes Specialist
Nurse
Derbyshire Children's Hospital
Derby Hospitals NHS Foundation
Trust, UK

Elaine Domek
Paediatric Nurse Practitioner
James Paget University Hospitals
NHS Foundation Trust
Norfolk, UK

Amy Dopson
Child Health Tutor
University of Surrey, UK

Mandy Doran
Childhood Bereavement Councillor
Deputy Head of Family Support
(Bereavement)
Senior Nurse
Rainbows Hospice for Children
and Young People
Loughborough, UK

Sharon Douglass
Clinical Nurse Specialist in
Children's Pain Management
Nottingham Children's Hospital
Nottingham University Hospitals
NHS Trust, UK

Joanna Doyle
Senior Nurse Manager, Children's
Community Nursing Service
Aneurin Bevan Health Board, UK

Helena Dunbar
Consultant Nurse for Paediatric
Respiratory Diseases
Leicester Royal Infirmary NHS
Trust, UK

Jo Dursley
Staff Nurse, Children's Emergency
Department
Derby Hospitals NHS Foundation
Trust, UK

Julie Eaton
Clinical Nurse Specialist, Paediatric
Oncology
University Hospital of North
Staffordshire, UK

Shaun Edwards
Staff Nurse, Neonatal Intensive
Care Unit
Derby Hospitals NHS Foundation
Trust, UK

Claire Fellows
Junior Sister/Clinical Skills
Facilitator, PICU
Birmingham Children's Hospital
NHS Foundation Trust, UK

Emma Fitzsimmons
Staff Nurse
Nottingham Children's Hospital
Nottingham University Hospital
NHS Trust, UK

Ellie Forbes
Clinical Coordinator/Trainee
Senior Nurse Practitioner
Royal Hospital for Sick Children
Edinburgh, UK

Helen Frizell
Lead Educator, Maternal & Child
Health
Basingstoke & North Hampshire
NHS Foundation Trust, UK

Caroline Galloway
Play Specialist, Children's Gastro
Unit
Nottingham Children's Hospital
Nottingham University Hospitals
NHS Trust, UK

Emma Gamble
Paediatric Urology Nurse
Specialist
Children's Renal and Urology Unit
Nottingham Children's Hospital
Nottingham University Hospitals
NHS Trust, UK

Catherine Gibney
Play Specialist, Oncology Day Care
Nottingham Children's Hospital
Nottingham University Hospitals
NHS Trust, UK

Liz Gormley-Fleming
Senior Lecturer Children's Nursing
Principal Lecturer LTI
University of Hertfordshire, UK

Claire Hardy
Play Specialist, Children's Renal Unit
Nottingham Children's Hospital
Nottingham University Hospitals
NHS Trust, UK

Julie Harvey
Epsom & St Helier University
Hospitals NHS Trust, UK

Janet Holmes
Paediatric Orthopaedic Nurse
Specialist
Nottingham Children's Hospital
Nottingham University Hospitals
NHS Trust, UK

Shelley Jepson
Lead Nurse, Paediatric
Nephrology
Nottingham Children's Hospital
Nottingham University Hospitals
NHS Trust, UK

Peter Johnston
Paediatric Clinical Educator,
Community Children's Nursing
Acorn Centre
Ballymoney
Northern Ireland, UK

Chris Jones
Senior Lecturer in Clinical Skills
(Child Health)
Birmingham City University, UK

Julia Judd
Advanced Nurse Practitioner
Southampton University Hospital,
UK

Laura Kane
Staff Nurse, PICU
Nottingham Children's Hospital
Nottingham University Hospitals
NHS Trust, UK

Sue Keeble
CNS Children and Young
Persons's Urology and
Continence Service
London, UK

Sara Keetley-Betts
Infection Prevention and Control
Matron
Nottingham University Hospitals
Trust, UK

Debbie Kilman
Modern Matron/Deputy Lead
Nurse, Children's Services
Cheltenham General Hospital,
UK

Sue Lawrence
Senior Lecturer, Clinical Skills
Birmingham City University, UK

Sandra Lawton
Nurse Consultant, Dermatology
Queen's Medical Centre
Nottingham University Hospitals
NHS Trust, UK

Angela Lee
Paediatric Nurse Consultant for
Trauma and Orthopaedics
Royal Berkshire NHS Foundation
Trust
Reading, UK

Alison Legge
Clinical Development Nurse, Trent
Regional Cleft Lip & Palate Service
Nottingham, UK

Joseph Manning
Research Fellow/Honorary
Paediatric Intensive Care Nurse
School of Nursing, Midwifery &
Physiotherapy
University of Nottingham;
Paediatric Intensive Care Unit
Nottingham Children's Hospital
Nottingham University Hospitals
NHS Trust, UK

Tim McDougall
Nurse Consultant/Clinical Director
(Tier 4 CAMHS)
Cheshire & Wirral Partnership
NHS Foundation Trust, UK

Virginia McGivern
Complementary Therapy Nurse
Specialist
Nottingham Children's Hospital
Nottingham University Hospitals
NHS Trust, UK

Lin McGraw
Matron, Paediatrics
Queen Mary's Hospital for Children
Surrey, UK

Molly McLaughlin
Paediatric Renal Critical Care
Nurse
Children's Renal & Urology Unit
Nottingham Children's Hospital
Nottingham University Hospitals
NHS Trust, UK

Ann McMurray
Asthma Nurse Specialist
Royal Hospital for Sick Children
Edinburgh, UK

Patricia McNeilly
Teaching Fellow, School of Nursing
and Midwifery;
PhD Candidate, School of Sociology,
Social Policy and Social Work
Queen's University Belfast, UK

Roni Middleton
Deputy Sister, Children's Burns
and Plastics Unit
Nottingham Children's Hospital
Nottingham University Hospital
NHS Trust, UK

Anna Mycock
Junior Sister, Paediatric
Neurosciences
Nottingham Children's Hospital
Nottingham University Hospitals
NHS Trust, UK

Diane Norton
Senior Lecturer, Department of
Family Care and Mental Health
University of Greenwich, UK

Janet Orr
Associate Lecturer, Child and
Adult Health Nursing
Faculty of Health
University of Plymouth, UK

Alyson Packham
Named Nurse Safeguarding
Queen's Medical Centre
Nottingham University Hospitals
NHS Trust, UK

Alison Parnham
Clinical Nurse Specialist
Nottingham CityCare Partnership,
UK

Jeanette Pearce
Resuscitation Officer/Clinical Skills
Facilitator Paediatrics
Resuscitation Department/
Paediatric Department
Gloucestershire Hospitals NHSFT,
UK

Clare Pedley
Senior Sister, Emergency
Department
Birmingham Children's Hospital
NHS Foundation Trust, UK

Jacqueline Randle
Associate Professor, Clinical
Skills Lead for Masters of Nursing
Science
School of Nursing
Midwifery & Physiotherapy
University of Nottingham, UK

Sheila Roberts
Senior Lecturer, Children's Nursing
University of Hertfordshire, UK

June Rogers
PromoCon Team Director,
Disabled Living NW
Manchester, UK

Katie Rogers
Clinical Educator, East Midlands
Children's and Young Persons'
Integrated Cancer Service
Nottingham University Hospitals
NHS Trust, UK

Helen Rollé
Advanced Children's Emergency
Nurse Practitioner
Derby Hospitals NHS Foundation
Trust, UK

Ruth Sadik
Senior Lecturer in Child Health
Faculty of Health and Social Care
University of Chester, UK

Jo Sims
Head of Family Support
Rainbows Hospice for Children
and Young People
Loughborough, UK

Janine Stanway
Health Visitor
Derbyshire Healthcare NHS
Foundation Trust
Austin/Sunnyhill Surestart, UK

Alison Taylor
Paediatric Practice Development
Nurse
Western Sussex Hospitals NHS
Trust, UK

Kelly Thompson
Student Health Visitor
(Children's Nurse)
Derbyshire Healthcare NHS
Foundation Trust, UK

Jackie Vasey
Senior Lecturer, Child Nursing
University of Huddersfield, UK

James Vass
Ward Manager
Wellcome Trust Clinical Research
Facility
Birmingham Children's Hospital,
UK

Natalie Vaughan
Clinical Lead Infection Prevention
and Control
Nottingham University Hospitals
Trust, UK

Kerry Webb
Clinical Development Sister, PICU
Nottingham Children's Hospital
Nottingham University Hospitals
NHS Trust, UK

Carli Whittaker
Critical Care Educator, PICU
Nottingham Children's Hospital
Nottingham University Hospitals
NHS Trust, UK

Jo Williams
Advanced Nurse Practitioner, ENT
Birmingham Children's Hospital
NHS Foundation Trust, UK

Matthew Williams
Paediatric Diabetes Specialist
Nurse
Nottingham Children's Hospital
Nottingham University Hospitals
NHS Trust, UK

Karen Williamson
Hospital Children's Nurse
NHS Shetland, UK

Catherine Wills
Staff Nurse
Nottingham Children's Hospital
Nottingham University Hospitals
NHS Trust, UK

Ali Wright
Gastrostomy Nurse Specialist
Nottingham Children's Hospital
Nottingham University Hospitals
NHS Trust, UK

Elizabeth Wright
Advanced Nurse Practitioner
Southampton University Hospitals
NHS Trust, UK

Symbols and abbreviations

❶	warning/stop
⚠	warning
▶	important
▶▶	don't dawdle
<	less than
>	more than
±	plus/minus
~	approximately
↑	increased
↓	decreased
ABCDE	airway, breathing, circulation, disability, exposure to ensure full examination
ACBT	active cycle of breathing techniques
AD	autogenic drainage
AFO	ankle–foot orthosis
AGE	acute gastro enteritis
AIRS	adverse incident reporting system
ANTT	aseptic non-touch technique
APAGBI	Association of Paediatric Anaesthetists of Great Britain and Ireland
ARDS	acute respiratory distress syndrome
AVPU	alert, voice, pain, unresponsive
BCV	biphasic cuirass ventilation
BE	base excess
BG	blood glucose
BiPAP	bilevel positive airway pressure
BLS	basic life support
BMI	body mass index
BNFC	British National Formulary for Children
BP	blood pressure
bpm	beats per minute
Ca	calcium
CO_2	carbon dioxide
CAF	common assessment framework
CAMHS	Child and Adolescent Mental Health Services
CAPD	continuous ambulatory peritoneal dialysis

CBT	cognitive behavioural therapy
CCN	children's community nursing
CCPD	continuous cycling peritoneal dialysis
CD	controlled drug
CDC	child development centre
CE	Conformité Européene (European Conformity)
Ch	Charrière—the outer circumference of the catheter in mm
CHD	congenital heart defect
Cl	chloride
cms	centimetres
CMV	cytomegalovirus
CNS	central nervous system
CPAP	continuous positive airway pressure
CPR	cardiopulmonary resuscitation
CRT	capillary refill time
CSF	cerebrospinal fluid
CSII	continuous subcutaneous insulin infusion
CSSD	Central Sterile Supply Department
CSU	catheter specimen of urine
CT	computerised tomography
CVAD	central venous access device
CVC	central venous catheter
CVI	Certificate of Visual Impairment
CVL	central venous line
CVP	central venous pressure
CVVH	continuous veno-venous haemofiltration
CVVHDF	continuous veno-venous haemodiafiltration
CXR	chest X-ray
CYP	children and young people
DCSF	Department for Children, Schools and Families
DIC	disseminated intravascular coagulation
DKA	diabetic ketoacidosis
DM	diabetes mellitus
DoH	Department of Health
DVT	deep vein thrombosis
EBM	expressed breast milk
ECG	electrocardiogram
EIA	equality impact assessment
ENT	ear, nose and throat
EPO	Emergency Protection Order

EPUAP	European Pressure Ulcer Advisory Panel
ETT	endotracheal tube
EVD	external ventricular drain
FB	foreign body
FBC	full blood count
FEV_1	forced expiratory volume per second
FFP	fresh frozen plasma
FG	French gauge
FiO_2	fractional inspired oxygen concentration
FRC	functional residual capacity
FVC	forced vital capacity
GA	general anaesthetic
GCS	Glasgow Coma Scale
GI	gastrointestinal
GP	general practitioner
H+	hydrogen
H_2O	water
H_2CO_3	carbonic acid
HAS	human albumin solution
Hb	haemoglobin
HCO_3	bicarbonate
HCP	health care professional
HCW	health care worker
HDU	high dependency unit
HEI	Higher Education Institution
HME	heat and moisture exchange
HPS	hospital play specialist
h	hour
HR	heart rate
HSWA	Health and Safety at Work Act
IBS	irritable bowel syndrome
ICP	intracranial pressure
IgE	immunoglobulin E
IM	intramuscular
IMF	immunofluoroescence
IMCA	independent mental capacity advocate
IO	intraosseous
IPCT	infection prevention and control team
iu	international units
IV	intravenous

K	potassium
kPa	kilopascals (unit of pressure)
LA	local anaesthetic
LFT	liver function test
LP	lumbar puncture
LSCB	Local Safeguarding Children Board
MAP	multi-agency action plan
MCP	multi-agency care package
Mg	magnesium
MHRA	Medicines and Healthcare Products Regulatory Agency
min	minute
mmHg	millimetres of mercury
MODY	mature onset diabetes mellitus of the young
MRI	magnetic resonance imaging
MRSA	methicillin-resistant *Staphylococcus aureus*
MSU	mid-stream urine
MUST	Malnutrition Universal Screening Tool
Na	sodium
NaCl	sodium chloride
NAI	non-accidental injury
NBM	nil by mouth
NCA	nurse-controlled analgesia
NCCPC-PV	non-communicating children's pain checklist-postoperative version
NG	nasogastric
NGT	nasogastric tube
NICE	National Institute for Health and Clinical Excellence
NIV	non-invasive ventilation
NMC	Nursing and Midwifery Council
NPA	nasopharyngeal airway
NPA	nasopharyngeal aspirate
NPSA	National Patient Safety Agency
NPUAP	National Pressure Ulcer Advisory Panel
NSAID	non-steroidal anti-inflammatory drug
NSPCC	National Society for the Prevention of Cruelty to Children
NTE	neutral thermal environment
O_2	oxygen
OPA	oropharyngeal airway
OPEP	oscillating positive expiratory pressure devices

PaCO$_2$	artial pressure of carbon dioxide in arterial blood
PaO$_2$	artial pressure of oxygen in arterial blood
PCA	patient controlled analgesia
PCV	packed cell volume
PD	peritoneal dialysis
PDR	postural drainage
PEA	pulseless electrical activity
PEG	percutaneous endoscopic gastrostomy
PEP	positive expiratory pressure
PEWS	Paediatric Early Warning Score
PGD	patient group direction
PHDU	paediatric high dependency unit
PIC	peripheral intravenous cannula
PICC	peripherally inserted central catheter
PICU	paediatric intensive care unit
PIPP	Premature Infant Pain Profile
PN	parenteral nutrition
PONV	post-operative nausea and vomiting
POP	plaster of Paris
PPE	personal protective equipment
PPP	Paediatric Pain Profile
PPP	post-procedural play
PR	per rectum
psi	pounds per square inch (pressure unit)
PSV	pressure support ventilation
PVC	pressure volume catheter
PYMS	Paediatric Yorkhill Malnutrition Score
RAST test	radioallergosorbent test (allergy blood test)
RBC	red blood cells
RCN	Royal College of Nursing
RCNI	Royal College of Nursing Institute
RIDDOR	reporting of injuries, diseases and dangerous occurrences regulations
RR	respiratory rate
RRT	renal replacement therapy
RTA	road traffic accident
s	seconds
SaO$_2$	oxygen saturation of arterial blood
SC	subcutaneous
SCIDS	severe combined immune deficiency syndrome
SENCO	special educational needs co-ordinator

SIMV	synchronized intermittent mandatory ventilation
STD	sexually transmitted disease
TAC	team around the child
TFT	thyroid function test
TLC	tender loving care
TPN	total parenteral nutrition
TPR	temperature, pulse and respirations
TRALI	transfusion-related acute lung injury
U&Es	urea and electrolytes
UK	United Kingdom
UNCRC	United Nations Convention on the Rights of the Child
USS	ultrasound scan
UTI	urinary tract infection
VAD	vascular access device
VAP	ventilated acquired pneumonia
WHO	World Health Organization
yrs	years

Chapter 1

The principles of patient assessment

Initial observation of the child/young person

Background
A great deal of information can be gained when we first encounter a child and their family/carers, which may assist in assessment and appropriate communication processes. In addition to undertaking assessment of vital signs to assist in diagnosis, care planning and support needs, all health personnel should develop skills of observation and effective use of all their senses when undertaking their work.

Equipment
• Eyes, ears, hands, and nose.

Procedure
Look at your patient's physical condition:
• Are they breathing normally/breathless/a poor colour?
• Are they hot, distressed, hungry, thirsty, obviously in pain?
• Are they moving as you would expect for their age?
• Are they well hydrated?
• Are they overweight/underweight?
• Is their appearance consistent with their age?
• Can they hear you/see you?
• Do they have a rash, bruising, or unexplained marks on their body?
• Is their hygiene attended to?
• Do they seem happy/anxious/withdrawn, etc.?
• Are they dressed appropriately for the weather/environment?
• Signs of good or poor hygiene.
• Signs of alcohol/drug use.
• Signs of infection or ketosis.

If being seen at home, consider:
• Environment—temperature, facilities for child's needs/developmental level, toys, etc.
• Observe their interactions with others.
• Listen to your patient and their family/carers:
  • How they communicate—language and fluency, any 'special' words or names they use.
  • Listen for clues about interests and personalities (without being overly intrusive or familiar), e.g. favourite team, sports, TV, music, subjects at school, hobbies, activities, etc.

Practice tip
• Make sure that you consider cultural differences in behaviour—for example, shaking hands and/or body contact may be inappropriate in some situations, and eye contact is considered rude in some cultures.

Pitfalls
• Making judgements based on personal values.
• Making judgements based on 'first impressions'.

User and carer involvement

Involving patients and the public in health care is mandatory.
- The Health and Social Care Act[1] expects that health service users and their carers will be engaged in discussion and consultation about the provision of services.
- All health care providers are required to provide ways to involve patients in decisions about the organization.
- It is important that patient and carer involvement becomes embedded in the culture of the organization, avoiding tokenism.

'Getting the Right Start', The National Service Framework for Children and Young People[2] sets out the expectation that children, young people and parents/carers are able to participate in designing health services to ensure they are delivered around the needs of the user. In addition, children and young people must be given opportunities to make informed decisions about their health care journey.

In order to participate:
- Children and young people should be given access to information which is appropriate to their level of understanding.
- The skills of the multi-professional team should be utilized to ensure that information is provided in a variety of formats. Hospital play specialists, for example, are experts in presenting information using art, craft, and multi-media tools. Children have been involved in the development of health services by engaging them with theatre workshops, creative design and other such fun activities.

Hospital youth work teams are crucial to facilitate young people's participation in health services. The National Youth Agency reports that young people can be engaged in activity workshops that enable them to voice their ideas and feedback concerns about health services. Activities and meetings should take place in areas in which young people feel at ease, ideally outside a hospital environment. It is also good practice to identify peer mentors to represent young people's interests.

The expertise of patients and their carers should be recognized and utilized to educate and support other families. The Expert Patient Programme has been developed to facilitate this.

Paediatric nursing staff should be aware that programmes for family support, particularly for those with long-term conditions are available.

Associated reading
National Youth Agency (2008). *Nottingham University Hospital: Project Report*. Available at: ℘ http://www.nya.org.uk.

[1] Department of Health (2008). *Health and Social Care Act Part 1—The Care Quality Commission*. HMSO, London.
[2] Department of Health (2003). *National Service Framework for Children. Standard for Hospital Services*. HMSO, London.

History taking

Background

History taking, physical examination and investigation make up the assessment process. History taking is the first stage of the diagnostic and decision-making process, and should be carried out in all cases of a child/young person presenting to a health care provider—it will be the main determinant of care.

Pathophysiological, psychological, social, and spiritual history should be recorded as appropriate, and can be carried out by any member of the children and young people's health care team with the necessary knowledge of child development and communication skills.

Approaches to history taking

- Privacy and confidentiality should be considered.
- Check whether the child and family speak the majority language—access interpreting services if necessary.
- In acute situations the A, B, C, D approach (as per Advanced Paediatric Life Support guidelines) should be adopted.
- In all other situations personal or organizational philosophy should guide data collection.
- Gain access to child's health record.
- Utilize organizational model of care as a framework for history-taking. Most children's nursing models incorporate usual activities of daily living, the child/young person's ability to carry out daily routines with or without assistance, and the role that others play in assisting daily living.
- In all instances the history-taker should remember that the child/young person remains the focus of the history and that the parents are subsidiary data providers.
- Documentation giving signs, symptoms, feelings and understanding should be written using the actual words of the information provider.

Content of history

Current problem

- Time of onset, duration and previous presentations.
- Is there known contact with people with similar problems/infectious illness?
- How did problem develop?
- Does anything aggravate or relieve the problem?
- Has the problem prevented nursery/school attendance?
- Prescribed/over the counter medication.
- Current height/length and weight.

Family history

Often taken by medical personnel.

- Previous pregnancies/still births/miscarriages.
- Familial illnesses especially those with genetic causation.
- Consanguinity of parent's relationship.
- Neonatal history.
- Composition of genogramme.
- Recent foreign travel data.

Development
- Known developmental delay.
- Progress relating to normal milestones.
- Immunization and screening test results.
- Sexual development and activity.

Social history
- Composition of current and previous family units.
- *Child care providers*: name all.
- Parental occupation.
- School or nursery attendance.
- Eating and sleeping patterns.
- *Pets*: types and names.
- Housing issues.
- Smoking habits of child/family.

Psychological history
- *Mood and feelings*: use questionnaire if appropriate.
- Hobbies, interests, and group activities.
- Friendships/relationships.
- Perceived difficulties and coping mechanisms.

Practice tips
- Safeguarding issues should be considered at all times.
- Observe child and family members for non-verbal congruence with what is being said.
- Every child under the age of 3yrs should be seen in minimal clothing during the assessment period, which can be achieved during weight procedures or examination.
- Create some time to see the child away from their parents so that they can, if they wish, discuss sensitive issues without parental presence.
- Young people should be given the option of having parents present during history taking.
- Telephone interpretation services can be arranged/purchased via most health service providers—check your local policy.

Pitfalls
- Children around the age of 3yrs become very modest and undressing can be traumatic.
- Young people/parents may only partly disclose what they believe to be sensitive information, if privacy is compromised, e.g. if in an open area and/or only shielded from others by curtains, etc.

Associated reading
Bickley L (2009). *Bate's Pocket Guide to Physical Examination and History Taking* (International edn). Williams and Wilkins, London.
Kessenich C (2008). The art and science of history taking. *J Nurse Practit* **4**(4), 304–5.
Resuscitation Council (2010). *Paediatric Advanced Life Support*. Available at: ℔ http://www.resus.org.uk.

Vital signs/examination

Key concepts

What are the differences between **vital signs** and **examination**?

Vital signs are important physiological observations comprising: heart rate, temperature, respiratory rate, and blood pressure. Vital signs are necessary in order to establish how unwell the child is and to determine what interventions or treatments are required to stabilize the child.

Examination requires careful inspection and palpation of the child. This is usually done sequentially from head-to-toe.

The two are complimentary to each other and should be done in synchrony. However, the practice of undertaking the vital signs or the examination in a child who is unwell is no mean feat! How you approach the child will very much depend on the age, cognitive understanding and emotional understanding of the child. It is essential to know not just the normal values for the child, but equally their normal behaviour and normal appearance prior to approaching them. Previous history, previous experiences, and fear of the unknown can all impact on your ability to carry out the examination and take the child's vital signs accurately.

Procedure

When undertaking vital signs and examination, a structured approach is crucial to ensure that nothing gets missed. A base-line or set of vital signs and examination can then be completed and documented in a logical, sequential order.

This should be done using the:
- **A**irway
- **B**reathing
- **C**irculation
- **D**isability
- **E**xposure, as recommended by the Resuscitation Council.[1]
- **A**—is the airway clear, compromised, or obstructed?
- **B**—work of breathing, accessory muscle use, respiratory rate, oxygen saturations, colour.
- **C**—pulse, palpate pulses peripherally and centrally, temperature, capillary refill time, blood pressure, fluid intake, and urine output.
- **D**—responsiveness using are they Alert, responding to Voice, responding to Pain, or Unresponsive, pupil size and Don't Ever Forget Glucose.
- **E**—look front, back, and head-to-toe for bleeding, bruises, breaks, and burns.

Practice tips

(📖 Procedure, p.6)

- The approach should be done each time a child is assessed irrespective of frequency of process.
- One should not move on to the next letter without ensuring that the previous letter has been attended to.
- Build up trust and a rapport with the child and their family first. Explain to them what you are doing.
- *Look*—at the child, at the equipment, and at the environment.
- *Listen*—to the child, to the parents/carer.
- *Feel*—touch the child, use your instincts, draw upon your experience.
- If you are not sure, go back to **A**.
- Document what you find and what you have not found or if you did not do one of the steps. For example, if you did not expose the child because they were too distressed or you could not get an accurate oxygen saturation recording because they were moving around, make sure that you record these details.
- If you are not sure or concerned tell someone and/or get help.

Common pitfalls

- Not starting with **A**.
- If you do not know what is normal for that child, then there is no baseline or frame of reference.
- Failure to recognize when a compliant child is a sick child.

Associated reading

Oliver A, Powell C, Edwards D, Mason B (2010). Observations and monitoring: routine practices on the ward. *Paediat Nursing* **22**(4), 28—32.

Royal College of Nursing (2007). *Standards for Assessing, Measuring and Monitoring Vital Signs in Infants, Children and Young People*. Royal College of Nursing, London.

[1] Resuscitation Council (UK) (2010). *Resuscitation Guidelines 2010: Paediatric Advanced Life Support*. Resuscitation Council, London.

Monitoring

Monitoring is the continued surveillance of your patient in order to detect changes in his or her condition.

Levels of monitoring

- The level of monitoring required will be based on your assessment of your patient's needs.
- Your assessment of the child/young person should determine what ongoing monitoring is aiming to achieve and result in a well-rationalized plan that shows the frequency and level of monitoring, which will be appropriate to identify changes in the child's condition.
- Assessment should ascertain how well the child or young person will tolerate electronic monitoring equipment and the application of probes that could potentially feel invasive and uncomfortable.
- The level of monitoring may be affected by the situation in which you are caring for your patient, e.g. environment, staff to patient ratio, etc.

Parents and carers may wish to be assisted to undertake some of their child's monitoring both in hospital, at home, and in other health care environments.

By instructing the parent/carer in what they should be looking for in their child, e.g. ↑ rate of breathing, signs of dyspnoea, ↓ oral intake, etc. they can be empowered to monitor their own child.

It is essential that professional staff remember their continuing responsibilities and accountability in such situations and always provide continuing and effective teaching, guidance and support to parents and carers.

Regular reassessment of parent/carer willingness, competence, and confidence to undertake any of their child's monitoring is essential.

Types of monitoring

Nursing staff and carers

Observation, assessment, and monitoring of the child's condition through personal contact may involve 1:1 nursing care or may involve regular visits to the child to check and record their vital signs, and/or their growth and development. Frequency of visits will be determined according to the child's condition, and the child and their carers' specific needs.

Monitoring with the use of medical devices

An ever-increasing range of electronic equipment is available to assist in monitoring the condition of neonates, children, and young people.

See the appropriate sections for more specific information on devices associated with particular elements of care.

Before using any device all personnel should ensure the following:

- They are trained and deemed competent in its use—if they are not, they should not be using it!
- They check, and adhere to, local systems of training, device classification and competence assessment.

- They are aware of and follow local risk assessment and management protocols.
- They are aware of and follow local incident reporting protocols.
- ❶ Remember—electronic monitoring is *not* a substitute for appropriate personal observation and assessment of your patient!

Associated reading

MHRA (2008). *Devices in Practice: a guide for professionals in health and social care.* MHRA, London.
Product literature catalogues for correct use of monitors.
Royal College of Nursing (2007). *Standards for assessing, measuring and monitoring vital signs in infants, children and young people.* RCN, London.

Professional decision-making in nursing practice

Background

Wherever a nurse works, at some point their professional practice will involve a process of decision-making. Any decision which a nurse undertakes needs to be a decision that is in keeping with the ethos of the Nursing and Midwifery Council (NMC) code of practice.[1] It needs to reflect systematic, logical, thinking and reflection based on sound professional knowledge and current evidence/research.[2]

Professional requirements and considerations

Decision-making should be a systematic, reflective, and knowledge-based process because such an approach is more likely to produce a resolution that is acceptable to the professionals and families involved.[3] Such a methodical process will:

• Be effective.
• Be reassuring.
• Limit personal bias.

When making decisions it is beneficial to follow a model or schema so that all aspects of the decision-making process can be seen to be clearly addressed (Box 1.1).

Practice tips

• Nurses should never use or manipulate a client/patient to achieve an objective, however apparently noble the intended objective.
• Patients/clients and their families should not be treated as collectives, but as individuals with unique requirements.
• All decisions should be based on the best available ethical model to resolve and/or elucidate the issue.
• The ethical approach should be used consistently from day to day.

Pitfalls

• Nurses think that they are too busy to be systematic about ethical and professional decision-making.
• Sometimes the decision undertaken is painful and uncomfortable for the healthcare team and structures should be in place to support staff.

Remember

• The process of decision-making should be seen as cyclical rather than linear—the introduction of the resolution should lead to the assessment of the efficacy of that decision and if needed further amendments should be introduced—which themselves are based on changes following subsequent professionally ratified decisions.
• All decisions concerning a child and his/her family need to also involve them. Children have a right to be involved in decisions about their care.

Box 1.1 Professional decision-making model

1. Observation
2. Information gathering
3. Evidence sifting
4. Research evaluation
5. Analysing choices
6. Fostering discernment
7. Encouraging reflection
8. Implementing
9. Evaluation

Points 1 and 2

Professional decisions are not likely to be undertaken if professionals are not aware of issues and/or problems. Therefore, a culture of continuous professional observation and reflection needs to be encouraged. Networking, attendance at conferences, and study-days, and reading professional literature all support a reflective and inquiring mind. Clinical practice engenders many instances of decision-making. When decisions need to be undertaken all relevant information concerning the case should be gathered from all possible sources. This includes relevant ethical theory, not only clinical procedures and professional perspectives.

Points 3 and 4

From all the information gathered, bearing in mind moral principles, a process of prioritization and evidence sifting will be undertaken. This, together with current evidence and research will need to be evaluated for relevancy and appropriateness.

Points 5, 6, 7

There is always more than one possible resolution to a quandary/problem. Looking at several possible resolutions is a thorough and systematic approach. This methodical approach encourages reflection upon previous decisions made and considerations about personal and professional values and the various moral perspectives that can be employed.

Points 8 and 9

Once a decision is undertaken it will need to be implemented. Implementation needs to be transparent and open to scrutiny.

Associated reading

Alderson, P. (2008). *Young children's rights: exploring beliefs, principles and practice*, 2nd edn. Jessica Kingsley Publishers, London.
United Nations (1989). *United Nations Convention on the Rights of the Child*. UN, Geneva.

[1] NMC (2008). *The Code: Standards of conduct, performance and ethics for nurses and midwives*. NMC, London.

[2] van Hooft S (1999). Acting from the virtue of caring in nursing. *Nursing Ethics* **6**(3), 189—201.

[3] Fry S, Johnstone M-J (2002). *Ethics in Nursing Practice—A Guide to ethical Decision-making*, 2nd edn. International Council of Nurses, Geneva.

Multi-disciplinary team working

In order to provide quality care to children and young people, healthcare professionals must work effectively as part of a team. Professionals within different disciplines each have their own skills and expertise. The key to effective team-working is to recognize the role of fellow professionals, and to utilize individuals' contributions to patient care.

An understanding of different professional roles within teams is essential.

The inquiry into heart surgery at Bristol Royal Infirmary[1] made clear recommendations in terms of child health care teams:

• Collaboration is essential.
• Professionals need to cross boundaries in order to be effective.
• Teams need to share responsibility in order to provide quality care for patients.

This inquiry was instrumental in identifying standards for multi-professional team-working within children's services, and the National Service Frameworks that followed (Department of Health, 2004) went on to set those standards.

Leadership within teams is crucial. However, it is important to recognize that the most senior professional is not always responsible for leading a team; indeed, professionals with a range of skills within a team should be encouraged to lead on different projects.

Several authors have identified skills and behaviours that demonstrate good team-working. In 2002, Borril and West[2] recognized key elements of effective team-working. These include; the development of rewarding and meaningful roles within a team, identification of shared goals, performance feedback and identifiable individual contributions. The authors highlight the importance of a range of skills that must be provided by professionals with a common goal of providing quality care to children and young people. A key skill for nursing staff is to understand the role of different professionals, and refer problems on in a timely and appropriate manner. For example, a paediatric nurse may recognize that a family needs financial support to cope with the demand of having a child in hospital and/or a child with a long-term health problem. The appropriate action would be to refer this to the team social worker.

In addition to understanding team structures, it is important to acknowledge that dynamics within a team can have an effect on patient care. Nurses, particularly those in management roles must be conscious of their influence on more junior members of staff. Giving all team members an opportunity to voice their opinion, as well as a culture of openness and challenge is crucial. In order to be effective, team members must have the ability to listen, recognize the role of others, and above all, ensure the patient remains at the centre of care.

Belbin (1993)[3] has been influential in recognizing different roles within a team. The author suggests 9 roles which are important within an effective team, and the characteristics of each team member ranging from coordinator to implementer. The author recognizes that each role is crucial and this is an important message for teams to take forward: each individual has a part to play in improving the experience of patients and families within children and young people's health care.

Associated reading

Department of Health (2004). *National Service Framework for Children, Young People and Maternity Services*. DoH, London.

[1] Department of Health (2003). *Learning from Bristol: the report of the public inquiry into children's heart surgery at the Bristol Royal Infirmary 1984—1995*. Available at: ℘ http://www.bristol-inquiry. org.uk/final_report/index.htm (accessed March 2010).

[2] Borrill C, West M (2002). *How good is your team? A guide for team members*. Aston Centre for Health Services Organizational Research, Birmingham.

[3] Belbin M (1993). *Team Roles at Work*. Butterworth-Heinmann, Oxford.

The principles applying to clinical skills/procedures

Achievement of clinical competencies/ proficiencies

Background

Clinical competence is a requirement for all nurses and midwives registered with the Nursing and Midwifery Council (NMC). This is underpinned by legislation in the form of the Nursing and Midwifery Act 2001. This is essential in providing safe and effective care, whilst safeguarding the public.

Principles

The achievement of clinical competence is undertaken as part of an academic programme for those seeking initial registration or leading to a qualification recordable with the NMC.

Mentor standards

- Mentors must be registered on the same part or sub-part of the register as the students being assessed, and for the nurses part of the register be in the same field of practice.
- They must have developed their own knowledge, skill, and competence for at least 1yr beyond registration.
- They must have successfully completed an NMC approved mentor preparation programme.
- They must be designated as a sign-off mentor to sign off proficiency for a student at the end of a programme.

Mentor responsibilities

- Organize and co-ordinate student learning activities in practice.
- Supervise students in learning situations and provide constructive feedback on their achievements.
- Set and monitor achievement of realistic learning objectives.
- Assess total performance, including skills, attitudes, and behaviours.
- Provide evidence as required by programme providers of student achievement or lack of achievement.
- Liaise with others to provide feedback, identify any concerns about the student's performance, and agree action as appropriate.
- Provide evidence for or act as sign-off mentors with regard to making decisions about achievement of proficiency at the end of the programme.
- To work at least 40% of placement time with a student.

Student responsibilities

- Act in accordance with NMC guidance on professional conduct for nursing and midwifery students.
- Be familiar with the procedures for achievement of competence in relation to the educational programme being undertaken.
- Engage in productive relationships with mentors and colleagues in clinical practice placements.

- Access support from the Higher Education Institution (HEI) providing the programme being undertaken.
- Actively seek the full range of available clinical experiences to enable achievement by the required date.
- Ensure that those concerned with the monitoring and assessment of clinical practice are fully informed of any difficulties encountered which might compromise achievement of competence.

Practice tips

- Always ensure that students are fully familiarized with the clinical placement environment.
- It is helpful to formally discuss progress at appropriately timed intervals during the clinical practice placement, e.g. at the beginning of the placement, in the middle and at the end.
- Consider the use of co-mentors (associates) or 'buddies' as a way of safeguarding the student should the identified mentor not be available.
- Remember that the assessment of clinical practice is 50% of the overall assessment for pre-registration students.

Pitfalls

- If either the student or mentor has concerns, they should seek advice immediately to avoid non-achievement of clinical competence.
- If the student's fitness to practice is questioned on grounds of health, competence, or behaviour the university must be contacted immediately.
- Document all relevant information contemporaneously, following NMC guidelines to avoid a lack of clarity should any difficulty arise in the practice setting.
- Remember that the mentor is solely accountable for signing off proficiencies.

Associated reading

NMC (2006). *Standards to support learning and assessment in practice.* NMC, London.
NMC (2009). *Guidance on professional conduct for nursing and midwifery students.* NMC, London.

Policies

The care of children, young people, and their families lies at the heart of paediatric nursing.

Policies, procedures, protocols, and guidelines play a vital role in maintaining and improving the standard of care this vulnerable group receives by:

- Defining standards.
- Describing how they should be achieved.
- Describing how they should be monitored.
- Describing to patients and families the standard of care they should expect to receive.

No policy, procedure, protocol, or guideline should reduce the standard of care given. Such documents should be:

- Clear.
- Unambiguous.
- Consistent (both with the rest of the document and with other organizational/national documents).
- Effective.
- Evidence-based.
- Practical with achievable outcomes.
- In line with current best practice.

Definitions

- *Policy:* a course or general plan that sets out the overall aims and objectives in a particular area.
- *Procedure:* a method of performing a task which sets out a series of actions to be taken.
- *Protocol:* lays down in precise detail how the actions are to be undertaken.
- *Guidelines:* a set of principles that help the practitioner to decide on a course of action.

Developing a policy, procedure, protocol, or guideline

Who should be consulted?

- Staff who will be using the document.
- Local policy review group.
- Trust information governance manager.
- Clinical lead/head of department.
- All other relevant stakeholders including, where appropriate, children, young people, and their families.

How is the document developed?

- Check that a similar document does not already exist (saves duplication of effort and reduces the potential for inconsistency).
- Undertake consultation.
- Compile document.
- Undertake training needs analysis and agree process to address any needs identified.
- Perform Equality Impact Assessment.

What next?

Following local Trust policy on consultation, ratification, and approval of documents:

- Apply version control (practitioners can check that they are using the current version).
- Apply document control (allows monitoring of review dates to ensure that documents are reviewed on time).
- Disseminate and implement the document.
- Monitor compliance.
- Follow agreed regular review process for the document.

Remember

- Guidelines do not replace professional judgement and discretion.
- In a legal setting, practitioners may need to be able show that they have complied exactly with a protocol.

If you, the practitioner, believe that any policy, procedure, protocol or guideline fails to meet any of the necessary criteria, it is wise to address the issue at the earliest possible opportunity rather than be confronted with trying to make important decisions using ambiguous or contradictory information in an emergency situation or when time is short.

Seeking consent

Background

Consent to treatment must be sought of the patient and/or their legal carer before any medical or health care procedure can commence. Most commonly, it is parents who give legally binding consent for their child's health care treatment—consent by proxy. This consent must always be given with the child's best interests paramount. The consent to treatment and care may be given verbally or non-verbally. Increasingly, in acknowledgement of the child's developing cognitive competencies, children are approached directly for their affirming consent (assent) to treatment. This is considered good health care practice and reflects the current understanding of the rights of a child in regards to a child's right to self-determination.

Legal and social requisites

- In England, Wales, and Northern Ireland, a child is automatically assumed as competent to give consent for their own treatment upon reaching the age of majority at 18yrs. In practice, this can be a lower age if the adolescent is considered emancipated, i.e. they are already married, are themselves parents, serve in the armed forces, and/or considered Gillick competent.
- In Scotland the legal age of capacity to make self-determining decisions is 16yrs.
- Children who are not Gillick competent and who are under the age of 16yrs cannot give legally binding consent or refusal to their treatment.
- According to the NMC all nurses have a responsibility to participate in discussions about the assessment of individuals to provide informed consent.

Practice

In order for informed consent of be legally valid the child (if Gillick competent) and/or the parent or guardian must be capable of demonstrating that they:

- Comprehend the nature of the intervention.
- Understand the implications of the decision that they have undertaken.
- Have given their consent/refusal freely, i.e., they are under no undue pressure.
- Have considered the major possible side effects to the intervention and that any inherent risks in the procedure/treatment have been explained to them.

Obtaining a child's assent to treatment should always be considered because the process itself helps the child develop an awareness of their disease process.

Children should be told about their treatments as this approach is more likely to promote compliance and the child's sense of control.

As the child matures it takes control over decisions concerning informed assent for its treatment and care. Giving informed consent/assent is normally a shared parental decision-making process with the immature neonate having the least input and the mature adolescent having the greatest input.

Giving informed assent/refusal is an interactive evolving process that helps develop the child's sense of responsibility for its health and well-being.

Problems in practice

- A parent may give consent to a procedure on behalf of a child, but the child can vehemently refuse such treatment and/or intervention. This issue is especially problematic with the older child. To resolve it, requires tact, and an understanding of the child and its family. Health care workers should always be guided in their decisions by the legally binding principle of the *best interests of the child*.
- A child may have different levels of mental capability and capacity depending on the subject area, and this may influence the result of the assessment by health care workers of the child's mental capabilities (Gillick competence).

Remember

- All children and/or their legal guardians (usually parents) should be asked for their consent to medical or nursing treatments, interventions, and procedures.
- A parent may refuse treatment for their child and the child may concur with this decision, but if the medical team consider this decision not to be in the child's best interest they may seek legal advice to overturn the parent's and child's decision.
- Both consent to treatment and refusal of treatment needs to be recorded in the patients' records.

Associated reading

Alderson P. (2008). *Young children's rights: exploring beliefs, principles and practice*. 2nd edn. Jessica Kingsley, London.
Alderson, P. (2007). Competent children? Minors' consent to health care treatment. *Soc Sci Med* **65**, 2272–83.
Cornock M. (2007). Fraser guidelines or Gillick competence? *J Children's and Young People's Nursing* **1**(3), 142.
Department of Health (2001). *Consent: A Guide for Children and Young People*. HMSO, London.
Department of Health (2001). *Consent: Working with children*. HMSO, London.
Gillick v. West Norfolk and Wisbech Area Health Authority [1986] AC 112.

Confidentiality

Background

It is one of the fundamental pillars of professional conduct that health care workers, including all nurses and nursing students, maintain as confidential all matters pertaining to the lives, treatments, and prospects of the patients that they work with. The primary rationale for this position is the assumption that patients and clients are more likely to divulge the necessary information for their treatment and care if they are assured that nurses will keep as private and intimate the information they receive in confidence.

Legal requirements and considerations

In the UK all registered nurses and nursing students are legally bound to work within the NMC Guidelines,[1] which states that:
- You must respect people's right to confidentiality.
- You must ensure people are informed about how and why information is shared by those who will be providing their care.
- You must disclose information if you believe someone may be at risk of harm, in line with the law of the country in which you are practicing.

This position is justified by adherence to Article 8—The right to respect for private and family life—of the European Convention of Human Rights (UK 1998). The article states that:
- Everyone has the right to respect for his private and family life, his home, and his correspondence.
- There shall be no interference by a public authority with the exercise of this right except such as is in accordance with the law and is necessary in a democratic society in the interests of national security, public safety or the economic well-being of the country, for the prevention of disorder or crime, for the protection of health or morals, or for the protection of the rights and freedoms of others.

Families as social units of care are due assurances of confidentiality but children as individuals are also due their own assurances of confidentiality. This is because children under the Children Acts (1989, 2004) the United Nations Convention of the Rights of a Child[2] and the Lord Scarman and Fraser Recommendations (1985) all confirm the child's autonomous status in proportion to its developing individuality and capabilities. The UNCRC[2] specifically protects and upholds the right of all children to privacy and self-determination.

Practice

- Nurses should never discuss outside of their practice areas information about children or their families obtained in the course of their work.
- No discussion about children and their families should take place in a public area where it can be overheard.
- All documents pertaining to a child and their care should be kept in a safe and secure place.
- Information about a patient and his/her family should only be shared with other professionals on a 'needs-to-know' basis.
- Any disclosure of information to any party concerned should *normally* be subject to permission from the child and/or their legal carer.

Problems in practice

- Nurses may feel uncomfortable maintaining information and/or aspects of care confidential concerning children or adolescents.
- Occasionally it is necessary to share information about a child against their wishes, especially where abuse is suspected.
- Gillick competence and Fraser Guidelines tend to supersede all other legal recommendations. In reality the law concerning the authority of children to make autonomous decisions for themselves is unclear and currently contradictory.

Remember

- Patients/clients have the right to control access to their own personal health information. This may include families controlling information about their children, but also children and adolescents may wish to keep information about their care confidential and not have it disclosed to family or adult carers.
- A child who is deemed Gillick competent is able to prevent their parents viewing their medical records.

Associated reading

DoH (2003). *NHS Confidentiality—Code of Practice*. HMSO, London.
Gillick v. West Norfolk and Wisbech Area Health Authority [1986] AC 112.
HM Government (1989). The Children Act. HM Government. HMSO, London.
HM Government (2004). The Children Act. HM Government. HMSO, London.
NMC (2009). *Record Keeping—Guidance for nurses and midwives*. NMC, London.
UK Parliament (1998). *Data Protection Act*. HMSO, London.

[1] NMC (2008). The Code: Standards of conduct performance and ethics for nurses and midwives. NMC, London.

[2] UN (1989). United Nations. Convention on the Rights of the Child. UN, Geneva.

Safeguarding children

Policy for safeguarding children has developed dynamically over the past decade. Legislation and policies are in place that enable and empower health professionals to safeguard and promote the welfare of children.

Lord Laming's progress report, *The protection of Children: A progress report*[1] confirmed that robust legislative, structural, and policy foundations are in place, but commented: 'Much more needs to be done to ensure that services are as effective as possible to achieve positive outcomes for children'.

In May 2009, the government responded by publishing The Protection of Children in England Action Plan.[1] Progress has already been made to address the recommendations in the publication of the revised Working Together to Safeguard Children March 2010.[2] This document contains both statutory and non-statutory guidance.

When attempting to safeguard children, health care professionals must be aware of and have a duty to follow relevant legislation and policy. Everyone shares responsibility for safeguarding and promoting the welfare of children and young people irrespective of individual roles.

Legislative framework

Children

The Children Acts 1989[3] and 2004,[4] respectively, provide a comprehensive legal framework for the care and protection of children.

A child is anyone who has not yet reached their 18th birthday. If a child has reached 16yrs of age, is living independently, or is in further education, is a member of the armed forces, is in hospital or in custody, does not change his or her status or entitlement to services or protection under the Children Act 1989.

Local Safeguarding Boards

Safeguarding and promoting the welfare of children requires effective co-ordination in every local area. The Children Act 2004 required each local authority to establish local safeguarding children board (LSCB).

Safeguarding and promoting the welfare of children is defined as:
• Protecting children from maltreatment.
• Preventing impairment of children's health or development.
• Ensuring that children are growing up in circumstances consistent with the provision of safe and effective care.
• Creating opportunities to enable children to have optimum life chances and enter adulthood successfully.

Health care professionals have a duty to safeguard and promote the welfare of the child and prioritize the child's safety over and above the health care professional relationship with other family members.

Policy framework

Guidance has been given nationally in the publications: *What to do if you're worried a child is being abused*,[5] and the NICE guidelines *When to suspect child maltreatment*.[6]

The Principles of Safeguarding policy include:
• Listening to and believing the child.
• Discuss any concerns with line manager/or other senior colleague.

- Refer to local authority children's services social care.
- Record all aspects contemporaneously.
- Continue until your concerns have been addressed.

Identifying, and assessing harm, abuse, and neglect

- The Children Act 1989[3] introduced the concept of *significant harm* as the threshold that justifies compulsory intervention in family life, in the best interest of children. The local authority has a legal duty to make enquiries where there is reasonable cause to believe a child is suffering or likely to suffer harm.
- *Abuse and neglect* are forms of maltreatment. Children can be abused in a variety of settings by a variety of people, including persons known and unknown to them. There are four categories of abuse:
  - *Physical abuse* may involve hitting, shaking, throwing, poisoning, burning or scalding, drowning, suffocating or otherwise causing physical harm to a child. Physical harm may also occur as a result of fabricated or induced illness by a parent or carer.
  - *Emotional abuse* is the persistent emotional maltreatment of a child significant enough to cause severe and persistent adverse effects on the child's development.
  - *Sexual abuse* involves forcing or enticing a child or young person to take part in sexual activities, whether or not the child is aware of what is happening. Sexual abuse may include contact and non-contact activities. Women and children as well as men commit acts of sexual abuse.
  - *Neglect* is the persistent failure to meet a child's basic physical and/or physiological needs, which may result in the serious impairment of the child's health or development.

Assessing needs

The framework for the assessment of children in need and their families[1] underpins the process of assessing needs, planning services and reviewing the effectiveness of service provision at all stages of work with children and families. The dimensions of the Common Assessment Framework (CAF) are based on these in the assessment framework. (See 📖 Common assessment framework, p. 28 and Fig. 2.1). Practitioners need to be aware of the wider issues that may impact on a child's welfare:

- Substance and alcohol misuse.
- Domestic abuse.
- Poor mental health.
- Poverty and debt.
- Relationship factors.
- Poor housing/homelessness.
- Poor parenting.
- Poor physical health and disability.
- Teenage pregnancy.
- Poor school attendance.
- Parents with a learning disability.

What to do if you suspect a child is being abused or neglected

Discuss the case with line manager, senior colleague, or supervisor.

- If concerns remain you could also, without necessarily identifying the child, discuss your concerns with a senior colleague in another agency, e.g. social care, in order to develop a wider understanding of the child's needs and circumstances.
- In general discuss the concerns with the child (age appropriate) and parents, and seek their agreement to the referral, unless you consider such a discussion would place the child at an increased risk of significant harm. The child's safety and welfare must be the overriding consideration.
- If you still have concerns, you should refer the child to children's social care; following up the telephone call with a written referral with 24–48h (as per local safeguarding procedures).

What happens following a referral to children's social care services?

- Social care should acknowledge receipt of the written referral within 1 working day. If you have not heard within 3 days, contact children's social care worker again.
- Following receipt of a referral, social care complete an initial assessment within 7 days.
  - An initial assessment may identify a child as being 'in need'.
  - When no actual or significant harm is identified the social worker discusses with the child, family, and colleagues to decide on the next steps, and this may identify a need for other services, in which case the social worker leads a core assessment and co-ordinates the provision of services, records discussions, and outcomes.
  - If actual or likely significant harm is identified, a strategy discussion, involving local authorities and other relevant agencies to decide whether to initiate a S47 enquiry (Section 47 of Children Act 1989).[3] Social care leads a core assessment and other agencies including health contribute. The Children Act 1989 places a statutory duty on health professionals to cooperate.
  - A child protection conference will be convened within 15 working days with family or other professionals and a plan is agreed to ensure the child's safety and welfare. Health professionals invited to an initial conference will be expected to provide a report.
- Initial Child Protection Conference, if significant harm is identified the child becomes subject to a child protection plan under one or more of the categories of abuse. The recommendations are implemented and reviewed within 6 months of the initial child protection conference, until the concerns are resolved.

What happens when the child is the subject of a child protection plan?

- Core group meets within 10 working days of the initial child protection conference. Members include key worker (social worker), family, and relevant agencies. The group plans how to deliver the recommendation of the protection plan. Specialized services will be commissioned.

What happens when the child needs immediate protection?

- Where there is a risk to the life of a child or likelihood of serious immediate harm, an agency with statutory child protection powers (e.g. local authority, police, and NSPCC) should act quickly to secure the immediate safety of the child. Health professional may identify immediate concerns and need to act promptly.
- Planned emergency protection will take place following an immediate strategy discussion. Legal advice is usually sought before agencies initiate legal action. Action can be in the form of Emergency Protection Order (EPO), Court order, or Police protection can be used in exceptional circumstances where there is insufficient time to seek an EPO.

Points to note

- Give consideration to race and ethnicity of the child and family, and how these should be taken into account is fully assessed throughout the safeguarding process. This includes the needs of the other children within the same household or establishments.
- The child's wishes and feelings should always be ascertained, and regard given to the age and understanding when making decisions about what services to provide.

Associated reading

Department for Education and Skills (2006). *Every child matters. Information Sharing: Practitioner's guide*. DfES, HMSO.

[1] HM Government (2003). *Every child matters*. HMSO, London.

[2] HM Government (2010). *Working Together to Safeguard Children*. Department for Children, Schools, and Families, HMSO, London.

[3] HM Government (1989). *The Children Act*. HM Government, HMSO, London.

[4] HM Government (2004). *The Children Act*. HM Government, HMSO, London.

[5] Department for Education and Skills (2006). *What to do if you're worried a child is being abused*. DfES, HMSO, London.

[6] National Institute for Health and Clinical Excellence (2009). *When to suspect child maltreatment*. NICE, London.

Common assessment framework

Background

Health professionals must be able to recognize when a child's health or development is or may be affected, when a child is suffering, or may be likely to suffer significant harm. Information can be gathered and analysed within the three domains of the assessment framework, which covers:

• The child's developmental needs.
• The parent's or carer's capacity to respond to those needs.
• The wider family and environmental factors.

The CAF is a shared tool for use across all agencies. This tool requires informed, explicit and written consent from the child, and/or family. The CAF should identify at the earliest opportunity children who have additional needs and should provide them with a co-ordinated multiagency support plan to meet their needs within universal, targeted and, if appropriate, specialist services.

❶ LSCB will have processes in place to ensure the CAF is implemented locally. The CAF is not a tool to be used if there are safeguarding concerns about a child's safety and wellbeing. Any such concerns should be referred to the Children and Young People's Services

The Common Assessment Framework triangle (see Fig. 2.1) is a tool that facilitates and promotes:

• Holistic and child-centred care with a firm focus on the child's development using a solution focused approach.
• A plan based on strengths, as well as weaknesses.
• An interagency culture of understanding and trust.

Process

There are four main stages in undertaking a common assessment:

• To identify needs early.
• To assess those needs.
• To deliver integrated services.
• To review progress.

After this initial assessment it may be possible for a single agency to create an action plan and review it with the family.

Alternatively it may be necessary to hold a 'Team Around the Child' (TAC) meeting where a team of practitioners, facilitated by the lead professional, comes together to decide how they can support a child and the family. All agencies are expected to develop and deliver a multi-agency action plan (MAP). It is essential that the child and family are present at these meetings. Where this is not possible their views must be included.

Identified outcomes also need to include roles, responsibilities, timescales, and review date.

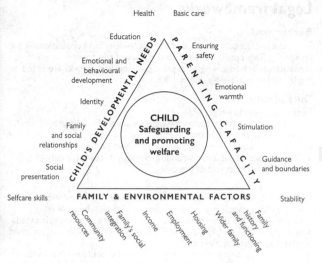

Fig. 2.1 The Common Assessment Framework Triangle.

Role of the lead professional

It is the role of the lead professional to:
- Act as a single point of contact for the child and family.
- Ensure the child and family is central to any discussions.
- Co-ordinate the delivery of the MAP.
- Build trusting relationships with the child and family.
- Reduce overlap and inconsistency in the services received.

Documentation

Local areas will have devised their own version of documentation for completion. Professionals are advised to check what documentation is used locally.

Associated reading

[1] HM Government (2003). *Every Child Matters* HM Government, HMSO.

[2] HM Government (2010). *Working Together to Safeguard Children*. Department for children, schools and families, HMSO.

Legal frameworks

Background

There is a professional requirement to act lawfully both professionally and personally. This entails adhering to the laws of the country in which you are working. The following legal principles and frameworks are based on the laws of the United Kingdom (UK).

Duty of care

Duty of care exists when:
- It is foreseeable that a claimant would be affected by the actions or omissions of the defendant.
- There is sufficient proximity between the two parties.
- A court considers it fair, just, and reasonable to impose a duty of care in all the circumstances of the case.

Duty of care
- Is owed to patients as soon as a health care worker takes responsibility for providing care, e.g. the nurse going on duty assumes a level of responsibility for all the patients on the ward, not just those allocated.
- Includes what is said, or not said if failure to give that information could adversely affect the patient.
- Is a duty to protect patients from harm. Staff should always act within the limits of confidence and competence and seek more experienced help when required.

UK law *does not* currently require doctors and nurses to act as 'Good Samaritans' and stop to assist someone in need of medical attention if that person is not one of their patients. If they do stop to help, a duty of care will exist as soon as they assume responsibility for the person's care.

Negligence

Negligence occurs when
- A duty of care was owed.
- The duty of care was breached.
- The breach of duty of care either caused harm to the patient, or was a significant contributory factor.

When deciding if a health care worker has been negligent or not, consideration is given as to whether they were acting in line with reasonable opinion (The *Bolam* test). Any person acting in a particular capacity must exercise the skill expected of someone claiming to have that skill/expertise. Inexperience or being a student is irrelevant as, if there is any doubt or uncertainty, help and guidance must be sought.

Consent

See 📖 Seeking consent, p. 20.
- This is a process, rather than a task.
- Requires time, information, and understanding.
- Provides the health care professional with a defence to the criminal charges of assault and battery and, providing sufficient information has been given, the civil charge of negligence.

- The person giving the consent must be competent to do so, have sufficient information to inform their choice, and not be pressurized or coerced into making a decision.
- All people over the age of 16yrs are presumed to be legally competent under the terms of the Mental Capacity Act 2005.
- Holders of parental responsibility are defined within the Children Act 1989,[1] and the Adoption and Children Act 2002.[2] Parental responsibility ceases when the young person becomes 18yrs old.

Record keeping

See 📖 Documentation, p. 35.

Records should provide evidence of decision-making and the supporting rationale. Records are an essential part of a patient's care and may be relied upon at a later stage. Health care workers should adopt the attitude that their records will be scrutinized at some point and ensure that they create accurate, objective, and contemporaneous accounts. Schedules for the retention of records are provided by the Department of Health.

The Children Act 1989[1]

- Introduced the principle of the 'welfare of the child is paramount'.
- Defines parental responsibility as having 'all the rights, duties, powers, responsibilities, and authority' that go with being a parent and defines who holds it (amended by the Adoption and Children Act 2002).[2]
- Parental responsibility is always held by natural mothers and both parents if married at the time of the child's birth. If a married couple later divorce, both parties still retain parental responsibility.
- The situation for unmarried couples varies within the different countries of the UK, although each has legal processes for unmarried fathers to acquire parental responsibility. For example, since December 2003 in England and Wales, unmarried fathers who are named on the birth certificate as being the father automatically have parental responsibility, but this is not a retrospective decision. Health care staff need to be familiar with the specific law of the country in which they work.
- Parental responsibility enables identified adults to make decisions on behalf of a child, or young person under the age of 18yrs, e.g. where to educate the child, where to live, agreeing to medical treatment. In the majority of situations, the need to make many of those decisions will diminish as the legal capacity of the young person increases.
- Applies to children and young people up to the age of 18yrs.
- Established clearer safeguarding processes.

Children Act 2004[3]

- Provides the legislative basis for *Every child matters: change for children*[4] and for better information sharing.
- Promotes integrated planning, commissioning, and delivery of children's services.
- Promotes better accountability of local authority children's services.
- Created a statutory requirement for LSCBs.
- Established a Children's Commissioner for England who is required to promote the views and interests of children and young people in line with the United Nations Convention on the Rights of the Child.

- Introduced the development of Children's Trusts arrangements to create frameworks that will help improve outcomes for children and young people.
- The five key outcomes are: being healthy, staying safe, enjoying, and achieving, making a positive contribution, and achieving economic well-being.

Human Rights Act 1998[5]

- Sets out a series of rights or articles to which all people are entitled.
- For health care staff, the following are the most notable:
  - Article 2—the right to life 'No one shall be deprived of his life intentionally'.
  - Article 3—the prohibition of torture 'No one shall be subjected to inhuman or degrading treatment'.
  - Article 8—the right to respect for private and family life 'Everyone has the right to respect for his private and family life.' This includes the right to self-determination and links with giving or withholding consent by a competent person.

Mental Capacity Act 2005[6]

- Applies to all person over the age of 16yrs, but it does not overrule any aspect of the Children Acts.
- Applies only in England and Wales.
- A person is assumed to have capacity unless it can be proved otherwise.
- A person must not be treated as unable to make a decision unless all practicable steps to help them do so have been taken without success.
- A person is not to be treated as unable to make a decision merely because they make an unwise decision.
- Any act done or decision made, under the Act for, or on behalf of a person who lacks capacity must be done, or made, in their best interests.
- Before acting in a person's best interests, due regard must be given to selecting the course of action least restrictive on the person's rights and freedom of action.
- Legalizes advance decisions, although staff should establish that this decision still reflects the wishes of the person who made it as, if they have capacity, they could chose to withdraw the decision.
- The definition of advance decisions only allows for the refusal of treatment.
- Amended powers of attorney to include medical decisions.
- Advance directives and lasting powers of attorney can only be created by a competent person over the age of 18yrs.
- Established a new Court of Protection that can appoint a *deputy* to make decisions on behalf of a person lacking capacity.
- Created the post of Independent Mental Capacity Advocates (IMCA's) to be used when there is no-one other than a professional carer to consult about the person's best interests.

Young people with learning disabilities and who lack capacity for decision-making are protected by both the Children Acts and the Mental Capacity Act. Their parents would be able to make decisions for them until they are 18yrs. After that, the parents do not have parental responsibility. It is likely that they would continue to act under best interests, but there may be a point at which a court appointed deputy has to be requested. Consideration of this may need to form part of transition processes from children's to adult led services.

Learning from enquiries
- Learning from Bristol 2001:[7]
  - Identified communication and consent as a key issue.
  - Criticized the imbalance of power between professionals and patients that contributed to parental vulnerability and disempowerment.
  - Advocated partnership working.
- The Victoria Climbie Report 2003.[8]
- Serious Case Review Baby P Report 2009.[9]

Common features of these reports include:
- Identified failures around interagency communication.
- Failure to follow established procedures.
- Inexperience and lack of skill of individual staff.
- Lack of resources.
- Recommended change of management and accountability structure.
- Recommended an overhaul of safeguarding procedures.
- Altered professionals' awareness.

Health care staff should be vigilant and ensure compliance with requirements relating to the safeguarding of children. This includes aspects such as adherence to bruising protocols in non-ambulant children. Communication is a frequent issue in these reports. Staff should be aware of their own communication skills as well as those of others.

Associated reading

Dimond B. (2008). *Legal Aspects of Nursing 5th edn.* Pearson Education Limited, Harlow.
Gillick v West Norfolk and Wisbech Area Health Authority (1986). AC 112.
Herring J. (2008). *Medical Law and Ethics.* 2nd edn. Oxford University Press, Oxford.
United Nations (1989). *Convention for the Rights of the Child.* UN, New York (ratified by the UK in 1992).

[1] Department of Health (1989). *Children Act.* HMSO, London.

[2] Department of Health (2002). *Adoption and Children Act.* HMSO, London.

[3] Department of Health (2004). *Children Act.* HMSO, London.

[4] Department for Education and Skills (2006). *Every Child Matters: Information Sharing—A Practitioners Guide.* DfES, London.

[5] Department of Constitutional Affairs (1998). Human Rights Act. HMSO, London.

[6] Department of Health (2005). *Mental Capacity Act.* HMSO, London.

[7] Bristol Royal Infirmary Inquiry. (2001). *Learning from Bristol: the report of the public inquiry into children's heart surgery at the Bristol Royal Infirmary 1984–1995.* HMSO, London.

[8] House of Commons Health Committee (2003). *Victoria Climbié Inquiry Report.* HMSO, London.

[9] Department for Education (2010). *Haringey Local Safeguarding Children Board Serious Case Review, 'Child A', March 2009.* HMSO, London.

Health and safety

Background

The law states that any environment in which health care workers are practising must be safe, both for staff, clients, and visitors/carers.

Each practitioner must recognize their own responsibility to promote and maintain the safety of the environment, and all people within it. They should familiarize themselves with appropriate legislation, national and local policy, and should access training and updates provided by their employer in order to practice safely within current protocols.

Regulations

The Health and Safety at Work Act (1974) identifies the responsibilities of both employers, and employees in providing, and maintaining safe environments. Other regulations have been added, which provide detail on responsibilities relating to other health and safety issues.

The basis of all regulations/guidelines is the need to risk assess environments and activities, in order to:
- Identify hazards.
- Identify individuals at risk.
- Evaluate risk.
- Consider how risk can best be safely minimized and managed.
- Record assessment and all activity.

Untoward incidents

All environments need a robust system for reporting and investigating untoward incidents.

Reporting and recording incidents, and near misses is vital to provide information which will enable trends to be identified, and strategies developed to minimize future risk.

Reporting procedure

- Report incident or near miss to senior manager.
- Fully complete an incident form (for some incidents, e.g. an incident involving medication it may be necessary to complete more than one type of form—check local policy).
- Notify Health and Safety Officer.
- Consider immediate practice review issues in immediate team, while awaiting recommendations/requirements from incident form analysis.
- Action recommendations/requirements following incident analysis.

Serious incidents or near misses will need to be more widely reported to appropriate agencies, e.g. Environmental Health Department, Public Health Department, Medicines and Health care Products Regulatory Agency (MHRA), etc.

Associated reading

http://www.mhra.gov.uk.
http://www.hse.gov.uk.

Documentation

Background

Documentation is used to communicate the care provided, and provides a legal record, which can function as evidence when care is questioned or deemed unsatisfactory. Documentation may be used in criminal or other court proceedings.

Documentation should:
- Promote high standards of care delivery.
- Promote continuity of care.
- Enhance communication between health professionals, other agencies, and children, and their families/carers.
- Provide comprehensive and accurate account of care delivery, and management.
- Assist in identification of condition changes and/or problems.

Procedure: principles and requirements

- As a registered practitioner, you are accountable for all the documentation you complete.
- Patient documentation should be kept securely and confidentially.
- All your records must be:
  - Accurate.
  - Clearly written in black, indelible ink.
  - Written in terms which will be easily understood.
  - Dated and timed.
  - Relevant.
  - Exclusive of jargon or abbreviations (other than those which are clearly explained or locally endorsed as acceptable).
  - Objective and factual—do not include subjective or potentially offensive material.
  - Signed, with each signatory's name and designation on each document.
  - Inclusive of patient's details—name, case/hospital number (other details as required according to area of care, and local policy).
- All documentation written by students should be checked, and endorsed though countersignature by their mentor/supervisor.
- Records should provide:
  - Full accounts of assessments and plans of care.
  - Information regarding the patient's condition.
  - Interventions provided.
  - Evidence of safe and accountable practice.
  - Arrangements for continuity of care.
  - Communications with child, family, other health professionals, and agencies.

❶ Remember—in a court of law, care is not considered to have been given unless it has been documented.

Associated reading

NMC (2010). *Record keeping: guidance for nurses and midwives.* NMC, London.

Developmental considerations

Background
Knowledge and understanding of child development is at the heart of every activity that is carried out by a children's nurse. Understanding patterns of physical development; how children make sense of things, and how they develop relationships with others is essential in engaging in meaningful therapeutic relationships with children, young people, (CYP) and their families.

Broad areas of development include
- Physical development.
- Cognitive development.
- Social development.

Development occurs in predictable sequences of development but the timing may differ between CYP. There is a range of ages in which normal development occurs. Knowledge of normal developmental milestones enables recognition of and response to any deviations. A specific understanding of children's interpretation of health, illness, and their internal bodies enables developmentally appropriate preparation, and participation in management, and decision making. Children's nurses need to find out what is already known by CYP as the starting point in further developing CYP's thinking. Other considerations:

Key considerations
Infant
- Stranger anxiety.
- Strong attachment to main carer.
- Can remember unpleasant experiences.
- *Erikson:* trust vs mistrust.
- *Piaget:* sensorimotor.

Toddler
- Egocentric.
- Animism.
- Negative.
- Limited understanding of time.
- *Erikson:* autonomy vs shame and doubt.
- *Piaget:* sensorimotor—preoperational.

Pre-school
- Worry about injury and fear bodily harm.
- Conscious of their bodies.
- May view pain as punishment.
- Animism.
- *Erikson:* initiative vs guilt.
- *Piaget:* pre-operational.

School age
- Understand purpose and effect.
- Interested to find things out.
- Value their friends.
- *Erikson:* industry vs inferiority.
- *Piaget:* concrete operational.

Adolescent
- Autonomy.
- Identity.
- Concern about body image.
- Peer group are important source of support.
- *Erikson:* identity vs role confusion.
- *Piaget:* formal operational.

Implications for practice

Infant
- Parents/usual carer to assist in care, and main source of comfort.
- Avoid unpleasant procedures near bed space.

Toddler
- Prepare for resistance, and negative behaviour.
- Demonstrate the behaviour required.
- Use distraction techniques.
- Keep equipment that may be perceived as frightening out of view.
- Preparation time should be close to procedure.

Pre-school child
- Like explanations about what is to happen.
- Likes rhyming and repetition.
- Use plasters.
- Be clear that no aspect of treatment is punishment.
- Let them participate where possible.

School age child
- Explanations of what is being done, and what the effect will be, e.g. pain management, invasive procedures.
- Encourage co-operation and participation, facilitate decision making.
- Enable them to take increasing responsibility.

Adolescent
- Explanations including benefits of treatment.
- Ensure privacy.
- Promote active decision making.
- Opportunities for interaction with peers and for self-expression.
- Help parents shift responsibility and autonomy for care management.

Associated reading

Bee H, Boyd D. (2010). *The Developing Child*, 12th edn. Pearson Education Inc., Boston.
Moules T, Ramsey J. (2008). *Children's and Young People's Nursing*, 2nd edn. Blackwell Publishing, Oxford.

Psychological aspects of health and wellbeing

Background

Children's emotional health, and psychological wellbeing manifests in what they say, and what they do. There is a growing recognition that mental, and physical health are of equal importance, and that interventions to prevent mental health problems, and intervene early when children are struggling is crucially important.

Why is emotional health and psychological wellbeing important?

Most mental health problems begin early in life, disrupting education and social development, and limiting life chances. Untreated psychological problems are linked to poor physical health, educational failure, family and social problems, crime, and anti-social behaviour. As well as health services, this generates a future cost burden on social services, schools, and the youth justice system.

All nurses and other children's professionals share a responsibility to ensure that every child is given every opportunity to reach their fullest potential and to enjoy good psychological well-being.

How can nurses help?

Nurses who have been trained can provide a range of therapies and treatments. Deciding which approach to use depends on the developmental stage of the child, the evidence base for use, and the specific wishes of the child, their family, or carers.

Non verbal or expressive therapies involving play, music, or dance may be appropriate for younger children, whereas adolescents, or teenagers may prefer and benefit from talking therapies, such as cognitive behavioural therapy (CBT) or family therapy.

Child psychotherapy can be used to help the child explore emotions, and relationships, or learn how to change things which are contributing to poor emotional health, or compromising overall wellbeing.

Individual strategies that focus exclusively on children are rarely effective. In addition, it is important to consider the influence of family, friends, and wider society when making sense of a child's difficulties and supporting them to make changes. Many factors that combine to produce poor outcomes for children are outside their direct scope of influence to change. It is therefore important that nurses work with parents, teachers, and peers to bring about positive psychological changes for children.

Peer relationships become increasingly important as children get older. Group support can be facilitated by nurses to help children, and young people discuss problems, identify with others, and share ways to resolve conflict or difficulties.

Interpersonal skills

The most valuable tool that nurses can draw on to support children to develop emotional health and psychological wellbeing is their own 'self'. Nurses should pay attention to what they say and how they say it, and how they react to children in their care.

For example, when supporting a child who is angry, the nurse's voice should be lowered and sentences should be short, simple, and lack abstract. This is because children who are upset, distressed, or unhappy sometimes have difficulty with information processing. The nurse should manage their own emotional responses and be aware of their non-verbal behaviour.

Wherever they work, attention to these core skills can enable nurses to manage and contain a range of complex challenges and difficulties within a busy, emotionally charged, and demanding environment.

Reducing stigma

All nurses share a responsibility for helping to reduce the stigma associated with mental health and illness. This requires a co-ordinated effort focused on public mental health and prevention of poor emotional health through universal interventions.

For example, whole school approaches that address emotional intelligence and skills to understand and manage feelings, and resolve conflict can lead to reductions in bullying, and improve attainment in schools. They are also crucially important in tackling the negative attitudes and behaviours that reinforce stigma about mental health. School nurses are in key positions to be reducing stigma champions.

As well as prevention, nurses play key roles in supporting recovery for children who may already be struggling. Targeted and selective intervention is aimed at reducing impairment associated with the severity, complexity, persistence of the mental health problem they are living with.

Support for nurses

Supporting children who are traumatized or helping those who have suffered abuse or loss can be emotionally demanding. Like all people, it is important that nurses recognize that they have limits. Awareness of our own strengths, vulnerabilities, and weaknesses affects the way in which we intervene and support children.

Working with children with a range of difficulties may evoke strong feelings in us. It is therefore essential that nurses have access to support and supervision in relation to their appraisal and management of what can often be highly emotive work. For example, if the nurse is aware that they have strong views about bullying because they experienced this themselves, they can factor this into how they support a child who is being bullied or bullying others.

Associated reading

Dogra N, Leighton S. (2009). *Nursing in Child and Adolescent Mental Health*. Open University Press, London.

Family-centred care

Background

Official recognition of the individual needs of the child, and the benefits of including the family in health care, and treatment of children in hospital was due mainly to the *Platt Report*.[1]. The Platt Report concluded that many of the practices involving the hospitalization of children were detrimental to both the child and its family. One of the limitations of the Platt Report was that it only took into account the psychological effects of a child's separation from the security and stability of its family.

Successive National Health Service reports now take into account the wider sociological implications of child health:
- The Children Acts (1989, 2004).[2,3]
- Welfare of Children and Young People in Hospital (DoH 1991).[4]
- Audit Commission (1993).[5]
- Patients Charter (DoH 1996).[6]
- Every Child Matters (Department for Children, Schools and Families 2003).[7]
- Children's National Service Framework (DoH, 2004).[8]

All the evidence advocates the involvement of parents/carers and families in caring for children, giving individuals choices about the health care they receive. In today's multicultural environment, children's nursing is about communication, education, and working with parents/carers and families to achieve the best outcome for the child.

Family-centred care is a partnership in which families and health care providers work together to promote the role of parents/carers in the care of their children. The transfer of knowledge, skills, and attitudes enables health care workers and families to bring together their expertise for the good of the child and their family. In today's society families present themselves in a range of social relationships, assumptions should not be made about family values and traditions. Health care providers need to be aware that families sometimes constitute hostile environments that do not conform to family norms.

Family-centred care

A child's ill-health is a traumatic and frightening experience for the whole family. Caring for the family is often fraught with difficulties as individual beliefs and values about health care often collide with both practical and financial issues. Caring for the family as a whole must involve parents in decisions about care, respect for individuals, and consideration of the needs of all the family. The main focus in all negotiations with family members is that the child and their needs are at the centre of health care services. Family-centred care as a philosophy is often badly defined and practically challenging. Health providers within children's services need to place the emphasis of care on the child and family's strengths, within the context of child health and well-being.

Parental involvement/parental participation

Family-centred care has been widely accepted as an integral part of health care services that put the child at the centre of care with parental involvement in decision making that keeps family environments as normal as possible. Health professionals need to be aware of how family dynamics influence parental perceptions of health care and its effects on individual members of the family. Parents have a life-time of knowledge about their child; they recognize changes in behaviour that many health professionals would dismiss as the norm. Parental participation involves partnership and collaboration between the health care team, and parents that promotes the welfare of the family, as well as the child. Parents are often best placed to identify their child's needs so collaboration between parents and health care providers is essential.

[1] Ministry of Health (1959). *The Platt Report.* HMSO, London.

[2] Department of Health (1989). *The Children Act.* Stationary Office, London.

[3] Department of Health (2004). *The Children Act: making provision for services provided to and for children and young people and for the establishment of a Children's Commissioner.* HMSO, London.

[4] Department of Health (1991). *Welfare of Children and Young People in Hospital.* HMSO, London.

[5] Audit Commission (1993). *Children First: A Study of Hospital Services.* HMSO, London.

[6] Department of Health (1996). *Patients Charter.* HMSO, London.

[7] Department for Children, Schools, and Families. (2009). *Every Child Matters.* HMSO, London.

[8] Department of Health (2004). *Children's National Service Framework for Children, Young People and Maternity Services.* HMSO, London.

Culturally appropriate care

Background

The Code for Nurses and Midwives requires all practitioners to work in a non-discriminatory way, to communicate, and share information effectively (NMC, 2008).[1] Therefore, the provision of culturally appropriate care is a basic requirement of all practitioners and not an optional skill.

This requires both sensitivity to the cultural background, beliefs, practices, and expectations of patients, and clients in their care, and also the knowledge and skills to accommodate differences, and provide culturally safe and appropriate care.

Culture

- Culture refers to the beliefs and practices common to any particular group.
- Culture can be seen as an inherited *lens* through which individuals perceive and understand the world that they inhabit and learn to live with it.
- Growing up within any society is a form of *enculturization* whereby the individual slowly acquires the cultural *lens* of that society.
- It is learned from birth.
- It is shared by all members of the same cultural group.
- It is an adaptation to specific activities related to environmental and technical factors.
- It is a dynamic, ever-changing process.

Health belief systems

Culture and illness are intrinsically linked; cultural heritage influences how we behave when well or sick and our expectations of health care. When children and their families require care, they will act and react within the context of their particular family, community, and societal culture.

- We all hold personal views regarding health and illness, why we got sick, when we did, and what is needed for us to get better. Unless these beliefs are recognized and acknowledged they can influence practice adversely if they differ from those held by the patient.
- The nurse also has their professional culture with its beliefs, values, and practices.
- The patient's culture is based on the patient's life experiences of health, and illness, and their personal beliefs, and practices.
- Then there is the culture of the setting in which they meet (hospital, community, family setting).

All three need to be accommodated to provide culturally appropriate care (see Fig 2.2).

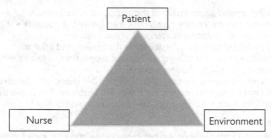

Fig 2.2 Elements for consideration when planning cultural care.

Assessment tools

To provide culturally appropriate care an assessment of need should be carried out. In addition to obtaining information regarding daily needs the following questions can help to understand the child, parents, and families health beliefs, and expectations:
- What do you think caused the problem?
- Why do you think it started when it did?
- What do you think your child's illness does to her/him?
- How severe is your child's illness? Will it have a short or a long duration?
- What kind of treatment do you think your child should receive?
- What results do you hope to receive from this treatment?
- What are the major problems that your child's illness has caused for you?
- What do you fear most about your child's illness?

(Kleinman's (1978) 'eight questions', cited in Fadiman (1998)[2]).

Practical aspects of care

- *Dietary preferences and prohibitions:* ensure you ask about these and order appropriately. Removing meat from a plate for a vegetarian is not a viable option. Do not assume food preferences based upon a stated religion, someone may say they follow a religion, but not adhere to any particular diet, always ask. Also consider where meals are eaten—in a public space or privately?
- *Hygiene:* is a bath or shower preferred? What about hand-washing before and after meals, or preparation before prayers.
- *Communication:* forms of address and correct pronunciation of names, be sensitive about personal space, and the use of eye contact, check understanding, and avoid the use of local idioms, which can be confusing.
- *Family structure:* who is the authority figure for granting permission for treatments and surgery? This may be an older relative or community figure based in another country.
- *Parenting styles vary:* some value independence of expression by their children, others expect respect for elders, and conformity to traditional gender roles. Avoid being unnecessarily judgmental if these vary from your own personal value system.

- *Gender sensitive issues:* including the appropriate use of touch, attitudes about accepting care from a member of the opposite sex and unwillingness to discuss matters of a sexual nature.
- *Self treatment strategies:* check if these have been used prior to admission or are still being used. Spiritual support may also be seen as a vital element in the healing process.
- *Customs and care at the time of death:* if possible check with the child and family what they require, but if they are unable to discuss this then seek information from appropriate community and spiritual leaders.

Pitfalls

- Without a sound relationship between culture and care, care can easily be fragmented into areas of difference, such as religion, food, or dress without trying to understand how these areas come together to form an integrated and meaningful whole.
- Making generalizations about specific cultural groups can lead to assumptions, stereotyping, and discrimination.
- Culture is constantly changing, evolving, and relying on information that is now considered out of date is incompatible with the provision of culturally appropriate care.

Practice tips

- Accommodate differences willingly and competently. Don't be afraid to ask—you can't know everything!
- Show respect by being available and accessible.
- Have information available in other languages, which explains the terminology used by health care professionals.
- Have contact details of advocates, translators, local leaders whose support the family may desire.
- Don't take over roles or impose your own beliefs or agendas.

Associated reading

Helman C. (2007). *Culture, Health and Illness,* 5th edn. Hodder Arnold, London.
Mootoo JS. (2005). A guide to cultural and spiritual awareness. *Nursing Standard,* **19**(17).
Watt S, Norton D. (2004). Culture, ethnicity, race: what's the difference? *Paediat Nursing* **16**(8), 37–42.

[1] NMC (2008). *The Code: standards of conduct, performance and ethics for nurses and midwives.* NMC, London.

[2] Fadiman A. (1998). *The spirit catches you and you fall down. A Hmong child, her American doctors and the collusion of two cultures.* Farrar, Straus, and Giroux, New York.

Care negotiation

Background

Over the past few decades it has been recognized in legislation, policies and strategies that it is in the best interests of the child or young person, if their parents or those with parental responsibility—and where possible, they themselves—are involved in decisions about their care.

Most children and young people, their families, and the professionals involved in their care do not unquestioningly accept decisions dictated by someone else. For the nurse caring for children and young people, care negotiation may be involved in anything from a complex lengthy formal process (e.g. co-ordinating a multiagency care package (MCP) for a technology-dependent child who is due to be discharged from hospital) to something brief and informal (e.g. trying to persuade a reluctant young person to have a blood test).

Procedure

Those involved in negotiation need to develop mutual understanding, trust and respect to achieve the best outcome. The method of 'principled negotiation' can be applied in a variety of contexts, to increase the likelihood of achieving an amicable and effective outcome. It involves 4 steps:
• Separate the people from the problem.
• Focus on interests, not positions.
• Invent options for mutual gain.
• Insist on using objective criteria.

Separate the people from the problem
People experience a variety of emotions, may come from different backgrounds, and have differing values, beliefs, and viewpoints. Parents who have struggled to secure help for their disabled child frequently describe it as a being 'like a battle' to get what they need. They may feel isolated, unsupported, frustrated, angry, guilty, and worried about the future. Professionals could respond to these parents by being defensive or by blaming one another. It is good for participants to express their feelings, but having done this they need to 'move on' and work together side by side to reach a solution to a problem, rather than go on fighting each other.

Focus on interests, not positions
Focus on the benefits that each of the participants could achieve through successful negotiation. It is essential that the people involved avoid making assumptions about what the other parties may want; it is far better if everyone communicates openly so that each of the parties can understand one another's hopes and fears.

Lack of clarity about one another's roles, and poor communication between different agencies, are continuing barriers to good multiagency working in supporting children and families. The introduction of single shared assessment, planning, and recording tools for use within a framework of co-ordinated meetings, planning, and review (along with shared training) is aimed at breaking down these barriers.

Invent options for mutual gain
After the problems or issues have been identified, and people's hopes and fears have become clearer, the participants need to work together to create and identify a range of possible options before deciding on what option to pursue. Participants need to discuss the potential consequences of each alternative course of action.

Insist on using objective criteria
Use of some objective standard ensures reason and logic are applied to reaching a solution, rather than it being driven by emotions. The criteria that will be applicable will depend upon the situation. Relevant criteria will include child protection legislation, national best practice guidelines, and standards, and local policies, protocols, and guidelines.

Practice tips
- For effective negotiation you need to be able to imagine how someone else may be feeling, and to seek to understand their point of view.
- You need to be clear about what is and what is not negotiable in this situation. Seek advice from appropriate colleagues if you are unclear.
- Remember that, as a professional, you are not negotiating on your own behalf but on behalf of your team or organization.
- Remember that outcomes that may not seem particularly important to you may be (or appear to be) vital to others involved in the process.
- Before a meeting it may be helpful to draw up a list of all the things you would like the other person or people to do and rank them in order of priority.
- Sitting beside someone, rather than opposite them, can help them feel you are there to help them to reach a solution, rather than to oppose them.
- Always keep in mind while negotiating what will happen (legal sanctions, financial implications, medical consequences) if the parties cannot reach an amicable agreement.

Pitfalls
- Negotiation may be protracted. This leads to frustration for everyone involved. Agree to clear time limits and stick to them.
- The participants may not reach an agreement. All involved need to be informed and aware of what will actually happen (sanctions, consequences, enforcement actions) if they fail to reach an agreement.

Associated reading
Fisher R, Ury W. (1981). *Getting to Yes: Negotiating Agreement Without Giving In*. Penguin, London.

Nursing models

Background

A nursing model provides nurses with a framework for assessing a patient's needs and enables nurses to plan the care that meets those needs. They promote patient centred care and enable continuity of care. They are based on values that the model's author believes are important to nursing. They also influence the paperwork used on a patient's initial assessment.

Examples of nursing models

Roper, Logan, and Tierney

This model is based on 12 activities of daily living:

- Maintaining a safe environment.
- Communication.
- Breathing.
- Eating and drinking.
- Elimination.
- Washing and dressing.
- Controlling temperature.
- Mobilization.
- Working and playing.
- Expressing sexuality.
- Sleeping.
- Death and dying.

On admission, what is normal/usual for the patient in relation to these activities is assessed. Any changes that have led to the admission are also considered. The patient's level of independence is assessed throughout their admission and the care plan updated accordingly.

Orem

The focus of this model is to promote the patient's independence. Orem, who developed this model, believes that patients want to be able to carry out their own care and, in doing so, will recover more quickly. Orem describes three types of needs people have:

- Universal self-care requisites, e.g. air, water, food, elimination, activity, and rest, solitude, and social interaction, hazard prevention, and promotion of normality.
- Developmental self-care requisites, which are either maturational or situational. Maturational needs involve promoting progress, e.g. adjusting to starting school. Situational needs arise from an effort to prevent harm caused by development, e.g. taking medication to prevent disease progress.
- Health deviation requisites, these needs are those which result from a patient's condition, e.g. a patient with diabetes must take insulin.

A self-care deficit occurs when a patient cannot fulfill these three needs on their own. Nurses must assess patients for self-care deficits and then provide total support, partial support, or education. This model is suitable for use in the community or rehabilitation wards.

Nottingham model

This model is specific to paediatric nursing. Children are assessed under 11 activities of living.

- Sleep and comfort.
- Control of body temperature.
- Washing/care of skin/dressing.
- Eating and drinking.
- Elimination.
- Communication.
- Breathing.
- Play and learning.
- Emotional and spiritual.
- Safety.
- Mobility.

Normal activity for the child or adolescent is ascertained, and any changes are assessed. Any problems that are discovered lead to a care plan being written. For example, if a child has asthma the details of this will be discovered when the patient's breathing is discussed. The nurse can then plan what care is required in response to this. Care plans will be updated in response to changing care needs. The involvement of the patient and carers in the assessment and formation of care plans is vital.

Pitfalls

- Initial assessments are not always updated regularly enough.
- Practice areas may use the same model of nursing for a long time, without reviewing its appropriateness for purpose/client group.
- Paediatric wards tend to use a model that is focused on children—the needs of neonates, and/or adolescents may require the use of different models.

Associated reading

Orem DE. (2001). *Nursing Concepts of Practice*, 6th edn. Mosby, Maryland Heights.
Roper N, Logan W, Tierney AJ. (2000). *The Roper Logan Tierney Model of Nursing based on Activities of Living*. Churchill Livingstone, London.
Smith F. (1995). *Children's Nursing in Practice—The Nottingham Model*. Blackwell Science, Oxford.

Care planning

Background

Care planning provides:
- A list of activities that the nurse engages in from the time of admission until discharge and is an integral skill required by all nurses.
- Essential documents that support the continuity of care providing a record of the individual care needs of the child and family along with the interventions required to meet mutually agreed goals.
- A reflection of actual and potential problems, devised in partnership with the child and family, and their level of involvement in the care process.
- An on-going process reflecting change in the care requirements of the child and family during their hospital/community care episode. In order to utilize care plans effectively the nursing process should be followed.

Care plans may be:
- Produced exclusively for the child and family, usually hand written.
- Core care plans, computer, or standardized care plans developed for specific problems not specific children. The nurse is responsible for deciding which aspects of the care plan apply, recognizing when problems have not been identified, adding the unique child and family needs to it, and detecting changes which may contradict following the care plan.
- Care pathways-written for specific conditions within an expected time frame to achieve expected outcomes. The children's nurse needs to be able to identify variance and plan care accordingly.

Procedure

Assessment

Collection and recording of subjective and objective data to include normal state and altered health status for the child with regard to activities of daily living. Significant information should be reported to relevant multidisciplinary team members as identified, e.g. tachycardia, decreasing level of consciousness, etc.

Problem identification

- Based upon analysis of information gathered during assessment.
  A nursing problem is a statement of the gap between the normal and presenting state.
- May be actual or potential. Actual problems exist currently and are evident from the assessment. Potential problems are those that could arise as a consequence of the actual problems identified.
- A statement of problem is formulated.
- Problems should be listed in order of priority more urgent problems determined first.

Planning
- Specific goals and interventions are identified to meet each problem statement.
- Should be negotiated with the child and family.
- Goals should be set for every nursing problem identified.
- Goals should be prioritized, and specific to the child and family; they should be specific, measurable, achievable, realistic, and attached to a time frame.

When writing a goal for a child the following should be considered:
- *Subject:* who is expected to achieve the goal?
- *Verb:* what actions must the person take to achieve the outcome?
- *Condition:* under what circumstances is the person to perform the action?
- *Performance criteria:* how well is the child to perform the criteria?
- *Time:* by when is the child expected to be able to perform the action?

Implementation
Plans are carried out, implementation involves receiving handover, prioritizing care, assessing and reassessing the care needs of the child and family then performing the interventions making changes as necessary.

Evaluation
Is an ongoing activity that continues for the duration of the child's stay in hospital, or as a recipient of nursing care needs in the community. Documenting the care given and the effect of the interventions undertaken must be carried out. Feedback of the effectiveness of the interventions should be an ongoing process.

Practice tips
Care plans should reflect the individual needs of the child and family, be an ongoing activity that contributes to the overall quality of care delivered to the child ensuring provision of holistic evidence-based care.

Pitfalls
Nursing care plans should:
- Only have the care that a nurse is legally and professionally able to administer to the child.
- Not be confused with the medical plan of care, be updated on a daily basis, and be individualized.
- Not be a medical diagnosis or prescription of a therapeutic treatment.

Associated reading
Barrett D, Wilson B, Woollands A. (2009). *Care planning: a guide for nurses.* Pearson Education, Essex.
NMC (2004). *Standards for proficiency for pre-registration nurse education.* NMC, London.
NMC (2008). *The Code: standards of conduct, performance and ethics for nurses and midwives.* NMC, London.
NMC (2009). *Record keeping: guidance for nurses and midwives.* NMC, London.

Working with families and carers

Background

Family-centred care focuses on the child or young person not in isolation, but within the context of their family unit, whatever form that may take. It is a central principle of good practice in children's and young people's nursing that family and carers are involved in meeting their child's health care needs. In the hospital context, this naturally extends to their presence and active involvement during clinical procedures.

❶ Negotiation is key. The level of involvement with which families and carers feel comfortable needs to be discussed early on so that everyone is clear. Many parents and carers, with a little investment of time, can learn clinical skills previously regarded as solely the nurse's domain. More children than ever are now nursed in the community, and many parents and carers are accomplished at performing complex procedures at home. True family-centred care therefore acknowledges the parent or carer as a member of the multidisciplinary team.

Some procedures are particularly emotive and challenging with regard to family presence. Resuscitation, some painful or invasive procedures, and breaking bad news can all provoke a high degree of distress for children, families, and staff alike. It can be very hard for parents and carers to separate their own emotional response from what is truly best for their child, especially during an emergency or distressing procedure.

Practice tips

- A parent or carer's involvement, however minor, makes a difference. Play and distraction are non-threatening contributions they can make.
- Respect a parent or carer's decision to leave during a procedure.
- For procedures requiring the child to keep still, ask parents or carers to help with supportive holding to increase their sense of control and the child's feelings of security.
- Good pain management is crucial during many procedures. Involve parents and carers in pain assessment.
- Do not call parents 'mum' or 'dad'; use their names.
- Be vigilant for warning signs of a parent or carer about to faint during a procedure, especially if blood is involved.
- If there is a language barrier, arrange verbal and/or written information in the family's native language prior to a procedure (if possible) to facilitate easier communication.
- Families know their children best!

Pitfalls

- ❶ *Beware of making your own value judgements:* avoid making assumptions about how much involvement a parent or carer should have.
  - This includes the possibility that a parent or carer will not want to be present for a procedure he or she has previously been involved with. Always treat each episode of care as if for the first time.
  - For older children, don't assume they will be happy for a parent or carer to be present during a procedure. Respect their autonomy.

- *Parents are parents first and foremost:* even if they are health professionals with clinical skills of their own do not pressure them to take a clinical role during a procedure.
- *Clinical procedures can be very stressful situations:* aggressive behaviour can result from a perceived lack of information. Update parents and carers regularly.
- *Remember some procedures cause stress for staff too:* it is usually helpful to take time to debrief after any distressing incident.
- *Ensure siblings are not forgotten:* seeing a brother or sister undergoing even a 'routine' procedure without explanation can be very frightening for a child.
- *Never make assumptions about relationships or family dynamics:* it can be embarrassing for everyone if you address a mother as a grandmother!

Associated reading

Hemphill AL, Dearmun AK. (2006). *Working with children and families.* In: Glasper EA, Richardson J. (eds) *A textbook of children's and young people's nursing.* Churchill Livingstone/ Elsevier, Edinburgh.

Smith L, Coleman V. (2010). *Child and family-centred health care: concept, theory and practice,* 2nd edn., Palgrave Macmillan, Basingstoke.

Teaching skills to children, young people, families, and carers

Background
In the context of care-giving, it can be both useful and helpful to teach skills that will enable both the child and young person, or those caring for them to effectively manage their own health and illness. This is a negotiated process and needs to be undertaken on an individual and family basis.

Principles

Planning
- Negotiate a suitable time and environment to teach the skill.
- Gather relevant materials and equipment.
- Prepare the sequence of tasks to be undertaken.

Introduction to demonstration
- Assess prior knowledge and understanding.
- Discuss with those whom you are teaching the aim of the skills session.
- Gain verbal consent for the skills session to take place.

Demonstration and explanation
- Choose mode of demonstration, e.g. manual or use of media, such as video.
- Provide information on the equipment being used.
- Explain the procedure both at the outset and throughout the demonstration.
- Ensure that explanations are clear, concise and at a level that is appropriate for those who are being taught.
- Demonstrate the skill in a logical sequence.
- Provide any relevant written or electronic sources that support the demonstration.
- Answer any questions to clarify understanding.

Practice
- Ensure that those being taught are happy to practice the skill following demonstration.
- Provide support and supervision as required.
- Allow an appropriate amount of time for further clarification and understanding.
- More complex skills may require a lengthier practice time and a greater degree of repetition before competence is achieved.

Test
- Revisit the aims to be achieved in undertaking the skill.
- Observe the skill being carried out.
- Give feedback to those carrying out the skill.
- Ensure that those undertaking the skill are happy to carry out the activity without supervision.
- Offer more practice if required.
- Document the competence of those undertaking the skill in accordance with local policy and NMC guidance documents.

Practice tips

- Be aware of the cognitive competence of those being taught, taking into account their age, intellectual, and fine motor development.
- For younger children utilize creative methods of demonstration, e.g. appropriate visual images and teaching models.
- Always be mindful of the fact that those being taught can change their mind about participation at any time.
- Take into account the individual nature of the process and be prepared to be flexible in approaching each situation.

Pitfalls

- Be aware of how stress in certain situations might compromise the learning experience.
- Explanations/teaching materials that are too complex or lengthy will be unhelpful, and therefore are likely to hinder the learning process.
- Don't assume that a parent, child, or young person will want to learn the skill.

Associated reading

Curzon LB. (2003). *Teaching in Further Education—An Outline of Principles and Practice*. 6th edn. Continuum International Publishing Group Ltd, London.

Quinn FM, Hughes SJ. (2007). *Quinn's Principles and Practice of Nurse Education*. 5th edn. Nelson Thornes Ltd, Cheltenham.

Communication

Communication rules

Background

Communication is defined as a process involving exchanges of verbal and non-verbal messages, to convey emotions, information, ideas, and knowledge. Priority in ensuring effective communication when caring for the child and their family is important for establishing a therapeutic relationship. Alongside this is the need for good communication with the multi-professional and agency teams involved with the child and family. There are many challenges to establishing and maintaining effective communication. This chapter aims to give some helpful tips and advice.

Procedure

- Start from a value that everyone is individual and will communicate differently.
- Introduce yourself to the child and family.
- Prioritize time for effective listening. This is hard to do and may require great effort.
- Consider the child's age, development, emotional, psychosocial, cultural, and spiritual needs.
- Utilize age-appropriate language when communicating with the child/ young person.
- Consider the child's illness and its effect on the child and family, e.g. a child with an exacerbation of their asthma may not be able to talk.
- Be clear and concise when talking, and avoid using medical jargon.
- Dependent on the child's age, liaise with their family regarding what terminology to use, e.g. what names do they use for genitalia, prior to explaining the procedure of catheterization.
- Involve family members important to the child in the communication process.
- Be aware of and involve the child's wider social network, e.g. school, nursery, Brownies, sports clubs.
- Consider technology use, e.g. texting, computers.
- Adopt and maintain a body position that is comfortable and conducive to the communication, e.g. being on the same level as a toddler, sitting next to a young person.
- Select the appropriate environment for communication, ensuring privacy, dignity, and lack of disturbances.
- Liaise with multi-professional colleagues and agencies to explore the availability of communication aids, e.g. crib cards when English is not the first language, dolls for play preparation purposes.
- Ensure the child's safety and be aware of local safeguarding procedures if there are concerns, e.g. if a child confides in you that they have been abused. (See 📖 Safeguarding children, p. 24.)
- Ensure your personal safety, informing your line manager and work colleagues of potential or actual conflict situations.
- Be open and honest. Be aware that you may not know all the answers.

- Be prepared to liaise with other professionals and colleagues, and direct the child and their family to further information.
- Consider the use of written literature to compliment verbal communication, e.g. leaflets, books, web site addresses.
- Be aware of reading difficulties and any other special needs that may require alternative resources, e.g. Braille translations, DVDs, computers.
- Document all interactions appropriately.

Practice tips

- Be creative when communicating with multi-professional teams, there are many alternatives to meetings in rooms, e.g. web cameras, meeting in alternative places, etc. However, consider any confidentiality risks.
- Do not be afraid or feel a failure when communication is not going well. Discuss this with your line manager, clinical supervisor, mentor, or work colleagues. Reflection is an effective way of looking at what is working and what could be better.
- Be aware of cultural and social differences of communication, e.g. in some cultures it could be seen as offensive to touch. Get to know the child and family, and establish agreed communication methods.

Pitfalls

- Effective documentation is integral to good communication. Spending time establishing communications is useless if not shared with others. (See 📖 Documentation, p. 35.)
- Communication is integral to safety. For example, during a critical care event, each team member needs to be clear about their role, otherwise life-saving interventions could be missed.

Associated reading

Donnelly E, Neville L (2008). *Communication and Interpersonal Skills*. Reflect Press, Exeter.
Glasper A, McEwing G, Richardson J (2009). *Foundation Skills for Caring Using Student Centred Learning*. Palgrave, Basingstoke.

Breaking bad news

Background

Bad news is defined as any information that adversely challenges an individual's view of their planned future.[1]

Within children's nursing there are many situations and circumstances in which such news is shared. It may be expected or unexpected. Giving and receiving bad news is a unique experience for all the individuals involved and is an essential aspect of professional practice.

Why is it important?

The way news is broken to families is often remembered clearly and can affect:

- Long-term adjustment to the condition.
- Future relationships with health care professionals.
- Compliance and adherence to medical management and treatment.

Approaches to breaking bad news

To aid practitioners in the complex task of breaking bad news models and frameworks have been developed. Commonly cited examples include Rabow and McPhee's[2] five-step mnemonic model ABCDE, Baile et al.'s[3] six-stage protocol SPIKES, and Price et al.'s[4] framework for supporting parents hearing bad news.

Procedure

These approaches emphasize the need for preparation, clear and effective verbal and non-verbal communication, listening, and observational skills to enable practitioners to respond sensitively to family members.

Local policies and procedures should be consulted.

Preparation

- Arrange a quiet, comfortable environment.
- Ensure privacy and minimize interruptions.
- *Prepare:*
  - Be knowledgeable about case.
  - Discuss with the doctor what is going to be disclosed.
  - Consider the emotional nature of the event.
- Consider the need for an interpreter.
- Ensure all information is collated and available, e.g. test results, information leaflets, contact numbers.
- Both parents should attend whenever possible.
- Consider social and cultural issues that may impact on family members' responses.
- Ensure all parties who need to be there are present.

Breaking bad news
- Determine what the family already knows.
- Be clear and honest in providing information, avoiding medical jargon or ambiguous language.
- Be compassionate and empathetic, and progress at the family's pace.
- Listen and observe responses so that subsequent support is relevant to individual family members.
- Understand the initial reactions that may be expressed, e.g. denial, anger, and bargaining.
- Check understanding of both the child and family.
- Offer to stay with the family after the disclosure of bad news, be guided by the needs of the child and family.
- Check the child and family have understood.

After the meeting
- Arrange follow-up meetings as appropriate to the individual needs of the child and family.
- Provide contact details and written information.
- Consider the information needs of other members of the family, e.g. siblings, grandparents.
- Debrief all staff involved.

Practice tips
- Breaking bad news is a skill that can be taught, but the experience of senior clinicians and nursing staff is invaluable. Seek their advice.
- Nurses may give bad news, but more frequently their role is a supportive one. Working in partnership is essential to ensure that parents and children receive information that is clinically accurate, culturally sensitive, developmentally appropriate, and respectful of the family's privacy and dignity.[4,5]
- All those involved should be appropriately trained in breaking bad news, have expert clinical knowledge, an understanding of the specific case, and where possible, a therapeutic relationship with the family.

Pitfalls
- Poor planning.
- Not taking enough time.
- Overly identifying with the family.

Associated reading
℘ http://www.childbereavement.org.uk/for_professionals.

[1] Buckman R (1984). How to break bad news: why is it still so difficult. *Br Med J* **288**, 1597–9.

[2] Rabow M, McPhee S (2000). Beyond breaking bad news: helping patients who suffer. *Student Br Med J* March, 45–88.

[3] Baile W, Buckman R, Lenzi R, et al. (2000). SPIKES—a six step protocol for delivering bad news: application to the patient with cancer. *Oncologist* **5**, 302–11.

[4] Price J, McNeilly P, Surgenor M (2006). Breaking bad news to parents: the children's nurse's role. *Internat J Palliat Nursing* **12**(3), 115–20.

[5] Price J, McNeilly P (2008). Breaking bad news to parents. In: Kelsy J, McEwing G, eds. *Clinical Skills in Child Health Practice*. Elsevier Ltd, Edinburgh.

End of Life decisions

Background

End of Life care should be treated as an individual and unique experience for each child and their family. The aim is to achieve a 'good' death and this will be defined differently by each family.

In some circumstances End of Life decisions may need to be made very quickly (e.g. if there is a sudden deterioration in condition); in others, however, the discussion of options, decisions, and plans can commence many years prior to death.

There is no set time for raising these issues with a family; it is dependent on the specific needs of the family and the trajectory of the child's condition. All families should be offered the information and support required to make these difficult decisions—some families may choose not to act at this time, some may choose not to act at all.

Many health organizations now have policies, procedures, and documentation to aid in the process. It is important to note that terminology does differ—the documentation may be referred to as End of Life plans, Advanced Care plans, or Personal Resuscitation plans.

Procedure

Considerations

- Treatment options and expected outcomes.
- Symptom control options.
- *Preferred place of death:* home, hospital, or hospice. This decision will also be dependent on the medical choices made.
- The child and young person, as well as the family need to be included in all aspects of decision making.
- Age, development, and understanding of the child/young person's needs must be taken into consideration.
- For legal decisions, the parents must take responsibility—'Gillick' competence and the Mental Capacity Act needs to be considered. However, even when competence/capacity is not present the child/young person's wishes should be considered.
- *Cultural, spiritual and religious beliefs:* a family's belief systems will impact on the decisions they make.
- Organ donation.

Practical information

- *Team work/communication:* the child and family must be at the centre.
- *Good and fast discharge planning:* considering all eventualities and support for child and family.
- *Provision of information for the child and family to enable informed choices:* ensure that this is given in clear, easily understood language. An interpreter should be used if required; do not rely on the extended family to interpret.
- *Relay information to children and families in an open and honest way:* it is important to avoid proffering false hope.

Practice tips

- Ensure good communication between all professionals and services involved with the child/young person/family.
- The availability of services varies from area to area. This needs to be considered when decisions are being made.
- Timing of discussions to meet the family need is important.
- Documented decisions prior to death will usually assist the Child Death Review Process.
- Within some belief systems 'end of life' is not an appropriate term as it is viewed that life does not end, but passes into another phase.
- End of life decisions are often intrinsically linked with 'do not resuscitate'. However, it is important to acknowledge, that for some families, the decision to attempt resuscitation is part of the plan.
- Accurate documentation and record keeping is essential.
- The family will require ongoing support whilst making these decisions—both during the end of life phase and after death.
- Families may wish to consider other elements at this time; this could include last wishes, holidays, and funeral planning.
- There is a need to accept that children and their families may change their mind on any element of care. These decisions need to be accommodated wherever possible.

Pitfalls

- Professionals need to ensure that their personal views do not influence the decision-making process.

Associated reading

♫ http://www.act.org.uk.
♫ http://www.childhospice.org.uk.
Department for Children, Schools, and Families (2010). *Working Together to Safeguard Children— A guide to interagency working to safeguard and promote the welfare of children.* HMSO, London.
Liverpool Care Pathway for the dying patient (2009). [Online]. Available at: ♫ http://www.mcpcil. org.uk/liverpool-care-pathway/documentation-lcp.htm Local Policy/procedures.

Communicating with other health professionals

Background

People can communicate through both verbal and non-verbal cues; however, verbal communication through conversation is the most common method. Within health care there are an extensive range of health professionals who may be involved in the care of the child/young person and their family, depending on the healthcare needs and the interventions they require. It is important to remember the need for the child/young person and their family to be involved in their care, and hence effective communication is imperative.

It is important to note that, in many cases, there will be other professional agencies involved in the care of the child/young person, e.g. social services, education. Therefore, further consideration needs to be given to whether these agencies need to be involved in the communication process.

Rationale

The Nursing and Midwifery Council (NMC) code states that nurses have a responsibility to share information and work collaboratively with colleagues, respecting their knowledge, skills, and expertise, and acknowledging the valuable contributions that they can make to the care of the child/young person.

Procedure

- Ensure all information is recorded in the patient's records in a clear, concise, and accurate manner (see 📖 Documentation, p. 35).
- Ensure all pertinent information is shared with the relevant healthcare professionals.
- Devise a record of the professionals involved in the child's care, including their name, title, and contact number.
- Ensure confidentiality is maintained.
- *Ask yourself:*
  - Who needs to know?
  - Why do they need to know?
  - What do they need to know?
  - What is the most appropriate method of informing the professional?
  - Who will be responsible for informing the professional?
- Gain consent of child and family to share information with the relevant professionals who are involved in the child's care, especially if the professionals are outside the health care domain.
- Encourage the young person/family member to record the names and titles of health professionals they are referred to.
- Health boards/Primary Care Trusts will have set policies/procedures in relation to communication and information sharing, and these should be adhered to.

Practice tips

- Through successful communication, information can be shared and professionals can pool their knowledge/skills to work collectively with the child/young person/family to provide the most appropriate care.
- Good communication facilitates a more effective package of care, prevents gaps or duplication of services or treatment, and promotes trusting relationships between professionals, as well as between professionals and the child/young person and their family.
- The need to safeguard children is a prime example of the requirement to share information and communicate effectively with relevant professionals (see 📖 Safeguarding children, p. 24).
- The need for effective communication when assessing, planning, implementing, and evaluating patient care should not be underestimated.
- The Data Protection Act (1998)[1] states that personal/sensitive information cannot be disclosed from one agency to another. However, information can be shared with the consent of the child/family.
- Tips to promote effective communication:
  - Regular team meetings.
  - Allocation of a Key worker.
  - Joint assessments and care planning.
  - Co-location.
  - Accurate record keeping, including emails, telephone calls, conversations, meetings, etc.
  - Promotion of networking to increase knowledge of the roles and responsibilities of other members of the health care team.
  - Commitment from staff to share information.
  - Patient-held records/shared records.

Pitfalls

The most common barriers to effective communication are:
  - Concerns regarding breach of confidentiality.
  - Lack of awareness/appreciation of other professionals roles.
  - Lack of awareness of other professionals involved in the child's care.
  - Poor working relationships between health professionals.
  - Lack of consistency, constant re-organization of staff.
  - Fear of loss of control.
  - Restricted opportunities to share information.
  - Limited time and resources.

Associated reading

Welsh Assembly Government (2005). *National Service Framework for children, young people and maternity services in Wales*. WAG, Cardiff.

[1] Data Protection Act (1998). The Stationary Office, London.

Managing violence and aggression

Background

Visitors, patients, and staff have seen an increase of violence and aggression within the NHS in recent years. Violence can be defined as the 'implicit or explicit behaviour towards an individual that challenges their safety, health or well-being'. Aggression can be defined as 'feelings of anger or antipathy resulting in hostile or violent behaviour'.

The Government introduced the Zero Tolerance campaign in 1999[1] and this, along with measures such as Conflict Resolution Training, has helped to reduce incidents of verbal/physical abuse within the NHS.

Procedure

Contributory factors to violence and aggression

When dealing with paediatric patients and their families, it is imperative that the staff are aware of underlying factors that could contribute towards aggression/violence. These may be caused by a number of extrinsic factors:

- Fear of hospitals.
- Previous experience.
- Bereavement of a family member.
- Money difficulties.
- Impatience.
- Frustration.
- Anxiety.
- Resentment.
- Drink, drugs, and inherent aggression.
- Mental health problems.
- Rising activity levels and workload.

Physical indicators of violence/aggression

May include:

- Angry facial expression.
- Agitation/restlessness/irritability.
- Pacing.
- Shouting.
- Threats/gestures.
- Withdrawal—reluctance/refusal to communicate.

Preventative measures

- Good communication in relation to all aspects of care.
- *Information screens*: e.g. informing service users of waiting times.
- Improved design of the working environment can offer significant therapeutic benefits to patients, and boost staff morale.
- The use of colour and light promotes well-being, and fosters a healing environment.
- Noise reduction.
- Early warning systems, e.g. the NHS Security Management Service has launched new guidance on the use of markers on patients' care records (see ▢ Practice tips, p. 67).

Management of violent or aggressive behaviour
- Ensure your own safety, ensure there is a clear exit.
- *Ensure the safety of others:* children/families/staff—remove them from the immediate area if necessary.
- *Maintain a safe distance from the aggressor:* preferably at arm's length.
- Be vigilant for equipment that could be used as a potential weapon.
- *Utilize good communication skills:* maintain eye contact without staring, maintain an open posture, speak in a clear, confident, calm manner.
- Try not to become defensive or argue with the individual.
- Listen to the individuals concerns/complaints without judgment.
- Ask open-ended questions to clarify the problem and attempt to offer realistic solutions.
- Call for assistance immediately if you feel the situation is escalating to a level you are uncomfortable with. Shout for help if necessary. Follow local policy in relation to dealing with aggressive behaviour, e.g. contacting hospital security/police/social services depending on the situation.
- Inform the nurse in charge of the unit.

Following the incident
- Ensure the safety of all patients, family members and staff.
- Complete an incident form as per local policy.
- Ensure debriefing/clinical supervision is available to all staff involved in the incident.

Practice tips
- Markers on patients care records will alert staff that they are at risk from either the patient or someone associated with them regarding physical violence or aggression.
- It is important to remember that the majority of patients and relatives are positive towards the care that they receive.

Pitfalls
- Poor communication can be a major contributory factor to an escalation of violence and aggression in the practice setting.
- ❶ Do not enter into an enclosed space that does not afford a clear escape route or from which you cannot be easily observed.

Associated reading
Duxbury JA (2002). An evaluation of staff and patients' views of and strategies employed to manage patients aggression and violence on one mental health unit. *J Psychiat Ment Hlth Nursing,* **9**, 325–7.
Nursing and Midwifery Council (2010). *Code of Conduct.* NMC, London.

[1] National Health Service Executive (1999). *NHS Zero Tolerance to Violence.* NHSE, London.

Effects of hospitalization

Background

There are well-documented effects of hospitalization on the physical, social and emotional well-being of the infant, child, or young person, as well as that of their parents and siblings. Whilst the average length of stay is only 2 days, the experience could affect their future attitude towards all aspects of health care.

For the past 50yrs the adverse effects of separation have been recognized. Bonding will be affected if an infant and parent are separated. For a toddler or young child, hospitalization will often lead to a period of regression and insecurity.[1,2] Key concerns for the older child and young person usually include isolation from peers, missed schooling, lack of privacy, and loss of control. Parents and carers may feel very anxious, guilty, and distressed about their sick child, in addition to being concerned about the welfare and reactions of their other children, missing work, and increased financial pressures.

Procedure

Promoting positive effects and reducing negative effects

- Involve the child and their family, whenever possible, in assessing their needs and in planning, carrying out, and evaluating their care. This should help to reduce the disruption in role/routine caused by hospitalization and help them to feel confident in continuing their care at home.
- Where possible make all efforts to keep the child and family together to reduce the potential negative effects of separation, e.g. providing parental accommodation where available or fold down beds at the child's bedside.
- Liaise with appropriate professionals (e.g. dieticians, community/ specialist nurses, health visitors, occupational therapists, pharmacists, physiotherapists, play specialists, psychologists, social workers, speech therapists and teachers) to ensure appropriate intervention and support is given to the child and their family.
- Provide explanations and support to the child and their family before, during and after investigations/treatments. Ensure the language used is appropriate for both child and family.
- *Promote play in order to:*
  - Create an environment where stress and anxiety are reduced;
  - Aid in assessment and diagnosis;
  - Help the child understand treatment and illness;
  - Provide an outlet for feelings of anger and frustration;
  - Help the child regain confidence and self-esteem;
  - Speed recovery and rehabilitation (see Chapter 6).
- *Procedural pain may be relieved by:*
  - Age-appropriate preparations;
  - Topical anaesthetic cream;
  - Distraction and relaxation techniques, such as singing, blowing bubbles, and guided imagery.

- Self-administration of inhaled nitrous oxide may be helpful in school age children and young people.
- Breastfeeding or giving sucrose solution during or just before procedures appears to reduce discomfort in infants. Sedation may occasionally be required (see 📖 Sedation, p. 250).
- Assess acute and chronic pain using age-appropriate tools. Use analgesia and non-pharmacological interventions.
- Implement standard infection control precautions to reduce the risk of transmission of microorganisms from both recognized and unrecognized sources of infection. (Refer to Chapter 7).

Practice tips

- Greet the patient and their family, and introduce yourself when they or you arrive in the clinical area. This helps them feel noticed and cared about, even if you do not have a lot of time available to speak to them.
- Never assume that a child or family will react in a certain way.
- Try to avoid judgmental beliefs and values that can be transferred to the child and their family.
- Recognize the uniqueness of each person, their past experiences and current coping strategies.
- Appreciate that some families have external pressures that make it difficult for them to stay with their child. Try not to make judgments.
- Some children/young people gain comfort from being able to bring in familiar objects, e.g. quilts, pillows, toys, pictures.
- For some children, particularly younger ones it can be useful to try to adhere as closely as possible to their normal routine in an attempt to reduce the impact of their hospitalization.
- Use the interpreter service to aid communication with patients and families with a hearing impairment who use signing, or those from non-English speaking backgrounds who do not speak or understand the English language competently.
- Do not expect a family member or friend to act as interpreter.

Pitfalls

- Poor communication between nurse, child, and family.
- Failure to allow adequate time to listen to a child and/or families concerns.
- Some children (and adults), desiring to please the healthcare professional who is asking them questions, may say what they think the professional wants to hear. Observation of whether their actions and demeanor are consistent with what they have said can be helpful.

Associated reading

Kuttner L (2010). *A child in pain: what health professionals can do to help*. Crown House Publishing, Bancyfelin.

Shields L (2001). A review of the literature from developed and developing countries relating to the effects of hospitalization on children and parents. *Internat Nursing Rev* **48**(1): 29–37.

[1] Robertson J, Robertson J (1989). *Separation and the very young*. Free Association: London.

[2] Bowlby J (1998). *Attachment and Loss. Volume 2: Separation, Anxiety and Anger*. Pimlico, London.

Communicating with the child or young person with special needs

Background

Children and young people with special needs use a wide range of verbal and non-verbal ways to communicate. Practitioners often struggle with this area of practice, particularly if they do not work with disabled children and young people on a consistent basis. All too quickly, they rely on parents to tell them how a child or young person feels. This can result in excluding them, leaving them with a feeling of helplessness and reliance at a time when they are striving to become more independent.

Procedure

Before you meet the child or young person

- Find out what you can about the child or young person's way of communicating before you meet them.
- If you don't have a good knowledge of their way of communicating be proactive! Consult with parents or carers, colleagues, written resources, and the World Wide Web.
- If you are going to meet the child or young person at home or it is a planned admission to hospital, consider sending them some information beforehand explaining who you are.

When you meet the child or young person

- Introduce yourself to the child or young person (even if they appear to have very profound or complex needs).
- Smile, be friendly, and address them by name. Young children in particular make their minds up about you in the first 15s.
- Use a calm, unhurried approach.
- Spend some time building a rapport with the child or young person, and use additional resources like play or drawings (if appropriate) to tap into their world.
- Speak to the child or young person on the same level—you may need to sit down.
- Give children and young people choice and control as much as possible. This reduces the power relationship between you, as an adult professional, and them.
- If you are having difficulties understanding them, say so; give yourself and them time.
- If you are unsure, check back with the child to see if your understanding is correct.

Practice tips

- See the child or young person first and their impairment second—they are the same as any other child.
- Start from the position that all children can communicate—it is your job to adapt your way of communicating to suit them.
- Communicating with children and young people takes time—time for you to get to know the child and their individual way of communicating.

Pitfalls

- Don't talk to others, e.g., parents or professionals, as if a child or young person isn't there.
- Don't finish children or young peoples' sentences for them (unless they want you to do this). Be patient.
- Avoid using jargon, double negatives, or asking two things at once.
- If you don't understand the child, don't rush in and ask the parent immediately, try again.
- Don't pretend you have understood the child or young person if you haven't; they will figure this out very quickly.

Associated reading

Goodwin M, Phillip-Jones T (2010). *The champion toolkit—participation and engagement with disabled children and young people,* Section 2. The Children's Society, Birmingham City Council and Disability Inclusion Community Education, Birmingham.

Marchant R, Gordon R. (2001) *Two-way street. Communicating with disabled children and young people.* Dublin: NSPCC, Joseph Rowntree Foundation, and Triangle.

Assessing the child/young person

Assessment of graphic trends in patient observations

Background

Accurate assessment of observations (vital signs) in children is essential. Although arrest is rare, deterioration (and improvement) can be rapid. Subtle changes in a child's condition can be a critical clue to identifying this. A trend in observations is provided by several sets of measurements over time; the information provided by the trend is of more use than that from an isolated set.[1]

The use of early warning scores can also help identify those children in the 'golden hour' before collapse and critical illness occurs;[2] an early warning score should be used as part of a comprehensive assessment. Measurement of observations is a fundamental skill, which should be part of a holistic approach to the child or young person's care. It is not simply a task to be done.

Equipment

- Clean, reliable, regularly serviced, and appropriate equipment for the age and size of the child.
- Thermometer and probes.
- Stethoscope.
- Saturation monitor.
- Documentation.
- Paediatric early warning score.

Procedure

- A full set of observations includes temperature, pulse, respiratory rate, blood pressure, capillary refill time, oxygen saturations, AVPU (Alert, Responds to Voice, Responds to Pain, Unconscious) score, and pain assessment. The first set recorded provides 'baseline observations'
- Ideal frequency for observations will depend on local protocol as well as the condition of the individual patient.
- Children on continuous monitoring should have hourly observations made as a minimum.[3]
- Ensure the chart is dated and timed for each set of observations.
- Clear, accurate, and consistent plotting of values on the observation chart is vital.
  - Values should be plotted using appropriate symbols, e.g. dots linked by straight lines (see Fig. 4.1).
  - Blood pressures should be documented as Xs or Vs linked by dotted lines.
- By observing graphic trends, patterns/influences can be recognized, e.g.:
  - An increase or decrease in temperature will affect heart rate.
  - A decrease in respiratory and heart rate can be noticeable linked to if a child is sleeping.

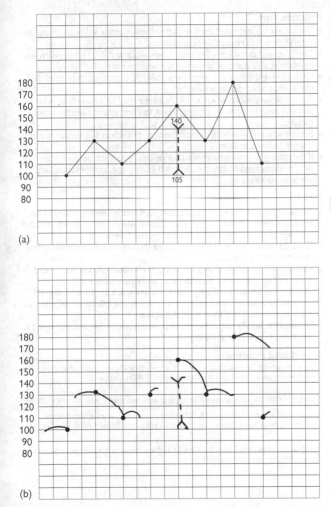

Fig. 4.1 Examples of correct (a) and poor (b) documentation of the same set of observations, Note how much more clearly the graphic trend would be when documented as in (a).

Practice tips

- Your own pocket sized card with paediatric normal values is useful as a reference when recording observations.
- Observe and document the child's behaviour and interaction with his/her family; this is a crucial part of the assessment.
- Listen to parents/carers who know their child best; do they think he/she is improving or deteriorating?
- Taking observations when a child is asleep may be easier than awake and will help to provide a comparison to complete the assessment picture.
- Ensure you know who to report findings to such as the senior nurse, doctor, outreach team.
- If delegating measurement of observations, you must be sure the person delegated to has the required knowledge, competence, and confidence to do so.

Pitfalls

- No equipment can replace eyes, ears, and touch; use monitors as an aid to assessment rather than a substitute. Always cross-check monitor readings of heart rate with a manual measurement.
- Consider the emotional effect of parental presence or absence when recording observations.
- Young children often object to having their observations taken, and stress or fear can easily elevate heart and respiratory rate.
- When using an early warning score, always score as you see, e.g. do not attribute an elevated heart rate solely to the effects of salbutamol in a wheezy child and then alter the score.
- Remember, legally speaking, proof an event has or has not occurred is dependent on documentation.

Associated reading

Pearson, GA. edn (2008). *Why Children Die*: A Pilot Study 2006; England (South West, North East and West Midlands), Wales and Northern Ireland. CEMACH, London.

[1] Aylott, M. (2006). Developing rigour in observation of the sick child. *Paediat Nurs* **18**(8), 38–44.

[2] Duncan H, Hutchison J, Parshuram CS. (2006). The pediatric early warning system score: A severity of illness score to predict urgent medical need in hospitalized children. *J Crit Care* **21**, 271–9.

[3] Royal College of Nursing. (2007). *Standards for assessing, measuring and monitoring vital signs in infants, children and young people*. RCN, London.

Assessing breathing and oxygenation

Assessing breathing and oxygenation

Background

Adequate oxygenation is essential for all tissues. Prolonged hypoxia will result in irreversible tissue damage, brain injury, multi-organ failure, and death. As children have a lower pulmonary reserve and a higher metabolic rate than adults, their oxygen requirements are more significant and generally supplementary oxygen should be given as soon as signs of hypoxia are recognized. Measurement of blood oxygenation is the only true method of accurately assessing a child's level of oxygenation. However, there are other signs and symptoms which when assessed may indicate a less than adequately oxygenated state.

Equipment

- Stethoscope.
- Oxygen saturation monitor and probe.
- Documentation.

Procedure

Colour

- Any deviation from the child's normal skin colour may be indicative of hypoxia.
- Detecting hypoxia visually is very difficult; by the time mucous membranes are cyanosed the child's oxygen saturation is likely to be <80%.

Respiratory

Observe for:

- Position of child and airway patency.
- Respiratory rate (Table 4.1):
  - Know the normal respiratory rates for all children in order to recognize abnormalities.
  - When undertaking respiration rate, count respirations for one minute as breathing may be irregular.
- Tachypnoea (rapid respirations to increase oxygen levels).
- Dyspnoea.
- See-saw respirations.
- Recession:
  - Intercostal, subcostal, or sternal show increased work of breathing.
  - Recession in children >6yrs old is alarming.

Table 4.1 Normal resting respiratory rate values for children

Age (yrs)	Respiratory rate
<1	30–50
1–2	25–35
2–5	20–30
5–12	20–25
>12	15–20

- Use of accessory muscles, e.g. sternocleidomastoid in the neck.
- Head bobbing in infants.
- Nasal flaring (to increase air flow into the lungs).
- Wheeze (lower airway obstruction).
- Stridor (upper airway obstruction).
- Grunting (severe respiratory compromise).
- Inability or difficulty in speaking/feeding.
- Exhaustion (irregular rate).

Auscultation
- Use paediatric stethoscope for accuracy.
- Listen bilaterally for pitch, intensity, and quality, and for a complete respiratory cycle.
- Abnormal sounds indicate disease.
- Diminished or absent breath sounds requires immediate action.

Chest movement and percussion
- Observe movement of chest wall for symmetry and effort.
- Percussion can identify areas of collapse (dullness), or other changes in resonance.

Pulse oximetry
See ⌨ Oxygen saturation monitoring, p. 334.
- Normal value 95–99% in a healthy child.
- When used in optimum circumstances pulse oximetry will detect hypoxia before clinical signs are evident.
- Accurate pulse oximetry measurements have been shown to match those of arterial blood gas values.
- Place probe on fingertip/toe/ear lobe of older child, or outer aspect of foot near base of small toe/on big toe/palm of hand near base of little finger in infant.
- Be aware of manufacturer's recommendations for probe use.
- Inaccurate readings are easily obtained through poor peripheral perfusion, oedema, nail varnish, movement, smoke, or carbon monoxide poisoning.

Behaviour
- Involve parents in assessing changes in behaviour.
- Hypoxia or hypercapnia → disorientation/agitation/drowsiness.
- Prolonged hypoxia → loss of consciousness.

Practice tips
- Poor oxygenation will affect other organs and systems in the body, therefore, assessment of oxygenation should be carried out alongside assessment of other systems, particularly the cardiovascular and the neurological system.

Pitfalls
- All observations should be interpreted in the context of the whole child/young person.
- Be aware of the limitations of using oxygen saturation monitors.

Associated reading
Resuscitation Council UK (2008). *Paediatric Immediate Life Support*, 1st edn. RCUK, London.

Assessing circulation

Background

Assessing and interpreting a child or young person's circulation accurately is a key skill for nurses to ensure children receive efficient and effective care and to quickly detect any deterioration. Circulation, or the cardiovascular system, is assessed, observations made, and the results interpreted alongside a comprehensive health history, and full physical examination of the child/young person.

Equipment

- Stethoscope.
- Aneroid or electronic sphygmomanometer.
- Documentation.

Procedure

Heart rate

- The heart rate, or the number of times the heart beats in 1min, is based on the number of contractions of the ventricles of the heart. Assessing the heart rate also gives an opportunity for assessing the strength and regularity of the beats (Table 4.2).
- Pulse palpation points include radial, brachial, femoral, or carotid, and less commonly the dorsalis pedis, the posterior tibial, the popliteal, or the temporal artery. Palpate with middle and ring finger, but not the index finger or thumb as they have their own pulse.
- For infants <2yrs auscultation of the apex of the heart is recommended; use a paediatric stethoscope placed over the 4th intercostal space.
- Count for 1min to ensure accuracy and detect abnormal beats.
- Know the normal values across all ages of children in order to recognize abnormalities. Tachycardia may indicate early hypoxia, but may also be as a result of conditions such as pain or fever.
- Grade the volume of the pulse where 0 is no palpable pulse to 3, an easy to palpate pulse not obliterated with pressure (normal).
- An absent peripheral pulse may be a sign of shock.
- As with all assessments, record all observations and report any abnormalities.

Table 4.2 Normal resting heart rate values for children

Age (yrs)	Heart rate (bpm)
<1	100–160
1–2	90–150
2–5	80–140
5–12	70–120
>12	60–100

Capillary refill time
- Apply pressure for 5s to sternum, forehead, or digit, release pressure and count in seconds until normal colour returns.
- Expected capillary refill time (CRT) is <2s, report readings >2s; this may be indicative of shock/dehydration.
- Be aware of cold peripheries (feel and compare peripheries to central temperature and escalate concerns where these differ).
- Also be aware of cold environment.

Blood pressure
See 📖 Measuring blood pressure, p. 82.
- Blood pressure (BP) measures the pressure within the arteries; the systolic (higher number) is the maximum pressure as the heart pumps blood into the artery, and the diastolic (lower number) is the pressure between beats as the heart relaxes.
- An essential, but anxiety provoking procedure for children.
- Due to compensatory mechanisms, hypotension is generally a pre terminal sign in children.
- Accurate and consistent cuff size according to the child's size is essential for accurate readings; a cuff too small may lead to over estimation of BP, a cuff too large may lead to under estimation.
- Manual (anaeroid sphygmomanometer) or electronic (oscillometric) devices are available, however, whilst electronic devices may eradicate human error, (providing manufacturer instructions are followed), they are sensitive to movement and do not detect pulse volume or rhythm.
- Estimated expected systolic BP:

$$(\text{Age in yrs} \times 2) + 80$$

Skin
- Good perfusion is indicated by consistent skin colour over the trunk and limbs.
- Poor perfusion indicated by pallor → mottling → peripheral cyanosis → central cyanosis (respiratory arrest imminent).

Practice tips
Other considerations may include:
- Is oedema present?
- What is the child/young person's urinary output?
- Does the child have clubbing of fingers or toes indicative of chronic hypoxia?

Pitfalls
- Individual recordings need to be interpreted in the context of the whole child.
- Do not be too reliant upon monitors.

Associated reading
Resuscitation Council UK, (2008). *Paediatric immediate life support*, 1st edn. RCUK, London.

Measuring blood pressure

Background

Blood pressure is generated by the heart beating, and is a measure of the pressure exerted on the artery walls as blood flows through the arteries.

Blood pressure measurement can be used to help diagnose chronic conditions such as chronic kidney disease or cardiac disease. It can also be used to assess a child's condition following or during treatment. Blood pressure should be measured at least once per hospital attendance to obtain a baseline measurement for each child.

- *Invasive BP* measurements such as arterial BP monitoring enable continuous direct readings to be obtained, via an arterial line connected to a monitoring system. This is commonly used in critical care areas, however, it is not practical or 'child friendly' for most environments.
- *Non-invasive* methods are more appropriate for clinics and general environments. Two types are commonly used:
  - Automated (oscillometric) methods provide readings with little intervention from the nurse. Pressure changes in the cuff are compared to blood pressure data stored in the machine and readings provided accordingly. The machines pump up to pre-determined levels, and if the child is mobile and/or upset several attempts may be made to obtain a reading. Some machines pump up higher with repeated attempts
  - Manual sphygmomanometers are more labour intensive for the nurse, requiring the interpretation of sounds heard either via stethoscope or Doppler ultrasound device. However, the nurse has more control over the reading and can increase accuracy and comfort of the patient accordingly.

Equipment

- Automated or manual sphygmomanometer. Within service date and with intact tubing.
- Correct cuff size for child/young person.
- Stethoscope or Doppler if completing manual blood pressure measurement.
- Documentation.

Procedure

- The child or young person should sit down for 3min before a reading is taken, as exercise can cause a false high reading.
- The child should be comfortable and the limb used for measurement supported and relaxed.
- Where possible an arm should be used for the reading.
- The same limb and cuff should be used to ensure each reading is comparable. Readings will vary slightly between limbs.
- The cuff should be selected to ensure that the inflation area/bladder covers at least 80% of the limb circumference:
  - Most modern cuffs have a range indicator to assist in selection.
  - If several cuffs fit, select the cuff with the longest width.
  - Cuffs that are too small will give an inaccurately high reading, cuffs too large will give an inaccurately low reading.

- When undertaking a manual BP:
  - Estimate systolic pressure by palpating the pulse, whilst pumping the cuff. The systolic pressure is determined when the pulse disappears.
  - Release the pressure.
  - Pump to 30mmHg over the estimated pressure once stethoscope or Doppler applied to ensure the most accurate reading possible.
  - Deflate the cuff at 2mmHg/s listening for the Korotkoff sounds appearing and then disappearing. Release all of the pressure within the cuff once the diastolic sound is heard.
  - Ensure the child is comfortable.
  - Record the reading to the nearest 2mmHg, do not round up or down, to ensure the most accurate possible record is made.
  - When a Doppler device is used with small children it may be necessary to use two nurses as this ensures accuracy, particularly if the child is moving during the procedure. The systolic reading only can be heard.
- The systolic pressure is the higher number and related to the contraction of the heart muscle. During manual measurement this is identified when the first pulse sounds are heard returning. This is known as Korotkoff Phase 1.
- The diastolic pressure is associated with the heart muscle relaxing.
  - Using a stethoscope it is identified by the disappearance of all noise (Phase 5 Korotkoff sound) in most patients.
  - Phase 4, when sounds appear to become muffled should be used in patients in whom the sounds do not disappear.
  - This is not heard when using a Doppler device.

Practice tips

- Treatment should not be commenced based upon a single blood pressure reading in isolation.
- Reading accuracy can be affected by distress, anxiety, discomfort, equipment functioning and environmental factors.
- Trends in blood pressure, consideration of other influencing factors and patient observations should always be considered.
- BP increases with the age and size of the child.
- Centile charts for blood pressure are available for reference to ensure the correct norm is used for comparison (see 📖 Associated reading, p. 83).

Pitfalls

- Children can be uncooperative and a reading may be difficult to obtain.
- Obtaining a manual reading, particularly using a Doppler, may require two people.

Associated reading

National High Blood Pressure Education Program Working Group on High Blood pressure in Children and Adolescents. (2004). The Fourth report on the diagnosis, evaluation, and treatment of high blood pressure in children and adolescents. *Pediatrics* **114**, 555–76.

Measuring temperature

Background

Increased temperature is one of the body's defence mechanisms against infection. A rise in temperature makes the body hostile to invading pathogens and enables it to repair itself more quickly by increasing the metabolic rate. Measuring temperature is an important aspect of nursing care in paediatrics, as an increase in body temperature can be indicative of illness. A decrease in body temperature, usually caused by prolonged exposure to cold, can also be dangerous, if left untreated. As such, it is important that when temperature is measured, it is done accurately, so that clinical decisions can be made upon the result.

There are various sites and types of thermometer appropriate for recording temperature. The main sites used are the axilla, tympanic membrane and sublingual. In some settings, e.g. the intensive care unit, arterial temperature may be measured; due to their specialist use and invasive nature they will not be discussed here. There are small differences in the body temperature 'normal range' between the different sites and it is therefore important to know what these are, for the interpretation of the result (see Table 4.3).

Table 4.3 Normal temperatures at different sites

Body site	Type of thermometer	Range	Fever (°C)
Axilla	Electronic	34.7–37.3	37.4
Sublingual	Electronic	35.5–37.5	37.6
Ear	Infrared	35.6–37.5	37.6

Adapted from Sahib El-Radhi A, Carrol J, Klein N (2009). *Clinical Manual of fever in children*, with permission from Springer-Verlag GmbH. © 2009.

Equipment

• Thermometer.
• Protective probe cover (for non-disposable thermometers).
• Detergent wipes (for cleaning equipment between patients).

Procedure

• The child and parent should have the procedure explained to them and their consent gained.
• If disposable chemical thermometers are used, follow procedures given here and hold in place for the time stated in the manufacturer's instructions.
• *Axilla*: ensure clothes are loose around the axillary area and the correct mode is selected on the thermometer, e.g. depending on the age of the child. Place the probe under the arm, ensuring it is central in the axilla and hold in place, with the child's arm down, until the thermometer bleeps (or as per manufacturer's instructions).

- *Tympanic*: holding the pinna, straighten the ear canal. For children less than 1yr of age, pull the pinna straight back, for those older than 1yr, pull the pinna up and back. Insert the probe into the ear canal and press the button to start the temperature measurement. Hold the thermometer in place until it bleeps.
- *Sublingual*: insert probe into the sublingual space (below the tongue). Keep in place until the thermometer bleeps.
- After recording the temperature, dispose of the probe cover, or if using the disposable chemical thermometers, dispose of these in the correct bins.
- Wash hands and clean the thermometer before proceeding.

Practice tips

- It is important that the appropriate site and thermometer are selected to enable the reading to be as accurate as possible. The site chosen will depend on the child's preference, age, and clinical condition. Some children may have a dislike, or fear, of certain types of thermometer, so this should be taken into account as far as possible. Infants should generally have their temperature recorded in the axilla. Tympanic thermometry is not appropriate due to the size and shape of their ear canal. In children less than 4 weeks old, temperature must be measured in the axilla with an electronic thermometer.[1]
- Record the temperature on the observation chart as soon as possible including the site at which the temperature was taken to enable better interpretation of the result.
- If the temperature recorded appears contrary to the child's clinical condition, repeat the measurement.
- If the temperature recorded is below the normal range, ensure more clothing, or blankets are applied to the child.
- If the temperature is above the normal range and it is the first time the child has had a fever, inform the medical staff. Provide antipyretic therapy if required.

Pitfalls

- The main errors in taking temperature are the result of the probe not being in place correctly or, with tympanic measurement, not holding the pinna in the correct position.
- It may be difficult to obtain an accurate temperature recording if a method is selected that the child is not comfortable with, as they may try to withdraw from the probe causing it to dislodge. Communication is key to ensure the child is prepared for the procedure and is comfortable with the method selected.

[1] National Institute for Health and Clinical Excellence (2007). *Feverish illness in children: Assessment and initial management in children younger than 5 yrs.* NIHCE, London.

Measuring weight, height, and body mass index

Background

An important indicator of a child/young person's health and well-being is regular growth. Measurements taken include weight, height, and head circumference. From the age of 2yrs Body Mass Index (BMI) can be obtained to plot the heaviness of the child relative to their height, indicating if the child is over or underweight. For children who require medication for an acute or chronic illness, weight (and sometimes height) is vital for correct drug calculation and dosages.

Equipment

- Electronic scales.
  - Should be calibrated.
  - Set in kilograms.
- Length board/mat <2yrs.
- Stadiometer >2yrs.
- Re-usable narrow paper/plastic tape (non-stretch material).
- Centile chart/body mass index (BMI) chart/parent held record.

Procedure

Weight

<2yrs

- Ensure scales are placed on a non-slip surface in a safe environment.
- Remove infant's clothes and nappy.
- Place a sheet of blue roll on scales and turn scales on to show zero.
- Place infant on scales safely, lie them down if unable to sit. If able to sit confidently ensure parents/carers/health care worker (HCW) stands close by.
- When the reading has settled, take the measurement, and plot.

>2yrs

- Remove child/young person's outer clothes and shoes. If child wears a nappy this must be removed.
- Turn scales on until zero.
- Ensure child/young person stands safely on scales.
- Take measurement when the numbers have settled, and plot.

Length

<2yrs

- Remove infants clothes and nappy.
- Place infant supine on the board/mat, ensuring the head is touching the head board.
- Straighten legs and measure, ensuring feet are flat.
- Take the measurement and plot.

Height

>2yrs

- Remove child/young person's shoes.
- Stand child/young person with feet against back of board/wall, facing forwards, with their line of vision parallel to the floor.

- Place the lever on top of the head and take the measurement from the indicator, and plot.

Head circumference
- Taken as the size of the skull is related to brain size.
- Measure at the point of greatest circumference.
- Measure across the occipital, parietal, and frontal prominences.

BMI
- Weight (kg) divided by height (m^2).
- Plot on BMI chart.

Practice tips
- If infant becomes upset, stop procedure, ask parent to settle infant, and reassure. Restart procedure when infant is settled.
- If unable to settle the child to gain a weight, consider weighing the parent alone and then the parent and child together, subtracting the parents weight from the total to give the child's weight.
- If there is a need to take regular measurements, it should be done so at the same time of the day.
- When changing from length to height, the child's height may be slightly less than the length in measurement.
- Advise parents it is recommended once feeding is established that babies should usually be weighed at around 8, 12 and 16 weeks and 1yr; at the time of routine immunizations.
- If there are no concerns, babies should be weighed no more than once a month up to the age of 6 months, then every 2 months between the age of 6–12 month, then every 3 months from the age of 1yr.
- If an infant/child drops 2 or more centiles without being unwell refer to the general practitioner (GP) or community paediatrician.

Pitfalls
- If growth is not measured at regular intervals, faltering growth may not be identified.
- If an infant/child is measured too regularly, it may appear they have grown a small amount since previous measurements, which may cause anxiety.
- A good explanation of the centile charts to parents are vital, as parents may be anxious if their infant/child does not follow a specific centile.
- In a hospital setting, in emergencies, there may not be time to weigh a child, and therefore either a broselow tape may be used, or the calculations:

$$0–12 \text{ months } (0.5 \times \text{age in months}) + 4$$
$$1–5\text{yrs } (2 \times \text{age in yrs}) + 8$$
$$6–12\text{yrs } (3 \times \text{age in yrs}) + 7$$

Associated reading
⌘ http://www.rcpch.ac.uk/Research/UK-WHO-Growth-Charts.
Information and formulae for weight calculation can be found at ⌘ www.resus.org.uk

Assessing nutrition

Background

The increasing awareness of the relationship between diet and health status has raised the profile of accurate nutritional assessment. Over the past decade, formal assessment tools have been evaluated for use with children/young people. Assessment of nutrition is vital for a number of reasons in this group:

- They need more energy as their basal metabolic rate is higher.
- They have less stored fat, reducing their ability to cope with illness.
- Intake must be adequate enough for normal growth and development.
- They are at risk of malnutrition.
  - Both underweight, and increasingly at risk of obesity.
  - Hospitalized children can be at further risk of malnutrition.

Equipment

- Nutritional assessment tool.
- World Health Organization centile chart.
- Fluid balance/nutritional chart.
- Scales, tape measure, stadiometer.

Procedure

- Obtain height/length, weight, head circumference, BMI (see
  📖 Measuring weight, height, and body mass index, p. 86).
- Ensure a thorough history and examination is taken.
- Establish child/young person's current food/fluid intake and pattern.

Principles for infancy

- Most babies will feed 3- or 4-hourly for the first 12 weeks, when they will start to sleep for 8h at night.
- Weaning should be commenced by/around 6 months old with fruit, vegetables, or rice-based foodstuffs.
- Cow's milk should not be taken until 1yr of age.
- To help to promote healthy weight gain, infants should be fed according to their expected weight (see Table 4.4).
- It is recommended all children 6 months–5yrs are given supplements containing vitamins A, C, and D, in the form of vitamin drops.[1]

Table 4.4 Birth weight + weekly weight gain = expected weight (EW)

Age in weeks	Weight gain (g/week)
*2—12	200
13—24	150
25—36	100
37—52	50

*Most breast-fed infants will regain their birth weight by week 2/14 days so these weeks are excluded from the calculation.

Principles for children and young people

- Weight can be approximated: 0–12months = (0.5 × age in months) + 4; 1–5yrs = (2 × age in yrs) + 8; 6–12yrs = (3 × age in yrs) + 7.
- Self-report questionnaires/diaries should be triangulated with information provided independently by parents.
- The encouragement of a balanced diet is vital.
- For nutritional requirements see Tables 4.5 and 4.6.

Table 4.5 Estimated nutrient requirements for infancy

Age (months)	Fluid (mL/kg)	Energy (kcal/kg)	Protein (g/kg)	Iron (mg/day)
1	180	180	2.1	1.7
3	150	180	1.6	4.3
6	130	150	1.5	7.8
9	120	130	1.5	7.8

Table 4.6 Estimated nutritional requirements for children/young people

Age (yrs)	Drinks (mL/day)	Energy (kcal/day)	Protein (g/day)	Sodium (g/day)
1–3	900	1300	15	2
4–6	1200	1800	20	3
7–10	1800	2000	28	5
11–14	2000	2500	42	6
15–18	2600	3000	55	6

Practice tips

- Nutritional requirements may alter in a hospital environment to accommodate the child/young person's condition such as in faltering growth, prematurity, cystic fibrosis.
- Involve parents, and include within the assessment the child's behaviour. Malnutrition will lead to lethargy.
- Nutritional assessment requires a multi-disciplinary approach; liaise with, e.g. the dietician, health visitor, community paediatrician.

Pitfalls

- Assessment methods may provide a challenge when applied to children/young people with profound physical and/or cognitive impairment.
- Whilst family-centred care should be paramount, in order to gain accurate information, the nurse may need to directly observe and monitor all the child/young person's intake in a hospital setting, and not just rely upon self- or parental reporting.
- Cultural preferences and practices can impact nutritional intake and will need to be acknowledged in assessing and managing nutrition.

Associated reading

http://www.stampscreeningtool.org/stamp.html.

http://www.clinicalguidelines.scot.nhs.uk/Dietetics/Nutrition%20Policy%20YOR-DIET-003.pdf.

Shaw V, Lawson M. (eds) (2008). *Clinical Paediatric Dietetics.* 3rd edn. Blackwell Publishing, Oxford.

Royal College of Nursing. (2006). *Malnutrition, what nurses working with children and young people need to know and do.* RCN, London.

Information and formulae for weight calculation can be found at www.resus.org.uk

[1] NHS choices. (2011). *Birth to five. Vitamins.* Available at: http://www.nhs.uk/Planners/birth-tofive/Pages/Vitamins.aspx (accessed 9 June 2011).

Assessing fluid requirements

Background

Assessing fluid requirements

Background

Fluid intake and output is greater in younger children compared to older children/adults. Any alterations can progress quickly and have significant effects. In critical illness/injury the normal mechanisms that control normal fluid balance—thirst, hormones, renal function, may be disrupted.

Normal daily fluid requirement can be calculated per patient and forms an important part of daily nursing care in all specialities. Calculation is based upon the individual's weight in kilograms. This calculation provides a standardized formulation for any patient that does not have altered health status. Alterations may need to be performed if the patient has ongoing illness or acute pathology, e.g.

- Dehydration (see 🕮 Assessing dehydration, p. 94).
- Diarrhoea.
- Nephrotic syndrome.
- Congestive heart failure.
- Electrolyte abnormalities.
- Diabetic ketoacidosis.
- Burns.
- Neurological pathology, e.g. head injury.

Equipment

- Scales.
- Fluid balance chart.

Procedure

The calculation for total fluid requirement for a 24-h period:

- 100mL per Kg for the first 10Kg.
- 50mL per Kg for second 10Kg.
- 20mL per Kg for all subsequent Kg.

Example:

- A baby weighing 12kg = 10 × 100mL = 1000mL
  2 × 50mL = 100mL
  Total for 24-h period   1100mL
- A child weighing 26kg = 10 × 100mL = 1000mL
  10 × 50mL = 500mL
  6 × 20mL = 120mL
  Total for 24hr period   1620mL
- Accurate fluid balance is vital in order to establish total volume in compared to total volume out, influencing clinical decisions and care.
- Volume in can include feeds (oral, enteral, parenteral), IV drugs, and fluids.
- Volume out can include urine, stool, vomit, aspirates, drain losses.
- Documentation should be as accurate as possible:
  - Descriptions such as 'small vomit' should be avoided.
  - Consider how to gain an accurate measure, such as having incontinence sheets *in situ* so that the dry weight of the sheet can be subtracted from the total, giving an accurate measurement of losses.

Practice tips

- For some patients fluid balance and the amount of fluid administered will need to be strict and include all drugs and infusions. Fluid maintenance for these patients may have to be adjusted to reflect this.
- It must be remembered that response to fluid treatment as well as ongoing fluid losses will remain individual to each patient. Therefore, fluid management may need to be recalculated and adjusted as therapy progresses.
- Fluid calculations for young babies are normally based upon birth weight. This also applies to any baby who has not yet regained birth weight.

Pitfalls

- The calculation of insensible fluid losses is very difficult. It is related to elements such as ambient temperature, humidity, pyrexia (if present), patient skin quality as well as calorific intake. Medical advice regarding this calculation should be sought for each individual patient.

Associated reading

Higgins C. (2007). *Understanding laboratory investigations*, 2nd edn. Wiley-Blackwell, London.
National Institute for Health and Clinical Excellence. (2009). *Diarrhoea and vomiting caused by gastroenteritis; diagnosis, assessment and management in children younger than 5 yrs.* Available at: http://www.nice.org.uk/nicemedia/live/11846/43817/43817.pdf (accessed 24 February 2011).
Willock J, Jewkes F. (2000). Making sense of fluid balance in children. *Paediat Nurs* **12**(7), 37–42.

Assessing dehydration

Background

Dehydration in infants and children can be caused by a variety of pathologies. Children are at greater risk of fluid loss due to factors such as an increased body surface area and increased extracellular fluid. Without treatment, dehydration can lead to shock, and severe metabolic acidosis, which may result in death. Common pathologies include:

- Diarrhoea.
- Vomiting.
- Diabetic ketoacidosis.
- Gastroenteritis.

Dehydration can be categorized into mild, moderate, and severe.

- Mild dehydration: ~0–5% fluid loss.
- Moderate dehydration: ~5–10% fluid loss.
- Severe dehydration: ~10–15% fluid loss.

Equipment

- Scales.
- Monitoring equipment, e.g. sphygmomanometer for BP.
- Blood sugar and blood ketones bedside testing equipment.
- Documentation, including for fluid balance (see 📖 Assessing fluid requirements, p. 92).
- Urine collection equipment (see 📖 Specimen collection and storage, p. 178).

Procedure

- Assessment of dehydration can be completed by observing both vital signs and clinical signs.
- It must be remembered that both vital signs and clinical signs individually can produce unreliable results, but collectively will produce a more dependable estimate of fluid loss and condition.

Vital Signs

- *Heart rate:* ↑.
- *Pulse volume:* ↓.
- *BP:* ↔ or ↓.
- *Capillary refill:* ↔ or >2s.
- *Skin colour:* pale/mottled/white.

Clinical signs

- *Weight:* ↓.
- *Mucous membranes:* dry.
- *Urine output:* ↓.
- *Fontanelle:* sunken.
- *Eyes:* sunken.
- *Skin turgor:* ↓.
- Lethargic.

Further investigations
- Blood tests may be requested to support clinical findings.
- The most common blood tests for management of dehydration include:
  - *Bedside Testing*—blood sugar, that may be altered due to poor fluid/diet intake or altered absorption (see 📖 Blood glucose monitoring, p. 98).
  - *Laboratory testing*—urea and electrolytes (U&E); testing sodium, potassium, bicarbonate, urea, and creatinine. All may be altered due to the shifting of fluid within intracellular and extracellular spaces, as well as the initiation of compensatory mechanisms for metabolic acidosis.

Weight loss calculation
5% dehydration = 5mL loss of fluid/100g of body weight.

Converting grams to a %
Original weight – current weight =?
? ÷ Original weight × 100 = % weight loss
Example: For a baby whose birth weight was 2750g and current weight is 2450g:
2750g – 2450g = 300g.
300g ÷ 2750g × 100 = 10.9% weight loss.

Practice tips
- Within the treatment of dehydration, the electrolyte disturbance should be corrected slowly, normally over 24/48 hours.
- Once stabilization has occurred oral feeds should be recommenced in addition to rehydration therapy. This is especially important if the baby is breast fed.

Pitfalls
- Consideration should include that clinical signs of dehydration may only be visible once 2–5% fluid loss has occurred.
- Be cautious initially; over-hydration can be as dangerous as dehydration.
- The issue of insensible losses needs to be monitored and fluid management may need to be amended during therapy to achieve homeostasis (see 📖 Assessing fluid requirements, p. 92).

Associated reading
Higgins, C. (2007). *Understanding laboratory investigations*, 2nd edn. Wiley-Blackwell, London.
National Institute for Health and Clinical Excellence. (2009). *Diarrhoea and vomiting. caused by gastroenteritis; diagnosis, assessment and management in children younger than 5 yrs*. Available at: 🔗 http://www.nice.org.uk/nicemedia/live/11846/43817/43817.pdf (accessed 24 February 2011).
Willock J, Jewkes F. (2000). Making sense of fluid balance in children. *Paediat Nurs* **12**(7), 37–42.

Assessing urine output

Background

Assessment of urine output is essential within a wider evaluation of a child's circulatory status and can alert to conditions such as dehydration, renal damage or obstruction. Practical techniques can differ according to the age of the child but the principles are the same: to assess whether fluid intake is sufficient to maintain adequate perfusion of the kidneys.

Oliguria (reduced urine output) is a worrying sign and anuria (no urine output) is a sign of decompensated shock. Reduced urine output is considered an 'amber' or intermediate risk sign for serious illness in young children[1] and indicates a significant circulatory problem. Polyuria (overproduction of urine) can be indicative of problems such as diabetes mellitus or diabetes insipidus.

In a seriously ill child, urine output should be calculated per hour. Normal output is >2mL/kg/h in infants, >1mL/kg/h in older children.

It can be assessed by:
• Direct measurement from an in-dwelling urinary catheter.
• Collection and measurement of volume of urine in a suitable container.
• Weighing nappies and subtracting the weight of a dry nappy.

Equipment

• Dependent on method of collection. Urine collection pad, bag, or container.
• Sterile pot and collection bottle if a sample is needed for infection screening or other laboratory tests.
• A clean plastic jug is suitable in most instances to measure urine although a syringe may be needed for smaller volumes.
• Gloves should always be worn when handling body fluids.
• Apron.
• Scales.
• 1g weight = approx 1mL of urine.

Procedure

• Don gloves and apron according to local policy.
• Collect urine via catheter, container, bag, nappy.
• Stand container on level surface and measure or weigh.
• Calculate output. Formula for calculating output per hour is:

$$\text{Urine passed (mL)} \div \text{weight (kg)} \div \text{no. of hours since last voiding} = \text{mL/kg/h}$$

• Dispose of equipment.
• Document and report findings as appropriate.

Practice tips
- Enlist parents' or carers' help. A non-toilet trained child may need to be positioned over an appropriate container for some time in order to catch a urine sample for ward or laboratory testing.
- Have a container ready at the time a baby's nappy is being changed in case you can catch an opportunistic urine sample.
- Write the dry weight on the nappy before applying it to the child.
- Get the child to play with some water or leave a tap running to encourage the urge to urinate.
- Don't forget other losses, e.g. stool, vomit, and gastric aspirates when considering total fluid balance (see 🕮 Assessing fluid requirements, p. 92).

Pitfalls
- If a child/young person has diarrhoea it can be hard to differentiate urine from stool losses.
- Small volumes mean every millilitre is important.

Associated reading
Willock J, Jewkes F. (2000). Making sense of fluid balance in children. *Paediat Nurs* **12**(7), 37–42.

[1] NICE (2007). *Feverish illness in children. Assessment and the initial management in children younger than 5 yrs: quick reference guide.* NIHCE, London. Available at: 🔗 http://www.nice.org.uk/nicemedia/live/11010/30524/30524.pdf.

Blood glucose monitoring

Background

Blood glucose monitoring measures the amount of glucose in the blood. The body requires a continuous supply of glucose in order to produce cellular energy. Blood glucose levels will vary depending on such factors as exercise, when a meal was taken and the content of that meal. There are conditions when close blood sugar monitoring is required, such as:

- Diabetes mellitus where more frequent blood sugar monitoring is associated with improved glycaemic control,[1] identifies trends, and informs adjustment of insulin doses.
- Children on total parenteral nutrition (TPN).
- Metabolic and endocrine disorders.
- Seizures.
- Unexplained change in consciousness level.
- Neonates.

Normal blood sugar ranges are:

- 4–8mmol (before food).
- May ↑ to 10mmol (after food).
- In neonates hypoglycaemia is defined as a blood sugar <2.6mmol/L.

Equipment

- Blood glucose monitor: calibrated and quality control checked as per manufacturer's instructions.
- Blood glucose strips.
- Lancet device (finger pricker).
- Lancets.
- Cotton wool.
- Sharps bin.

Procedure

- Wash and dry hands.
- Prepare finger pricking device as per user instructions.
- Prepare blood glucose monitor as per user instructions.
- Open the blood glucose strip (after checking the expiry date) and place into the blood glucose monitor, ensuring the strip batch number matches that on the screen. If it doesn't match the monitor may need recalibrating.
- Use cotton wool to clean the finger or heel (heels for babies <1yr) to ensure accuracy of the results. Only ever use water to clean the site as another substance may alter the result.
- Prick side of finger/heel:
  - When choosing a site rotate areas to avoid nerve end damage.
  - Avoid the index finger and thumb as older children will use these frequently.
- Massage the area to promote blood flow and obtain blood sample, using gravity to your advantage.

- Apply blood to sampling area of blood test strip. The blood glucose monitor will bleep or start counting down if it has a satisfactory sample.
- Use cotton wool to stop bleeding and ensure the child is comfortable.
- Dispose of lancet and strip in the sharps box.
- The result will read on the machine, which should be documented clearly with the time, and take action as necessary. Any action should also be clearly documented.
- If an error appears the blood sugar will need repeating, a quality check on the blood glucose monitor undertaken, and the machine potentially changing.

Practice tips

- Ensure a new lancet is used each test.
- A suitable depth gauge setting on a lancet device reduces pain.
- Capillary blood flow is increased if the site used is warm, therefore it would be ideal in advance, for example, to place a sock on an infant's foot.

Pitfalls

- Accurate calibration of the meter is vital if coding is required.
- Ensure a good blood sampling technique.
- There will be an inaccurate result if blood sample size is insufficient.
- There are various blood glucose monitors, strips, and lancets. You must be competent in using these in each instance.
- Results will vary slightly between blood glucose monitors, so if a patient has their own, use the same machine and document which machine is being used.

Associated reading

Great Ormond Street Hospital. (2010). *Blood Glucose Monitoring*. Available at: ℘ http://www.gosh.nhs.uk/clinical_information/clinical_guidelines/cpg_guideline_00258 (accessed 20 February 2011).

National Institute for Clinical Excellence. (2004). *Clinical Guideline 15 Type 1 diabetes: diagnosis and management of type 1 diabetes in children, young people and adults*. Available at: ℘ http://www.nice.org.uk/nicemedia/pdf/CG015childrenfullguideline.pdf. (accessed 20 February 2011).

[1] Scottish Intercollegiate Guidelines Network (SIGN) (2010). *Management of diabetes, A national clinical guideline*. Available at: ℘ http://www.sign.ac.uk/pdf/qrg116.pdf (accessed 20 February 2011).

Personal hygiene and comfort

Making a bed/cot/bassinet

Background

A clean, well-made bed will help to make a child feel comfortable and safe, and promote confidence in care quality.

Equipment

- Clean bed linen.
- Appropriate linen skip.
- Equipment to clean and tidy bed space area.
- Personal protective equipment (PPE) as required.

Procedure

- *Assess the child and family's needs:* is this the best time to do this task?
- Obtain consent from them to undertake any task.
- Explain the procedure.
- Ensure that you have all equipment you need to hand.
- Clear the area of any obstacles so that you can move around freely.
- Ensure the bed area is warm enough and draught free.
- Close cubicle door and/or draw screens/curtains around bed area.
- Wash hands and don PPE as determined by local infection control protocols.
- If possible adjust the bed height to a comfortable working height for those performing the task.
- Encourage the child to help if they can or wish to and are able.
- Consider whether it will be most appropriate to change the bottom sheet from end to end or from side to side.
- Roll soiled bottom sheet towards child un-tucking either from one end of the bed to the other or from one side of the bed to the other.
- Ensure the mattress is clean—clean as per local policy as necessary.
- Place the clean bottom sheet on the exposed part of the mattress and tuck in corners. Keep the other part of the clean sheet rolled up close to the child and the remaining soiled sheet.
- Assist the child to move over the sheet rolls.
- Pull out the soiled sheet—dispose into linen skip.
- Clean the remaining part of mattress as necessary.
- Unroll the rest of the clean sheet and tuck in.
- Ensure sheet is straight and taut.
- Place clean top sheet over child and dispose of top sheet and blanket into linen skip. Tuck in corners of clean top sheet and blanket, but then loosen them by pulling them up from the centre of the bed to provide more room for movement and comfort.
- Change pillow cases and place pillows in appropriate position for comfort and clinical condition.
- Return bed height to that most appropriate to child's needs.
- Ensure that child is comfortable.
- Clean and tidy area around bed space as necessary.
- Return linen skip to appropriate place—place linen bag for laundry collection when no more than 2/3 full, following any local protocols for labelling, etc.
- Dispose of PPE.
- Wash hands.

Practice tips
- Roll up sheets for disposal from outside edges to inner material to avoid dispersing dead skin cells and other debris into the surrounding environment.
- Remember to check for displaced equipment, toys, dummies, etc.
- Make sure that the child is safe before during and after procedure—utilize cot sides as necessary as per local protocol.
- Ensure that bed wheels are locked.
- Ensure that items the child may need are within reach—nurse call button, drink, activities, etc.

Bed bath

Background

Many children will need assistance with personal hygiene due to the level of their cognitive and motor skills, and/or their physical condition.

Parents should be encouraged to participate in their child's personal hygiene as much as they are able and if the child/young person wishes them to be. The child is much more likely to relax if their parent is performing their usual cares.

A bed bath can help main self-esteem and positive body image, and is an opportunity to check the child or young person's skin, alongside promoting cleanliness and comfort. Hygiene needs should be addressed whenever necessary to promote the child's comfort and safety, and when needed, a bed bath should be performed once every 24h.

Equipment

- *Clean clothing (child's own if possible):* encourage the child to choose what they wish to wear if they are able.
- Clean bed linen.
- Bowl of hand-hot water.
- Soap and 2 clean face cloths (child's own if possible).
- Disposable wipes.
- At least 2 towels.
- *Child's own toiletries and equipment:*
  - Comb/brush, hair accessories.
  - Toothbrush, toothpaste, or mouth care pack.
  - Additional toiletries—deodorant, etc.
- Blanket.

Procedure

- *Assess child and family's needs:* is this the best time to do this task?
- Examine skin integrity carefully at all stages and take appropriate measures to deal with any sore areas (see 📖 Pressure ulcer risk assessment and prevention, p. 136).
- *Consider safeguarding and protection issues:* encourage parents/carers to fully participate if appropriate and the child/young person wishes it, consider whether there is a need for another person to be with you.
- Obtain consent to undertake any task.
- Explain the procedure.
- Ensure that you have all equipment to hand so that you don't have to leave the child during the task.
- Clear area of any obstacles so that you can move around freely.
- Ensure the bed area is warm enough and draught free.
- If possible, adjust bed to a comfortable working height for those performing the task.
- Close door and/or draw screens/curtains around bed area.
- Wash hands and remove top cover, leaving top sheet in place. Place large towel(s) over top sheet and then remove top sheet from under it so that child remains covered.

- Pull covers back and remove into appropriate linen skip if soiled or place at the end of the bed.
- Help the child into most comfortable position and assist them (and/or parent) to do as much of this procedure as they wish and/or are able.
- Remove clothing under bath towel.
- If child has an intravenous (IV) line, drain, or wound, etc., remove clothing from unaffected side first.
- Undertake eye care (see 📖 Eye care, p. 110).
- Undertake dental care (see 📖 Dental care, p. 114).
- Refresh water as needed.
- Wash and dry face.
- Wash each arm separately, placing a dry towel beneath each one. Rinse and dry each arm, apply deodorant as/if required, and cover.
- Undertake finger nail care (see 📖 Nail care, p. 116).
- Wash, rinse, and dry top half of body, leaving bottom half covered.
- *Check water temperature:* change if cold or dirty.
- Ask if child/parent wishes to wash genital area. If not, put on gloves and wash these areas with a second cloth (or disposable wipes) from front to back. (For boys post-puberty retract foreskin and wash penis underneath it). Rinse and dry, re-cover child, remove and dispose of gloves, and wash hands.
- Change water.
- Wash legs as arms.
- Undertake toe nail care (see 📖 Nail care, p. 116).
- Assist or roll child on to side, place a towel under their back and wash, rinse, and dry.
- Put on gloves and wash, rinse, and dry bottom using second cloth or disposable wipe. Dispose of gloves and cloth as appropriate. Re-cover child and wash hands.
- If the child has an IV line, drain, etc., redress affected side first.
- Dress child. Position as appropriate for comfort and clinical condition.
- Brush/comb and dress hair (see 📖 Hair care, p. 108) as preferred by child.
- Ensure bed rails are in place if required.
- Ensure child has all items they may require within easy reach.
- Clear away used equipment.
- Document care and report concerns, e.g. broken skin, infestations, etc.

Practice tips

- Make sure that you are aware of, and respect, any religious/cultural rituals related to a child's care.
- Disrupt normal routines as little as possible.
- Do not encroach on parent/carer's role, but offer support.
- Encourage independence, but supervise.
- Use opportunities for health education.
- The sick/distressed child may regress in their development and, therefore, may need more assistance than you might expect.

Baby bath

Background

Babies do not need a bath daily, but will need their face, neck, hands, and bottom washing every day. Milk often spills into the creases around a baby's neck, and if not cleaned and dried often enough, it can begin to get very sore. It is necessary to clean and dry their bottom for the same reason, as nappy rash can become a problem.

❶ Never leave an infant or young child alone or unsupervised in water!

Equipment

- Cotton wool.
- Baby bath.
- Clean warm water.
- Towels.
- Clean nappy.
- Clean clothes.
- Apron and gloves.
- Baby soap (unless the baby has particularly dry skin).

Procedure

- Gather all the equipment together prior to commencing the procedure to maintain the safety of the baby.
- Wash your hands.
- Fill the bath (no deeper than 10cm).
- Ensure the temperature of the water is appropriate—check with a thermometer (32°C to 35°C).
- Lay out the clean clothes, nappy, and the towel on a flat surface where you will dress the baby after the bath.
- Wash hands, and put on apron and gloves.
- Clean the baby's face prior to undressing it. Use a clean piece of cotton wool soaked in clean water and clean the baby's eye, from the centre to the outside of the eye. Use a fresh piece of cotton wool for the other eye. Clean around the ears with another piece of cotton wool, and dry the face and ears.
- Undress the baby and ensure any stool is cleaned from the baby's bottom. Hold the baby firmly, but gently, resting the baby's head in the centre of your forearm and holding under the baby's arm with your hand. Gently place the baby into the bath.
- Cup your hand and pour water over the baby's head, avoiding getting the water in its eyes.
- Use cotton wool to clean under the baby's arms and bottom. To clean the baby's back, carefully turn it over, holding under both arms, with its chest resting on your forearm and your other arm free to clean the baby's back.
- Once the baby is clean, carefully remove it from the bath and place on the towel. Wrap the baby up in the towel and dry the head and body, paying particular attention to any creases, e.g. in the neck, arms, and legs.

- Once dry, put on the new nappy and the clean clothes. Ensure the baby is safe, then dispose of the water, dirty clothes and nappy, apron, and gloves.
- Wash hands at the end of the procedure.

Practice tips

- Ensure all the equipment is gathered prior to commencing the procedure, so that it does not need to be interrupted for any reason.
- If you have no thermometer, place your elbow into the water. If it is too hot for you to do this comfortably, add some more cold water until it is at the right temperature.
- ❶ Hold them firmly—wet skin is very slippery!
- Some babies will love bath time, while for others it cannot be over soon enough! Provide suitable play and distraction materials to soothe where necessary and to promote enjoyment. Stroke and sing!
- Ensure environmental temperature is adequate—babies can lose heat very quickly.

Hair care

Background

The way a child feels is often related to their appearance, particularly as they get older. Hair care can be complex; consideration needs to be given to the child's preferences.

Grooming an infant or child's hair provides an ideal opportunity to observe for general cleanliness and parasitic infestations, such as head lice. If a child is well enough, then obviously it will be preferable for them to follow their own hair-washing routine and practice.

Equipment

- Clean bed linen in case of spillage.
- Bowl of hand-hot water.
- Jug.
- Face cloth to cover the child's eyes if they request.
- Comb/brush.
- Shampoo/conditioner (medicated shampoo if required).
- Towels.

Procedure

- *Assess child and family's needs:* is this the best time to do this task?
- Obtain consent to undertake the task.
- Explain the procedure.
- Ensure that you have all equipment to hand so that you don't have to leave the child during the task.
- Clear the area of any obstacles so that you can move around freely.
- Remove bed head.
- Ensure the bed area is warm enough and draught free.
- If possible, adjust bed to a comfortable working height for those performing the task.
- Close door and/or draw screens/curtains around bed area if child/family wishes.
- The water should be hand hot. If the water cools down then it should be replenished. If the child is able to be involved in their care, ask him or her to confirm the temperature of the water.
- Assist the child to the top of the bed and support their head over the edge.
- Place a towel under the child's shoulders to avoid wetting sheets.
- Place the bowl under the child's head and pour water over head with jug.
- Next shampoo the hair then rinse with water until the water runs clear. The bowl of hand hot water may need to be changed several times to ensure all the shampoo has been rinsed out properly.
- Dry the child's hair using a clean towel or hair dryer if they request to do so.
- Change the bed linen if it has become damp in any way and reposition the infant or child comfortably.
- Comb or brush the child's hair.
- Style hair as the child wishes.

Practice tips

- Make sure that you are aware of the child's own preferences regarding hair styling.
- Make sure that you are aware of any religious/cultural rituals related to a child's hair care.

❶ Observe scalp and hair shafts for lice and/or lice eggs (nits). The belief that head lice are associated with poor hygiene is common, but ill-founded. Lice are equally likely to be found on clean or dirty hair. See Box 5.1 for methods of dealing with head lice.

Box 5.1 Dealing with head lice

- *Use a nit comb:* a fine-toothed plastic comb with spacing of less than 0.3mm
- Start at the middle of the front of the scalp
- Comb the hair from the roots to the very end of the hair
- After each stroke, examine the teeth of the comb for living lice
- Rinse the comb if you find any lice
- Continue combing section by section until you've done the whole head of hair, including the area just behind the ears and at the nape of the neck
- For wet combing, simply wash hair and apply conditioner before starting these steps. Afterwards, rinse out the conditioner and check hair again with the nit comb before drying
- With curly hair you may find that oiling the hair makes it easier to use the nit comb effectively
- *Chemical treatment* may be considered for medical prescription if live lice are found:
  - Apply lotion as instructed by manufacturer
  - Allow hair to dry naturally after application. Do not use a hairdryer
  - Treatment may be prescribed for re-application after 7 days.
- *Wet combing* of hair may be ordered to remove head lice without the use of chemicals: Wet the hair, apply conditioner, and then comb with a fine-toothed comb for at least 30min every 3rd or 4th day over a 2-week period.

Eye care

Background

Infants and children's eyes are delicate, protected by tears that maintain moistness and cleanliness in the eye. However, in the unwell or unconscious infant or child, drying of the eye may occur. This, in turn, can lead to infections of the eye.

Nurses need to be aware that infants and young children may resist anything coming towards their face, requiring gentle persuasion or play diversion to facilitate the performance of eye care.

Equipment

- Gauze pieces or cotton wool balls for each eye depending on organizational policy. Check your local guidelines.
- Gallipot for each eye labelled for use with the left or right eye.
- Sachets of 0.9% NaCl solution.
- Medicated eye drops/ointment if prescribed.

Procedure

- One to two nurses may be needed to carry out eye care depending on the infant or child's compliance, alongside the parent.
- If the child is able to help in any way they should be encouraged to do so.
- Explain procedure and gain consent.
- If in a communal setting, screens can be drawn around the bed if requested by the child. If they are in a cubicle, close the door and draw the curtains.
- The child will need to be placed in a supine position, using gentle restraint as necessary to safely perform the eye care without causing any harm to the eye or child.
- Wash hands.
- Empty a sachet of 0.9% NaCl in the gallipots for each eye making sure the gallipot is kept covered if not in use. A different gallipot should be used for each eye to avoid potential cross-infection. Open the gauze pieces/cotton wool balls.
- Gently clean one eye at a time using the appropriate NaCl solution for that specific eye with a soaked cotton wool ball or gauze pad from the inside of the eye outwards, discarding the cotton wool ball or gauze pad after one clean. This will be sufficient to prevent infection and keep the eyes moist.
- If the eye looks infected in any way report this to the medical team who may prescribe medicated eye drops or ointment.
- If the child wears glasses ensure they are cleaned regularly or assist them to clean themselves.

Practice tips

- Giving teddy or a doll some eye care may help with a child's fears.
- A reward system may also help if the child is reluctant to participate.

Mouth care and oral assessment

Background

Mouth care and oral assessment

Background

Good mouth care practice is used to:
- Prevent infection.
- Remove food debris and plaque.
- Control pain.
- Allow optimum conditions for adequate oral nutrition and fluid intake.
- Freshen the mouth and support well-being.

Nurses carrying out oral assessment should have an understanding of the mouth's normal structure in order to be able to recognize changes.

Parents and children would normally undertake mouth care without any input from a health professional. However, during illness and/or certain treatments, both child and family are likely to need additional advice, support, and intervention.

Equipment

- Oral assessment tool.
- Patient documentation.
- Toothpaste.
- Soft toothbrush.
- Mouth wash.
- Sponges (if necessary).
- Water.
- Towel.
- Spit bowl.
- Pen torch.

Procedure

An oral assessment will be essential in order to plan the best mouth care for the individual child or young person. Staff undertaking oral assessment should be trained in the use of the tool.
- Assemble all necessary equipment.
- Consider use of an appropriate oral assessment tool.
- Explain procedure appropriately to child/young person and parent(s).
- Obtain consent to carry out the procedure.
- Position child appropriately; ensure they are in a comfortable position.
- Involve additional personnel as needed to help the child to maintain position, and provide distraction/activity as appropriate.
- Wash hands and apply non-sterile gloves.
- Examine the following areas of the mouth:
  - Swallowing.
  - Lips and mouth corners.
  - Tongue.
  - Mucous membranes.
  - Gingiva.
  - Teeth.
  - Voice.
- Use pen torch to look inside the oral cavity, shine the light from side to side and top to bottom of mouth, covering all structures and observing any tissue changes.

- When the assessment is complete, remove and dispose of gloves as per local policy and wash hands.
- Findings should be recorded in the child's health record and reported to the appropriate health professionals as required.
- Determine what appropriate mouth care is needed to ensure the child's comfort and well-being.
- Pain relief should be considered following consultation with appropriate medical staff if mouth integrity is compromised on assessment.
- Support child and family to participate or undertake care independently, as and when appropriate.

For dental care see 🕮 Dental care, p. 114.

Practice tips

- Staff undertaking oral assessments should be fully trained and competent in the equipment use.
- All nursing staff should have a basic understanding of how treatment and medication can affect the oral cavity.
- All children should have an oral assessment done on admission to hospital.
- It is recommended that children receiving treatment and/or medication should have an oral assessment carried out at least once a week.
- Oral assessment will need to be carried out daily if the child:
  - Is neutropenic or immunocompromised.
  - Has an oral assessment score of 8 or above.
  - Has a history of oral problems pre- or post-treatment.
  - Where the mouth falls within the sphere of treatment.
- Children and parents should be given advice and education on mouth care on diagnosis, and throughout treatment.

Pitfalls

- Don't be tempted to use your fingers to help you carry out an oral assessment.
- Make sure the child and parent understand what you are doing and why. Without their co-operation there is no way you will be able to carry out an oral assessment.
- It's easy to assume that a child/family is undertaking basic mouth care independently. Make sure you don't take this for granted.

Associated reading

Costello T, Coyne I (2008). Nurse's knowledge of mouth care practices. *Br J Nursing* **17**(4), 264–8.
UKCCSG-PONF (2006). *Mouth Care for Children and Young People with Cancer: Evidence Based Guidelines.* Guideline Report Version 1.0 February 2006. Available at: 🔗 http://www.rcn.org.uk.

Dental care

Background

Good oral hygiene will reduce risk of infection, dental and systemic diseases, distress, and discomfort. Teeth should be brushed at least twice a day, morning and evening. Plaque formation begins 4–6h after brushing. Commence brushing routine with the eruption of the first tooth.

Equipment

- Soft, size appropriate toothbrush. (The size and shape of the brush should be such that it can easily reach all tooth surfaces.)
- Fluoride toothpaste.
- Tap water.
- Sterile water (for babies less than 1yr).
- Obtain mouth care pack from sterile supplies service.
- Foam sponges.
- Soft paraffin/petroleum jelly.

Procedure

- Explain the procedure.
- Gain consent from child and carer.
- Encourage involvement and/or self-care where appropriate.
- Gather supplies.
- Wash hands.
- Assess *current mouth condition:* note presence of *Candida*, ulcers, breaks in mucosa, saliva consistency, and condition of teeth, tongue, gingiva, and lips. Note pain or difficulty in swallowing or using voice.
- ❶ Consider using an assessment tool (see 🕮 Mouth care and oral assessment, p. 112).
- Gently brush teeth and gums with brush and toothpaste for at least 2min, using a tiny smear of toothpaste for babies and a pea-sized amount for children.
- To brush effectively: place the head of the brush against the teeth, tilting the bristle tips to a 45° angle against the gumline. Move the brush in small circular movements several times on all the surfaces of every tooth.
- Brush the outer surfaces of each tooth, upper and lower, keeping the bristles angled against the gumline.
- Use the same method on the inside surfaces of all teeth.
- Brush the chewing surfaces of the teeth.
- To clean the inside surfaces of the front teeth, tilt the brush vertically. Make several small circular strokes with the front part of the brush.
- Encourage the child to spit after brushing, if they are able to. Do not rinse.
- Rinse mouth with water (sterile if under 1yr) if unable to spit.
- Apply soft paraffin/petroleum jelly to lips.
- Antibacterial mouthwashes and antifungal preparations may be prescribed for some children, e.g. those with oral *Candida* or mouth infection, the immunosuppressed child, those undergoing chemotherapy.

Practice tips

- Foam swabs are not effective for mouth cleaning. They are only helpful to moisten mouth or assist with rinsing.
- Infant toothbrushes are available that fit over a carer's finger to clean the teeth.
- Inserting the handle into a rubber ball may make it easier for the child to grip the brush.
- A child may find it difficult to control the pressure of their brushing. A brush with a flexible neck may help to absorb excessive pressure.
- Toothbrushes should be changed every 3–4 months, once the bristles begin to lose their natural position or following an infection.
- Children and carers will find different positions best for toothbrushing. Many find brushing from behind the most acceptable.
- It may be helpful to wedge/support the child between the knees of the carer.
- Tilt the child's chin so that their head is resting against the adult's chest or shoulder. In this position, you can see clearly into the child's mouth.
- As the child gets older, stand or sit behind them.
- Gently stretch on the cheek with toothbrush or index finger of the hand not holding the brush when brushing at the back.
- Techniques to encourage co-operation could include:
  - Counting teeth.
  - Demonstrating on a doll or another person—tell/show/do.
  - Story-telling, singing.
  - Positive encouragement and reinforcement.
  - Flavoured/stripey/'different' toothpaste.
  - Coloured/cartoon/musical/timer brushes.

Pitfalls

- Children under 7yrs are unlikely to brush effectively unsupervised.
- Rinsing reduces the benefit of fluoride toothpaste.
- There is a risk with the use of mouth sponges of the sponge becoming detached from the stick, thus becoming a choking hazard.
- Brushing too forcefully can result in abrasions in tooth enamel or dentin, causing tooth sensitivity problems.
- Swallowing toothpaste and/or use of excessive amounts of toothpaste may increase the risk of enamel fluorosis—absorption of too much fluoride while the enamel of the teeth is forming. Although this will actually strengthen the teeth it may lead to teeth enamel becoming pitted and discoloured. It may be recommended that children under 7yrs of age use a low fluoride toothpaste.
- 'Bottle mouth' occurs when a child sleeps with a bottle in their mouth. Liquids that stays in the mouth continuously can cause rapid decay.
- Thumb sucking and pacifiers are normal habits for newborns, but are not recommended beyond 36 months because they may lead to serious problems of jaw malformation and tooth displacement.

Associated reading

🔗 http://www.dentalhealth.org

Nail care

Background

Nails are a good indicator of health, it is therefore important to regularly check a child's nails whilst performing their basic hygiene cares. Look for signs of abnormalities, e.g. white marks, discolouration of the nails, etc.

Infants and children's nails are soft and thin, they can cause damage to the face if the infant or child is in the habit of scratching. Therefore, it is important to keep the fingernails well-trimmed. Nails need to be trimmed correctly.

Equipment

- Warm water.
- Soap.
- Towel.
- Infant/child nail scissors and/or soft emery board.

Procedure

- Explain the procedure and gain consent.
- One nurse and/or the parent can easily provide nail care depending on the infant or child's compliance.
- Encourage the child to help in any way they are able, if they can do so.
- Wash the child's hands with a mild soap.
- Soak the hands in warm water for a few minutes and dry properly.
- If the child's nails are long cut them using nail scissors, pushing the pad of the infants or child's finger away from the nail as you cut, in order to avoid cutting the finger.
- Observe nails and surrounding tissue for signs of damage, inflammation, discoloration, thickening, or infection. Record and report as appropriate.
- If the child's hands appear dry it may be appropriate to use a simple hand cream.

Practice tips

- If it's very hard for the child to keep still and you are reluctant to use scissors, you could use a soft emery board.
- ❶ Remember, observation of the nail bed is helpful when assessing perfusion and it is inadvisable for a sick child to wear nail polish.

Assessment of pain

Background

Accurate pain assessment is the foundation on which effective pain management is built. The nurse's role is fundamental to the assessment and management of pain. As such it is pivotal that nurses caring for children have a good knowledge base. Pain management in this population is widely recognized as challenging and complex due to factors such as the child's age, cognitive ability, perception of pain, severity of illness, and previous painful experiences.

Whilst self-reporting of pain is the gold standard of pain assessment, many children are unable to verbally communicate their pain; including premature infants, neonates, toddlers with limited vocabulary, and children with a cognitive impairment. Therefore, physiological and behavioural indicators of pain are often needed to supplement self-report (see Boxes 5.2 and 5.3).

Equipment

- The Association of Paediatric Anaesthetists of Great Britain and Ireland (APAGBI) and Royal College of Nursing Institute (RCNI) provide evidence-based recommendations for pain assessment tools suitable for children of different ages and cognitive abilities.
- Behavioural and physiological scales are used for infants and children unable to verbally communicate.
- There are many visual scales for school aged children to assess quality and quantity of pain experienced.
- Young people often prefer the visual analogue scale of 1–10.
- As there are so many tools available, to avoid confusion a single tool should be chosen for each age group, appropriate to the clinical setting (see Box 5.4 for examples).

Procedure

Utilize the QUESTT approach to pain assessment:
- **Q**uestion the child.
- **U**se a pain rating scale.
- **E**valuate behaviour/physiological changes.
- **S**ecure parents' involvement.
- **T**ake the cause of pain into account.
- **T**ake action (i.e. determine and use pain management methods) and evaluate results.

Practice tips

- Obtain an accurate pain history.
- Take the type and cause of pain into account (acute, chronic or recurrent).
- Involve parents/carers in all aspects of pain assessment and management.
- Utilize the QUESTT approach.

Box 5.2 Physiological indicators of pain

- Tachycardia
- Hypertension
- Tachypnoea
- Elevated blood glucose
- Pallor

Neonates and infants may have these symptoms and/or:
- Apnoea
- Bradycardia
- Desaturation
- Palmar sweating

Box 5.3 Behavioural indicators of pain

- Loss of appetite
- Restlessness
- Sobbing
- Lethargy
- Lying 'scared stiff'
- Guarding the area
- Pulling away
- Withdrawal
- Changed behaviour
- Irritability
- Unusual posture
- Screaming
- Reluctance to move
- Aggressiveness
- Disturbed sleep
- Crying
- Grimacing
- ↑clinging

In addition to these indicators, children with a cognitive impairment may also demonstrate the following behaviours:
- Lip smacking
- Arched back
- Head banging
- Rocking
- Biting own fingers/knuckles

- Use an appropriate pain assessment tool in conjunction with observing behavioural and physiological signs of pain. Combining behavioural assessment with changes in physiological signs is more indicative than using one method alone.
- Record the pain assessment tool chosen.
- Record pain assessment score and document interventions.
- Re-assess regularly and liaise with colleagues regarding further options (e.g. anaesthetist, pain team, and medical staff).

Box 5.4 Examples of pain assessment tools[1,2,3]

Premature infants and neonates
- Behavioural;
  - Premature Infant Pain Profile (PIPP)
  - Crying, Requires oxygen, ↑ vital signs, expression, sleepiness (CRIES)
  - COMFORT scale

Children and young people without a cognitive impairment
- Self report:
  - Wong and Baker,[4] FACES Pain Scale—valid for 3–18-yr-olds
  - Faces Pain Scale, revised—valid for 4–12-yr-olds
  - Pieces of Hurt Tool—valid for 3–8-yr-olds
- Behavioural: faces, legs, activity, cry, consolability (FLACC) valid for 1–18-yr-olds.

Children and young people with a cognitive impairment
- Behavioural:
  - Non-Communicating Children's Pain Checklist- Postoperative Version (NCCPC-PV)—valid for 3–19-yr-olds
  - Paediatric Pain Profile (PPP)—valid for 1–18-yr-olds
  - Revised FLACC—valid for 4–19-yr-olds

Pitfalls
- Changes in vital signs can be useful indicators that a child may be in pain, but pain signs can be conflicting and inconsistent, leading to difficulty in assessing the severity of the pain that the child is experiencing.
- Assessing pain by the use of physiological changes alone can be very misleading, as there are many events other than pain, which cause these changes.
- Even if the physiological indicators of pain diminish, pain may still be present as adaptation of the body's response to pain occurs after a period of time.
- It is important to note that pain behaviours may not always be obvious as they can be modified by factors such as the environment, fear, sleep deprivation, and cultural background. Each child's behaviour needs to be assessed individually as they may behave differently in different/ unfamiliar environments.

---

[1] Association of Paediatric Anaesthetists of Great Britain and Ireland (2008). *Good practice in postoperative and procedural pain.* Available at: ℘ http://www.apagbi.org.uk.

[2] Royal College of Nursing Institute (1999). *Clinical Practice Guidelines: The Recognition and Assessment of Acute Pain in Children Recommendations.* RCN Institute, London.

[3] ℘ http://www.rcn.org.uk/development/practice/pain.

[4] Baker C Wong D. (1987) QUESTT: a process of pain assessment in children. *Orthopaed Nurse* **6**(1), 11–21.

Pain management

Pharmacological pain management

Background
When considering pharmacological pain management, best practice is to utilize a combination of analgesic medications. This method of management (multi-modal analgesia) has a synergistic effect, as pain transmission can be blocked at several points along the pain pathway, resulting in an overall analgesic effect superior to that of one drug alone.

Analgesics should be prescribed and administered regularly, to prevent peaks and troughs in blood levels and the potential for 'break-through' pain. In addition, combination therapy has been shown to have an opioid sparing effect, i.e. the patient requires less opioid medication. Combining an intravenous or oral opioid with regular paracetamol and a non-steroidal anti-inflammatory drug (NSAID) such as ibuprofen or diclofenac sodium is a common method of achieving *balanced analgesia*.

Opiate use in neonates and children
The National Service Framework for Children and the World Health Organization (WHO) both highlight the fact that health care professionals are often reluctant to prescribe and administer opioids due to fears regarding addiction and side effects, in particular respiratory depression. In fact, in most healthy children, respiratory depression is uncommon. However, some children are more susceptible to the unwanted effects of opioids. These include children with poor respiratory function, infants, and neonates.

Neonates are particularly susceptible as they have:
- A large extra-cellular fluid compartment.
- Slower gastric emptying.
- Less fat and muscle as a percent of body weight.
- A higher body water content than that of older children and adults.
- Immature liver and kidneys.

All of these factors contribute to delayed excretion of drugs and a greater degree of accumulation of some drugs, including opiates. In addition, infants and neonates have a higher number of opioid receptors, which increases the risk of respiratory depression. Nevertheless, this does not mean that opioids should be withheld from this group of patients, just that they should be to be administered with caution and care.

Practice tips
- Provide pre-emptive, multimodal analgesia to achieve optimum pain prevention and management.
- When moderate to severe pain can be anticipated, analgesia should be prescribed and administered regularly, to prevent peaks and troughs in serum levels, and potential episodes of 'break-through' pain.
- Provide a child-friendly environment and utilize age-appropriate non-pharmacological measures.
- Involve the child's family in the management of their child's pain and support them in doing so.

Non-pharmacological pain management

Practice tips

Any measures that help treat pain and anxiety whilst reducing the need for pharmacological interventions, is an essential part of pain management. There are several non-pharmacological interventions that can be used with children, the most effective being parental presence along with age appropriate sensory measures and cognitive-behavioural therapies (CBT).

Encouraging positive coping strategies:
- Squeezing mummy or daddy's hand.
- Counting down.
- Deep breathing.
- Role-play.
- Positive statements (e.g. I can do this).
- Distraction—e.g. toys, books, blowing bubbles, children's videos, relaxing music, etc.
- Guided imagery.
- Heat and cold applications.
- Complementary therapies (e.g. massage and aromatherapy).

A multidisciplinary team approach is integral to implementing non-pharmacological measures and the role of the hospital play specialist/nursery nurse cannot be underestimated.

Neonates and infants can be sensitive to the adverse effects of analgesic medication. Therefore, any measures taken to reduce the need for analgesics must be recommended:
- Non-nutritive sucking.
- Tactile stimulation.
- Containment holding.
- Sucrose offers prompt and short-term analgesic effects.
- Breast-feeding mothers should be encouraged to breast feed during the procedure if feasible.

Associated reading

℠ http://www.rcn.org.uk/childrenspainguideline

Association of Paediatric Anaesthetists of Great Britain and Ireland (2008). *Good practice in postoperative and procedural pain*. Available at: ℠ http://www.apagbi.org.uk.

Buvanendran A, Kroin J (2009). Multimodal analgesia for managing acute postoperative pain. *Curr Opin Anesthesiol* **22**, 588–93.

Twycross A, Moriart A, Betts T (1998). *Paediatric Pain Management: a multidisciplinary approach.* Radcliffe Medical Press Ltd, Oxford.

Patient-controlled analgesia

Patient controlled analgesia (PCA) is a technique that gives the child control over the amount of analgesia they receive, delivered via a lockable pre-programmed pump. This method of administration can engage the child or young person in their treatment, giving them a sense of control, increasing their confidence, and helping to reduce anxiety.

- The child activates the system by pressing the button on a handset attached to the pump, which allows a small bolus dose of drug to be administered intravenously.
- Only the patient knows how much pain they are experiencing and, therefore, only the patient should press the button. This is a safety feature of the machine—as the child becomes sedated they are unable to press the button successfully.
- Morphine is the first line choice of opioid used in PCA infusions, but fentanyl is a useful alternative. Opioids reaches a peak effect in 4–5min, which is why the lockout interval is 5min, preventing the child from receiving more before the analgesia has time to be effective.
- This method of pain control is contraindicated for children who have previously shown adverse reaction to opiates, or have upper airway problems or head injuries.
- A background continuous dose infusion may be prescribed when PCA is in use.
- ❶ Staff caring for children using PCA must be suitably trained and assessed as competent.

Equipment

- Lockable infusion pump.
- Giving set with anti-syphon and anti-reflux valves.
- Opiate prescription.
- Drug chart.
- Pain assessment/observation chart.
- Oxygen saturation monitor.

Procedure

Selection criteria for the child/young person

- Identified and assessed as suitable for this technique.
- *The child or young person needs:*
  - The cognitive ability to understand the relationship between pushing the button and medication being delivered (if not see 📖 Nurse-controlled analgesia (NCA), p. 126).
  - To be aware that the expected outcome is pain relief and not necessarily the complete absence of pain.
  - Should have the manual dexterity to push the button of the device (if not see 📖 Nurse-controlled analgesia, p. 126).
- Equipment should be available and demonstrated on the ward, and parents advised not to press the button for their child.
- Staff must be knowledgeable and able to care for the child safely.
- Naloxone will be available on the wards to facilitate the reversal of the opiate should adverse effects occur.

- The pump should be programmed by appropriately trained personnel.
- The child and family should be provided with appropriate written and verbal information, in order to prevent inappropriate use.
- Non-return valves (e.g. Graseby PCA giving set) to be used if a dedicated cannula is not available to prevent the back flow of the opiate.

On collecting the child from theatre, recovery, or at the start of each shift change on the ward, check that:
- The PCA pump is working.
- The programme complies with opioid prescription.
- The syringe label complies with the opioid prescription.
- The opioid is also prescribed on the main prescription chart.
- Naloxone, anti-emetics, and concurrent regular analgesia is prescribed on the main prescription chart.
- The pump readings are recorded and checked.

Observe and monitor (as per your local policy):
- Heart rate.
- Respiratory rate and effort.
- Oxygen saturations.
- Pain score.
- Sedation score.
- Amount of opioid in the syringe.
- Record number of tries made by the child and the number of good tries.

Side effects of the infusion should be noted in the child's records and the pain team, ward doctor, and/or anaesthetist informed if:
- The analgesia appears inadequate.
- The child is unable to use the technique successfully.
- They are experiencing unmanageable side effects, such as nausea and vomiting, and pruritis (itching).
- If the child's respiratory rate falls below the prescribed rate indicated on the prescription chart, place the infusion on hold until the respiratory rate is above the prescribed rate.

Report any large discrepancy in the number of tries and the number of good tries, in combination with a poor pain score, to the pain team/anaesthetist. This may indicate a need to change the programme or may simply need re-education of the child on the use of the PCA.

Nurse-controlled analgesia

Infants and young children (less than 6yrs of age) would usually be prescribed NCA. It is a suitable alternative to a PCA for any child, regardless of age or cognitive ability, as it offers both the benefit of a continuous infusion and the flexibility of a bolus facility. Nurses can administer a bolus of analgesia prior to painful procedures or for breakthrough pain.

❶ Staff caring for children using NCA must be suitably trained and assessed as competent.

Entonox

Background

Pharmacology

Procedure

Advantages

Entonox

Background

Entonox is a ready-manufactured mixture of 50% nitrous oxide and 50% oxygen. The gas is contained in blue cylinders with blue and white quartered shoulders or is piped to the clinical area, recognizable by blue outlet hoses. The analgesic effects of nitrous oxide/oxygen are related to the nitrous oxide component of the gas.

Pharmacology

- Fat soluble gas eliminated completely by the lungs.
- Comparable effect to that of 10mg morphine.
- Carried by the blood to the central nervous system (CNS).
- Reaches the brain quickly, allowing rapid peak in analgesic effect usually within 2min.
- Not metabolized by the liver.
- Completely eliminated by the lungs, resulting in speedy reversal once administration has ceased.

Procedure

- The child must be able to comprehend and comply with the instructions on the use of the gas.
- Administered is via a user-demand valve system.
- Children often prefer to use a mouthpiece, rather than a mask.
- The tubing and/or mouthpiece should be renewed between patients.
- ❶ All personnel handling entonox cylinders and supervising self-administration of this gas should have the appropriate training.
- Ensure entonox is prescribed.
- Two health care professionals must perform the procedure; one to monitor the gas and the patient, the other to perform the intervention.
- Give supplementary analgesia prior to the procedure.
- Record the duration of the inhalation.
- Observe the child throughout the procedure to determine:
  - Conscious level.
  - Presence of side effects.
  - The effectiveness of the technique.
- Record any adverse effects and the effectiveness of the analgesia.
- Monitor the child until they are able to resume normal activities.

Advantages

- *Rapid onset:* child needs to inhale for 2min prior to procedure.
- *Patient controlled:* user-demand valve.
- Side effects and effects will normally dissipate rapidly when inhalation ceases.
- Flexible.
- Cost effective.
- Gives the child some control.
- Is a distraction.
- The extra oxygen in entonox increases peripheral circulation oxygenation in patients suffering from shock.

Suitable for short term pain relief for:
• Pain associated with the treatment of wounds.
• Pain associated with moving and handling patients.
• Pain associated with nursing and medical intervention,
  e.g. venepuncture/cannulation.
• Trauma, while awaiting for the effect of other pain relief to establish.

❶ The gas should not be administered to children with the following:
• Inability to comprehend or comply with the instructions.
• Situations where there is a risk of over sedation or impaired
  consciousness, e.g. head injuries, intoxication.
• Situations where there is a danger of inhalation of vomit or foreign
  bodies, e.g. maxillofacial injuries.
• Children that may have air-containing closed spaces,
  e.g. pneumothorax, acute intestinal obstruction.
• Existing bone marrow disease.
• First 16 weeks of pregnancy.

Precautions
• Toxicity may occur with prolonged use (maximum 1h per day over 5 days).
• With prolonged use, megaloblastic anaemia, peripheral neuropathy,
  leucopenia, or thrombocytopenia may occur due to megoblastic
  changes in the red cells and hyper segmentation of the neutrophils;
  check blood cell count.
• Entonox should be used with caution in patients with poor nutritional
  status as nitrous oxide can deplete the body's store of vitamin B12.
• Respiratory depression may occur if the child is on concurrent CNS
  depressants, e.g. opioids.
• Administration of other analgesic medicines may enhance the effect
  of the gas, but should not be withheld if a high degree of pain is
  anticipated.

Pitfalls
Side effects may include:
• Headache.
• Dizziness.
• CNS depression.
• Risk of asphyxia.
• Hypotension.
• Cardiac arrhythmias.
• Respiratory irritation.
• Raised intracranial pressure with prolonged use.

Associated reading
Pickup S. (2000). Procedural pain: Entonox can help. *Paediatric Nursing* **12**(10), 33–6.
Sealey L. (2002). Nurse administration of entonox to manage pain in ward settings.
  Nursing Times **98**, 46.

Regional and epidural local anaesthetics

These are widely used and accepted for peri-operative analgesia in children usually as an adjuvant to general anaesthesia (GA). Techniques range from simple local wound infiltration, blocks of single nerves, or plexuses to neuraxial blocks like spinal and epidural analgesia.

Regional anaesthesia modifies the neuro-endocrine stress response, providing profound post-operative pain relief; which reduces both the recovery period and length of hospital stay. By combining a continuous epidural infusion of a local anaesthetic with low-dose opiate, the pain transmission along the pain pathway is blocked, and offers unique benefits in the relief of acute and peri-operative pain.

Advantages
- It offers children pain-free post-surgical recovery.
- Offers a reduction in post-operative and post-trauma morbidity, particularly in the high-risk patient (i.e. children with respiratory disease, poor lung function and complex disability).
- Local anaesthetic blocks the conduction of nerves in the epidural space producing good pain control.
- High quality analgesia with minimal sedation allowing better lung expansion and improving the patient's ability to cough and clear secretions.
- In older patients there is a decrease in the risk of deep vein thrombosis.
- The reduced quantity of opioid drugs used decreases the degree of paralytic ileus after abdominal surgery.
- Nausea and vomiting may also be reduced in comparison to opioid infusions.

Indications for use
- Children undergoing major surgery, for example:
  - Major lower limb surgery.
  - Renal surgery.
  - Thoracic surgery.
- High risk children:
  - Cerebral palsy with ↓ lung function/prone to chest infections.
  - Cystic fibrosis.
  - Sensitivity to opioids.

Contraindications for use
- Lack of appropriately trained staff or heavy workload of staff.
- Patient/parent refusal.
- Sepsis/infection around epidural site.
- Allergy to local anaesthetics.
- Coagulation disorders.
- Spinal deformities.
- Existing neurological disease.
- Raised intracranial pressure.
- Extreme obesity.

Equipment

- Dedicated pump for use with epidural infusion.
- Yellow tubing.
- Epidural 'in use' sign.
- Yellow protocol/prescription chart.
- Continuous oxygen saturation monitor.
- Blood pressure monitor.
- All patients must have a patent IV cannula at all times.
- Yellow epidural labels to label giving set.

Procedure

Close observation and monitoring (as per local policy) of the following:

- Heart rate, respiratory rate and effort, and oxygen saturation level.
- Pain and sedation score.
- IV cannula.
- Blood pressure (BP) and urine output.
- Sensory and motor block.
- Site inspection and pressure area care.
- Temperature.
- Side effects, e.g. nausea, vomiting, pruritus.
- Complications, e.g. hypotension, respiratory depression, bladder dysfunction, epidural haematoma or abscess, or migration of catheter into a blood vessel.

Associated reading

Llewellyn N, Moriarty A. (2007). The National Pediatric Epidural Audit. *Pediat Anesthesia* **17**(6), 530–3.

National Patient Safety Agency (2007). *Safer Practice with Epidural injections and infusions.* Available at: ℘ http://www.npsa.nhs.uk/health/alerts.

Complementary therapies for children and young people

Background

Complementary medicine can be seen as therapies that can be given in combination with orthodox medical treatments.

Therapy is performed to suit the individual needs and condition of the child/young person, considering their emotional, physical, and psychological well-being.

Children and young people can be worn down by their illness, becoming stressed and anxious about being in hospital, and subsequent interventions.

The intention of using complementary therapies is to support the child and family through their treatment by offering them tender, loving care (TLC), symptomatic relief, emotional/spiritual support, and attempt to improve their quality of life.

This may be done by helping them to learn relaxation techniques, to alleviate anxiety and reduce pain (Box 5.5).

Box 5.5 Examples

Physical
- Massage
- Aromatherapy
- Therapeutic touch
- Reflexology
- Shiatsu
- Acupressure

Psychological
- Counselling
- Visualization
- Art therapy
- Hypnosis

Pharmacological
- Vitamins
- Homeopathy
- Dietary intervention

Undertaking massage

Massage consists of a series of kneading, stroking or percussive movements.

❶ Practitioners undertaking massage should be appropriately trained—there is some risk of causing limb/tissue damage if inappropriate technique is employed.

Equipment
- Aqueous cream or hand/body lotion.
- Towel.
- Relaxation music.

Procedure

- Ensure that the child/young person's medical condition does not contraindicate massage therapy.
- Provide the child and parent with appropriate information and explanation, and obtain a clear indication of consent.
- If possible try to create a warm, peaceful environment. Through creating the correct environment with soothing music, the child and their family find themselves in a relaxing atmosphere, and it will enhance the experience.
- Check comfort and lighting, i.e. not too bright.
- Ensure that consideration is given to the time, place, resources, and preparation of self, child, and family.
- Maintain dignity, privacy, individuality, comfort, safety, confidentiality.
- Monitor the child's response, recording, and reporting responses during and following the session. Ask for feedback, i.e. pressure, etc.
- Evaluate each session with the child/parent, ensuring that the aim of the session is being met, leaving the child comfortable on completion.
- Document each session on a care plan. Maintain accurate records.
- Work in respectful silence unless the child wants to talk.
- Do not massage if the child/young person has:
  - An infection, contagious disease, or high temperature.
  - A skin infection, bruising, or acute inflammation.
  - An inflammatory condition, such as thrombosis or phlebitis.
  - Unexplained lumps and bumps.
- Do not use oils to massage if there is oxygen therapy in use.

Practice tips

- The great thing about children and young people is that they will let you know if they are enjoying the massage!
- When you do get the opportunity to sit and talk. why not offer a hand or foot massage? It will be relaxing, and may help with pain relief.
- Cover areas not being massaged to keep patient warm.
- Warm the cream in your hands before starting the massage.
- Concentrate on the hands and feet.
- Keep contact at all times—use firm, gentle strokes.
- Be slow, steady, and rhythmic—take your time.

Pitfalls

- Many health care professionals lack confidence when it comes to massage, thinking they are not doing it properly.
- It can be difficult sometimes to find a quiet place to perform the massage.

Associated reading

Periodical—*Complementary Therapies in Clinical Practice.* Elsevier/RCN, London.

Rankin D (ed.) (2001). *The Nurse's Handbook of Complementary Therapies,* 2nd edn. Bailliere Tindall, London.

Vickers A (1996). *Massage and Aromatherapy: A Guide for Health care Professionals.* Chapman and Hall, London.

Moving and handling risk assessment

❶ During any handling task, if you need to lift more than 16kg (if you are female) or 25kg (if you are male), you should consider the child (or object if it's a box, etc.) to be fully dependent, conduct a risk assessment, and use manual handling assistance equipment.

❶ Ensure that you have been fully trained and assessed as competent in the use of any manual handling equipment you use.

Risk assessment should be carried out thoroughly, recorded, and reported appropriately, and its findings should direct the planning of care related to a child's mobility. (See 📖 Moving and handling, p. 520, for section on best moving and handling practice.)

Basic risk assessment should consider the following elements:
• **E** Environment.
• **L** Load.
• **I** Individual capability.
• **T** Task.
• **E** Equipment.

The ideal solution to a child's mobility problems is to aim to *assist the child to move themselves* by:
• Providing the most appropriate environment.
• Providing equipment to assist movement, e.g. walking frame, crutches, monkey pole, etc.
• Motivating the child though encouragement, play, etc.

However, in many cases this will not be possible, due to the child's age, condition, treatment requirements, etc. For these cases you should try to *minimize or remove as many of the risks associated with the required movement as possible*.

Particular considerations for manual handling risk assessment for infants, children and young people

• Differences in size of child and handler may mean that good posture may be difficult to maintain, e.g. handler may have to stoop, bend, etc. to reach a small child.
• It's an incorrect assumption that lifting a toddler or small child does not present a risk to the handler.
• Be conscious that child equipment may have been designed more with child's needs and safety in mind than with adult handlers' safety.
• Children may not comprehend the safety issues associated with moving and handling techniques, and be distressed by practices employed.
• Motivate the child through games, rewards, and encouragement.

All manual handling incidents/near misses must be reported using your organization's Adverse Incident Reporting System.

Associated reading

Health and Safety Executive (HSE) (1995). *Reporting of injuries, diseases and dangerous occurrences regulations* (RIDDOR). HMSO, London.

Pressure ulcer risk assessment and prevention

Background

Pressure ulcer risk assessment and prevention

Background

Pressure ulcers develop if localized area of tissue is destroyed as a result of soft tissue being compressed between a bony prominence and an external surface. The most common sites for children include:

- Sacrum.
- Buttocks.
- Heels.
- Ears.
- Malleolus.
- Lumbar spine.
- Occipital region in those <36 months.

Equipment

- Risk assessment tool.
- Preventative care plan.
- Pressure relieving mattress and cushion (support surfaces).
- Repositioning chart.

Preventative procedures

- Using a validated risk assessment tool, score each child for his/her individual risk of pressure ulcer development.
- Carry out this risk assessment within 2h of admission to hospital or on first community visit.
- Reassess weekly or more frequently if condition changes.
- If the child is identified as being at risk of developing pressure ulcers, devise and implement a preventative plan of action.
- Provide a mattress based on individual assessment that will reduce or relieve pressure.
- Record the *type* of mattress and cushion provided in the care plan.
- If the child is sitting out of bed, provide a cushion that will reduce or relieve pressure (with the exception of children sitting in moulded wheelchairs).
- Identify and implement a repositioning regime based on individual need and the level of equipment provided. This will be between every 2–3h.
- If the child is sitting out of bed, maintain the same frequency of repositioning in the chair, or alternate between bed and chair.
- Record all position changes on a repositioning chart.
- Ensure the regime and equipment provision is effective by assessing the child's skin during every position change using the skin tolerance test, looking for persistent erythema or non-blanching hyperaemia:
  - Press your finger lightly over the reddened area for 15s.
  - If the area blanches, it is not a category 1 pressure ulcer.
  - If the area is non-blanching, it is a category 1 pressure ulcer and additional preventative measures should be put in place.

Practice tips

- For children <36 months and in the supine position, the occipital region is the primary pressure point when nursed supine and the knees when nursed prone. The ears are also a common pressure site for this age group. Two-hourly repositioning of the head is recommended.
- While frequent repositioning may be contraindicated for children with haemodynamic or respiratory instability, consider upgrading the level of pressure-relieving mattress or the use of products such as pressure reducing pads applied over the bony prominence.
- Minimize shearing forces during repositioning by using sliding sheets for children over 8yrs old.
- Be vigilant to ensure no hard objects are pressing on the skin surface, such as monitor leads or intravenous lines, and avoid pressure from tubing, winged cannulae, or nasal prongs.
- Avoid the use of dressings on grade 1 pressure ulcers where the skin remains unbroken to ensure the area can be monitored.
- Use an appropriate assessment tool, such as:
  - Paediatric Yorkhill Malnutrition Score (PYMS) for children over 1yr of age.
  - Malnutrition Universal Screening Tool (MUST) for adults.
- Identify any nutritional deficits and instigate nutritional support to correct deficit and restore serum albumin levels.
- Where tissue damage is noted, grade this in accordance with the EPUAP (2009) Grading system.[1]
- Document all care provision and *do not assume that children do not develop pressure ulcers*.

Pitfalls

- If additional interventions do not take place on identifying grade 1 pressure ulcers, deterioration can occur rapidly.
- The application of dressings to grade 1 pressure ulcers is likely to cause maceration and skin breakdown.
- Pillows do not relieve pressure. Avoid placing under the child or between limbs. The use of more suitable devices should be explored.
- Using sheepskins or water-filled gloves to reduce pressure will be ineffective.
- The use of barrier creams should be avoided for children wearing nappies, as this will interfere with the absorbency at the nappy surface. Prolonged contact with urine or faeces on the skin may cause a topical fungal infection and increase the risk of pressure ulcer development.

Associated reading

Baldwin K. (2002). Incidence and prevalence of pressure ulcers in children. *Adv Skin Wound Care* **15**(3), 121–4.
Butler CT. (2006). Paediatric skin care: guidelines for assessment, prevention and treatment. *Paediat Nursing* **32**(5), 443–50.

[1] EPUAP (2009). *Prevention and treatment of pressure ulcers. A quick reference guide.* Available at: ℘ http://www.epuap.org.

Palliative care

Background

Palliative care supports children and their families/carers not just in the dying stages, but in the weeks, months and years before a child's death. It should commence at the point of diagnosis of a life-threatening/life-limiting illness through to End of Life care in the terminal stage and post-bereavement care.

Elements of palliative care

- Psychosocial, spiritual, emotional, educational, and social care needs.
- Access to specialist services as required.
- Education and training.
- Collaboration, co-operation, and communication between all disciplines and across all agencies involved in the child's care.
- Respite and short breaks.
- *Terminal stage:* 24h End of Life care.
- Bereavement support for family and siblings.

Practice tips

- Effective communication between the child and family, and across the multi-agency team along the palliative care journey is vital. The ethos should be of shared decision making.
- Caring for a child with a life-limiting or life-threatening condition impacts on the family as a whole, creating enormous strain on the parents, siblings, and wider family members. Care should be aimed at supporting the whole family.
- Be familiar with the ACT Care Pathway[1], which proposes a framework for all professionals and agencies to follow to ensure continuity of care and promote partnership working. It consists of three stages relating to a particular stage in the child's palliative care journey:
  - Diagnosis or recognition of a life-limiting condition.
  - Living with a life-threatening or life-limiting condition.
  - Recognition of end of life and bereavement.
- Parents of children with a palliative condition experience a loss of control throughout the palliative and terminal phase of their child's condition, as many decisions are made by professionals in their 'best interests'. They need to be empowered to take back this control and make informed choices with the appropriate professionals at the right time for them.
- End of Life care plans are a useful and necessary tool to enable families to plan and make choices in their best interests for their child. Advance care planning decisions evolve over time, through the development of trusting relationships. It is vital that named key professionals in the child and family's life address these issues.

- Length of illness may vary from days to years, and the child may survive into adulthood. Appropriate transitional arrangements to adult palliative care services must be in place. The ACT Transition Pathway[2] provides a framework for young people, families, and professionals to help them plan for and move on from children's palliative care services to adult services.
- Not all families want or need help at the beginning of their journey. However, it is important that they are aware of services available to enable them to make informed decisions as to when and how to access these.

Pitfalls

- Effective palliative care requires a broad multidisciplinary approach to care. This means for one child there may be many professionals and agencies involved in their care. As a result of this, much repetition around information giving regarding the child/young person's diagnosis, prognosis, symptoms, and choices occurs.
- There is confusion amongst professionals in terms of the terminology of palliative and terminal care. For this reason many families are only offered services when a child reaches the terminal phase of their illness.
- There is a lack of understanding between Do Not Resuscitate orders and End of Life Care Plans. End of Life Plans that have been drawn up efficiently and concisely in agreement between family and professionals cover all circumstances, wishes, and choices of the family including resuscitation status.

Associated reading

Pfund R, Fowler-Kerry S (eds) (2010). *Perspectives on palliative care for children and young people: a global discourse.* Radcliffe Publishing, Oxford.

[1] ACT Integrated Care Pathway for Children and Young People with Life-Threatening or Life-Limiting Conditions and their Families (2004). Available at: ℳ http://www.act.org.uk.

[2] ACT Transition Care Pathway: A Framework for the Development of Integrated Multi-Agency Care Pathways for Young People with Life-Threatening and Life-Limiting Conditions (2007). Available at: ℳ http://www.act.org.uk.

Care of the dying child

Background

Raising the subject of a child dying with a family can be extremely difficult for all concerned. However, when a judgement is made that a child is in the terminal stage of an illness, it is in the child and family's best interests to have some discussions regarding their wishes and choices at this time. This will include where the family wants the child to die. In some cases, however, death can happen very suddenly with little time for planning, but there are certain key principles that can be followed when caring for the dying child and his/her family.

Psychosocial needs

- The child should feel safe, loved, cared for, and comforted.
- Care should be consistent and supportive.
- Be sensitive to and recognize feelings.
- *Communication:*
  - Listen and allow the child to talk about what they want to, remembering they may or may not want to talk about death.
  - Work to ensure appropriate timing of communication whenever possible.
  - Use age-appropriate language.
  - Give verbal and written information that is specific, accurate, and honest.
  - Utilize available interpreting services.
- The child may have their own special wishes, e.g. writing a letter, making a video.

Physical needs

- Dignity and privacy are essential, but often the family do not want to be left alone. Don't avoid them—they may be longing to talk to someone. Discuss what *they* need and want with them.
- Follow infection control policies as necessary and appropriate.
- Adequate symptom and pain control is essential.
- Remember there will be physical changes in:
  - Elimination pattern.
  - Skin integrity.
  - Nutritional requirements.
  - Respiratory pattern.

Cultural needs

- Gain an understanding of family's wishes around religious and cultural beliefs. Respect religious considerations.
- Arrange a christening if required.
- Allow family members to be present to say goodbye.
- Arrange and discuss the post-mortem.
- This will be a coroner's case if child dies within 24h of admission or surgery.

End of Life Care Plan

Careful End of Life care planning, which is supported by the family, can enable them to cope better through their inevitable process of grief and bereavement. Involve them in:

- Decisions relating to cardiopulmonary resuscitation.
- Discussions regarding the discontinuation of inappropriate interventions.
- *Help them create a memory box:* photos, lock of hair, patient identification band.
- *Discuss the place of death:* hospital, home, hospice.
- *Discuss their choices and wishes:* e.g. care of body after death.
- Funeral arrangements.
- Support systems for family.
- Communication with other agencies and key professionals involved in the child's care to inform them of terminal stages.
- *Discuss organ donation:* if suitable for organ donation then procedures of counselling, consent, pastoral care, and support, preservation of organ for harvest must be maintained.

Family support

- After death allow parents to have as much time with the child as they want. Ask if they want to help lay child out, choose clothes, etc.
- Documentation needed:
  - Certification of death.
  - Notification of death form.
  - Register death within 5 days.
- Arrange bereavement counselling.
- Put in contact with self-help groups, e.g. Compassionate Friends, etc.
- Offer sibling support.
- Arrange outpatient follow-up appointment.

Pitfalls

- Sometimes children ask questions that have no answers.
- Sometimes we have to answer questions about death with 'I don't know'.
- Do not wait for the 'right time' to discuss death. Communicate honestly and openly.
- Avoid euphemisms such as 'not get better', be specific and concrete.

Associated reading

⌘ http://www.tcf.org.uk.

Sidebotham P, Fleming P. (2007). *Unexpected death in childhood: a handbook for practitioners.* John Wiley & Sons, Chichester.

Care of a child's body

Background

Where a child dies has an impact on how a child's body is cared for; this section will identify general principles that can be applied to all areas. It will always be essential to follow local policies and procedures, and contact other professionals as appropriate. The care and support the family receive at this time will have an impact on their ongoing bereavement process.

After a child dies: what happens next

- Contact the doctor. Whether the death is expected or unexpected; nothing should be removed (but infusions can be switched off), until seen by a doctor.
- Close child/young person's eyes and mouth as soon as possible following death.
- Ensure all measures possible are taken to reduce room temperature.
- Check if there is an existing End of Life plan/bereavement plan in place and follow.
- Identify spiritual and cultural needs. Contact spiritual or religious leader.
- Offer to contact family members if not present.
- Allow privacy for the family, and also time for the extended family and friends to visit.
- Once death has been verified, the child/young person should be washed or bathed, and dressed (last offices). The same care and attention should be taken as for a child who is alive.
  - Encourage parental involvement, offering appropriate information and support.
  - Collect everything you are going to need to avoid leaving the bathing area.
  - Do not remove anything from the child (e.g. jewellery, religious artifacts, long-term feeding tubes) without discussion with the family.
  - Use warm water and the child's own toiletries.
  - Ensure hair is presented how it normally would be.
  - Dress in clothes chosen by the family—do not forget underwear and socks.
  - Ensure all clothing removed is folded and returned to the family.
- Prepare the family for moving the child. This may be to the mortuary the funeral home, children's hospice, or home. Ensure parents have time to spend saying goodbye to their child prior to transfer. Ensure all documentation in order prior to the move.
- Inform all involved professionals/services of the death as soon as possible.
- Document all relevant information.
- Ensure the family has all necessary information and belongings prior to leaving.

Legal requirements

- It is a legal requirement that certification of death may only be carried out by a doctor (this would usually be the doctor who has attended the child during the child's last illness).
- Where death is unexpected the doctor will inform the coroner. A post-mortem may be required.
- All children's deaths must be reported to the local Child Death Overview Process.
- The family or a representative is required to register the death within 5 days.

Important information

- Explanations to family should be given at all stages and in all events. Ensure that this is given in clear easily understood language. An interpreter should be used if required; do not rely on extended family to interpret.
- Information given to families will not necessarily be absorbed, and may need to be repeated and/or written down.
- If at all possible, it is important for the family to have continuity of care and support at this time.
- Accurate documentation is essential.
- It is essential that cultural, spiritual, and religious needs are met around death; it may be beneficial to identify specific needs prior to death to enable planning to occur; e.g. if a child is required to be buried the same day.
- Remember this is the family's bereavement and not yours. However, it may be a very emotional experience, therefore, seek support for self and/or other staff members.
- Once again refer to local policy.

Associated reading

℞ http://www.act.org.uk.
℞ http://www.childhospice.org.uk.
Department of Child Schools and Families (2010). *Working Together to Safeguard Children—A guide to interagency working to safeguard and promote the welfare of children.* HMSO, London.
Local Policy/procedures.

Memory making

Background

The concept of memory making is carried out by all of us throughout life; however, when a parent is told that their child will not live, the recording of memories reaches a heightened importance.

Memory making can be facilitated by anyone who is involved with the family, but support from appropriate professionals can enhance the process. These may include play specialists, hospice workers, family support, and bereavement workers.

All family members should be involved in memory making—do not forget siblings.

At time of death

It may be very challenging to ask a newly-bereaved family if they wish for hand/foot prints and/or hair cuttings to be taken. However, this will be the last opportunity to obtain such a physical reminder of their child.

- *Hand and foot prints*: these can be captured in clay or paint depending on preference and availability. It is essential that the area is thoroughly washed following activity. If the death is anticipated it is preferable to obtain prints prior to death as this, in itself, will create a further memory for the family.
- *Hair cuttings*: if culturally appropriate, these should be taken from an area that is not obviously seen.

Memory box

Often memory making is focused on a memory box. There should not be a 'one size fits all' or a standard way to achieve the creation of a memory box—it needs to be a personal reflection of the person creating the box. Therefore, family members may each have a box that is very different and contains different items. Choosing and decorating an appropriate memory box to retain keepsakes in is an important part of memory making. Some ideas of what people may wish to include are:

- Photographs.
- Special toy or personal item, such as glasses, hearing aid.
- Drawings or written work.
- Item of clothing.
- Name bands/hospital cards.
- School reports.

Other activities

- *Sand jars*: different coloured sand is used to represent a memory then the jar is sealed.
- Making photo frames to display child photo.
- *Capturing other people's memories*: this can be achieved through funeral attendance cards and/or a special book bought to enable people to share their thoughts at the funeral/or when visiting.
- *Letter writing to the child*: can be sent with the child to the funeral or kept in the memory box.
- *Writing their child's story*: this may be soon after death or some time later.

- *Creating a space for reflection:* this is often in the garden and may include the planting of a small tree, bush, or water feature.
- *Hand and footprint memory tree:* all family members can contribute their hand/foot prints to this tree—this can be displayed on a wall.

Essential information

- Families need to understand to complete memory making at their own pace—it is not a race, there is no prize at the end!
- All memory making needs to be personal and individual to each family, it is important that their wishes and beliefs lead this work.

Associated reading

♫ http://www.childhospice.org.uk.
♫ http://www.winstonswish.org.uk.
Crossley D (2000). *Muddles, Puddles and Sunshine.* Hawthorn Press, Stroud.
Gilbert S. (2004). *Grief Encounter.* Grief Encounters Publications, London.

Incubator and Babytherm® care

Background

Neonates should be cared for within a neutral thermal environment (NTE). This can be defined as the environmental temperature at which (when their own body temperature is within normal limits) their metabolic rate is at a minimum and they are consuming minimal oxygen.

Choice of a suitable environment in order to promote maintenance of NTE for a neonate is essential to prevent thermal stress.

The enclosed environment of the *incubator* is likely to be the environment of choice for a neonate of less than 1.5kg, and/or a gestational age of less than 28–30 weeks, and other infants requiring particular care. Modern incubators have the ability to provide servo-controlled oxygen and usually have an integral oxygen monitor. Servo-controlled incubators are automatically regulated and can be set to the individual neonate's requirements prior to their arrival.

The less enclosed environment of the Babytherm®, with its overhead and gel mattress heat sources may be suitable for larger neonates and neonates needing ease of access, e.g. for investigations, treatment, etc.

Caring for a neonate in an incubator or Babytherm® will also support provision of the following:

* Oxygenation and humidification when clinically indicated.
* Accessible observation and assessment without the need to handle the neonate.
* Minimal handling.
* Isolation aiming to reduce the incidence of infection and imposing risks of the external environment.

A neonate being nursed in an incubator or Babytherm® should have their temperature monitored and recorded at least 4-hourly. If the temperature falls outside normal range, readings must be taken more frequently, documented, and recorded as appropriate, and the care/treatment plan reviewed.

Considerations when caring for a neonate in an incubator

* Incubators are generally set to maintain an initial temperature of 36.5°C. The set point can be altered according to the neonate's axilla temperature measurements. Remember that the optimum temperature range for the neonate is 36.7–37.3°C.
* It will take about half-an-hour for an incubator to reach this temperature once switched on.
* The optimum incubator temperature should be set and maintained according to age and gestation, and by assessing the NTE for the individual neonate to be cared for.
* Humidification should be added to the incubator environment if required—the need for this is determined by gestational age, days of life, skin condition, and underlying disease.
* Sterile water should be used for humidification and water level should be checked hourly and topped up as required.
* The incubator temperature should be checked and recorded hourly.

- Adjust set temperature according to the neonate's temperature, but only alter incubator temperature by 0.5–1°C every 15–30min to avoid extreme and sudden change in environmental temperature.
- Care should be carried out whenever possible via portholes, to avoid environmental heat loss.
- A neonate should not be left in an incubator with portholes open for longer than an hour.
- Clean incubator when in use as per local policy usually involving mild detergent and or hard surface wipes (alcohol-based) daily.
- Humidification chambers should be emptied and refilled with sterile water daily.
- Change the incubator for a clean one every 7 days.
- All cleaning, equipment changes, and set temperature adjustments should be appropriately recorded and reported.

Considerations when caring for a neonate in a Babytherm®

- A Babytherm® mattress will generally be set to an initial temperature of 37°C.
- It will take an hour to heat to the set temperature.
- The overhead heater will usually be switched on initially to Level 5. Each level is 10% higher or lower in temperature than the next.
- It will take half-an-hour for the overhead heater to reach the set temperature.
- Monitor and record the neonate's temperature at least 4-hourly. If temperature falls outside normal range, reading must be taken more frequently, documented, and recorded as appropriate and care/ treatment plan reviewed.
- Adjust temperature of mattress and/or overhead heater as indicated by neonate's own temperature.

Associated reading

Boxwell G. (2000). *Neonatal Intensive Care Nursing*. Routledge, London.
Cohen M. (2003). *Sent Before My Time: a child psychotherapist's view of life on a neonatal intensive care unit*. Karnac, London.

Play

Distraction

Background

Distraction is a tool that is used within the hospital setting to help take a child's mind off what is happening. The purpose of this technique is to divert the child's attention away from the procedure being undertaken in the hope that this will lower anxiety levels and enable the child to remain calm so resulting in better compliance to treatment.[1] Distraction can be utilized for a variety of procedures, e.g. the taking of blood, cannulation, removal of stents/catheters.

Equipment

The type of equipment used will depend on the individual child. A few examples:

- *Under 2yrs*: soothing musical toys, rattles, bells, picture projectors.
- *Pre-school*: bubbles, stories, interactive characters, bubble tubes (with fish), songs and rhymes, DVD's, music, musical instruments.
- *School age*: seek and find books, guided imagery, puppets, DVD's, interactive games, consoles, and books.
- *Young people*: conversation, seek-and-find books, consoles, DVD's, music, guided imagery, magazines.

Procedure

- Introduce yourself to the child and family, and gain consent.
- Take time to show the child and family around the area.
- It is important to build a good rapport with the child and family during this initial meeting.
- There are no set rules as to the best way to distract a child; however, it is important for one person to take the lead. (It can be confusing for the child if too many people are involved.)
- Each child will have their own needs and should be treated as an individual.
- Offer the child choices, e.g. where do they want to sit? What method of distraction would they like to engage with?
- Explain the medical procedure to be undertaken in age-appropriate terms. Explain how the distraction activity will assist with this.
- Once the distraction method has been chosen explain how this will work, then begin to engage the child in the activity.
- If you feel the distraction is not going well:
  - Try to encourage the child to relax by engaging them in some deep breathing exercises.
  - Try to divert their attention onto a different subject, e.g. by talking about things they like—school/pets.
- It is important to continue with explanations relevant to the medical procedure throughout as this helps to build trust.
- Re-evaluate throughout the procedure. If a child starts to become distressed a quick change of book or discussion topic will often help to re-engage them.
- If despite all efforts distraction does not provide an effective coping mechanism for a child, referral to a clinical psychologist should be considered.

Practice tips

- Procedures vary in length so it is important to have a variety of distraction tools on hand, especially for younger children.
- Offering limited choices can help facilitate a feeling of control over the situation.
- It is vital to choose distraction tools that are age appropriate.
- A conversation with a child or young person about a hobby, family, or school can be an effective distraction tool.
- Some children cope by shouting. (It is important to identify such coping mechanisms. Otherwise this could be misconstrued as an unsuccessful distraction effort when in reality shouting is the child's release and a mechanism which enables them to stay still enough for the procedure to take place safely).
- Good distraction will result in a less traumatic procedure for all involved.

Pitfalls

- Remember that distraction should be considered before any procedure begins.
- It is difficult to succeed with distraction if the child has been traumatized by a previous failed attempt.
- It is important to be honest with the child at all times. A successful procedure is not only one that has been completed, but one where the child feels positive at the end.

Associated reading

Jun Tai N. (2004). *Play in Hospital*. [Online] Available at: ℘ http://www.ncb.org.uk/dotpdf/open_access_2/factsheet_hospitalplay_cpis_20080131.pdf.

[1] Glasper A, Aylott M, Battrick, C. (eds) (2010). *Developing Practical Skills for Nursing Children and Young People.* Hodder Arnold (Publishers) Ltd, London, pp. 72–88.

Preparation and post-procedural play

Background

A child and family that have been well prepared for a procedure should be able to undergo it with a greater understanding; which should enable them to cope better during it. Preparation helps to eliminate fear and allows the child some control over the situation.

Post-procedural play is aimed at children who have had very little or no preparation for their procedure. The aim is to help the child understand their illness/treatment and encourage them to express their feelings within a controlled environment. It is important, however, to follow up all children who have had an invasive procedure in order to offer them the opportunity to engage in post-procedural play.

Equipment

See 📖 Equipment, p. 154, for the equipment list.

Procedure

Preparation

The following procedure will be based upon the example of a child who requires insertion of a central venous line (CVL):

- Preparation must be tailored to the child's level of understanding and age appropriate language should be utilized.
- It can be valuable to encourage siblings to take part in preparation as this can help to deal with any misconceptions the siblings may have.
- The involvement of a child's siblings can also further encourage the involvement of the child.
- Specialized dolls can be useful in order to familiarize the child with medical equipment, e.g. doll with a CVL attached.
- The hospital play specialist (HPS) can introduce the doll to the child and family. They can then play with it together.
- Patient/parents/siblings can be encouraged to engage in roll play, e.g. giving medicine, fluids into the CVL, or taking blood from it. This helps to empower the child and allows them to learn at their own pace.
- HPS can use the doll/role play as an aid to explain pending procedures/treatments.
- HPS should reassure and praise the child throughout the role play and give them as much control over the situation as possible.
- HPS will evaluate the situation and assess how much knowledge and understanding has been gained by this preparation.
- Further activities should be undertaken if the child requires further input (see other topics in this chapter).
- It is important to allow plenty of time for play and questions.

Post-procedural play

Circumstances surrounding a child admitted in an emergency situation may allow no time for preparation. Post-procedural play will enable the child to re-enact a procedure, ask questions and gain an understanding as to why things have happened to them.

- Post-procedural play (PPP) should be offered to all children routinely whether they have undergone preparation or not.[1]
- PPP can be used to help identify any fears/worries the child may have after a procedure has taken place.
- It can take the form of:
  - Discussion with the child/young person about their experience.
  - The use of tools, booklets, etc., to explain future steps in their treatment.
  - Role play with dolls and other equipment which allows the child to act out experiences they have had.
  - Making a diary where the child/young person can express themselves and their feelings.
  - *Normal play and art play*—important after invasive procedures in order to help children work through and express their thoughts and feelings.

Practice tips

- It is important to consider the age and ability of the child when undertaking preparation/post-procedural play.
- On occasion, preparation may need to be directed at the parents and or siblings of the child. A child may be too young to understand an explanation, but may find it enjoyable and learn from watching the process.
- ❶ It is important to use hospital equipment where appropriate/safe.
- Check the child's allergy status.

Pitfalls

- Not allowing time to evaluate and plan coping strategies for future procedures, e.g. relaxation techniques, breathing, etc.
- Not referring necessary medical questions to the appropriate multidisciplinary team member.
- An anxious child may need more than one session.
- It is common for children to dislike the smell of various hospital items, e.g. sterile wipes. This can be helped by offering something nice to smell, e.g. lavender bags.

Associated reading

[1] Glasper A, Aylott M, Battrick C. (eds) (2010). *Developing Practical Skills for Nursing Children and Young People*. Hodder Arnold (Publishers) Ltd, London, pp. 72–88.

Directed and hospital role play

Background

Play is vitally important for any child. It enables them to grow and develop physically, intellectually, emotionally, and socially, it also aids their communication skills. Through play and observation we are able to understand some of the child's worries, fears, and anxieties. When a child is in hospital they are placed in an unnatural environment. This can elicit many feelings not only for the child, but also their parents/siblings.

Hospital play can help bring an element of normality to children and their families, and can be used to help communicate and prepare children for impending procedures. Hospital equipment can be incorporated into many aspects of normal play. It is best to introduce this form of play in a non-threatening environment, such as the hospital play room, e.g. syringes can be used in water play or on the craft table with paint. This should help familiarize the child to a variety of hospital equipment, whilst also facilitating a trusting relationship between professional, and the child and family.

Equipment

There is a multitude of equipment that can be utilized, e.g.:
- Preparation dolls.
- Hospital equipment, i.e. syringes, gloves, wipes, etc. ⚠ Ensure allergy status of the child is checked prior to use of hospital equipment.
- Relevant booklets.
- Photograph albums.
- DVD's.
- Visit to a certain area (e.g. radiotherapy department).
- Feelings books.
- Personal diaries.

Procedure

The procedure will differ depending on the child and also the procedure they are being prepared for. For the purpose of this chapter, the following procedure is based on preparing a child for radiotherapy treatment:
- The main aim is to reduce any potential trauma and to empower the child so enabling various medical procedures to be carried out in a calm and controlled manner.
- It is important to build a relationship/rapport with the child and family.
- Explain the basics of the procedure to the child and family, and gain consent.
- A more in-depth process follows that will involve child participation.
- In relation to this example a visit to the radiotherapy department may be helpful. This will introduce the child and his/her family to the area, layout, the relevant professionals, and the different equipment they will come into contact with.
- If the child requires a mask for their treatment, it can be useful to encourage them to make and paint dough masks.

- It can also be useful to allow the child to play with the material that will be used for the radiotherapy mask, e.g. taking moulds of their hands. This can facilitate a true understanding of how these materials feel.
- For the radiotherapy treatment itself, it is important that the child lies still. Games like 'sleeping lions', which assist in this are helpful.
- The use of photograph albums, or DVDs are very good as a visual tool. They can depict other children/young people undergoing the same procedure and, as such, make a link with real life situations.
- A reward system, e.g. a personal sticker chart may be helpful as the child can show their achievements to others/countdown days to the end of treatment.
- The use of directed play is advantageous as it allows time to explain the procedure in a non-threatening environment and a way that the child can relate to/feel more at ease with.

Practice tips

- It can be helpful to provide the child/family with a personalized booklet, explaining the basics of the relevant procedure/s required.
- Feelings books/diaries are a further form of written communication that can be shared within the family. They can be useful for a child who does not feel able to verbalize their concerns especially for communicating these concerns to the health care professionals involved.
- A well-informed child/family is less likely to be traumatized by a hospitalization episode.

Pitfalls

- Not being completely truthful with patients about the treatment/ procedures they will undergo. If children/young person perceive that staff are not being honest they are less likely to trust them and potentially less likely to co-operate with future treatments/procedures.

Associated reading

Glasper A, Aylott M, Battrick, C. (eds) (2010). *Developing Practical Skills for Nursing Children and Young People.* Hodder Arnold (Publishers) Ltd, London, pp. 72–88.

Guided imagery

Background
Guided imagery is a way of helping children cope with invasive/painful treatments and procedures. It uses relaxation techniques along with the child's imagination to form a story or journey in the child's head. The image or story is guided by an adult and aims to help the child undergo treatment.

A play specialist can provide guided imagery in order to ease a child's anxiety. It can also be used alongside pharmacological measures as a form of pain management.

Procedure
For effective guided imagery the play specialist or professional should:
- Establish a rapport and trust relationship with the child and family.
- Provide the child and family with a full explanation of what guided imagery will entail, and what the experience will feel like and gain consent.
- Identify a focus for the image, e.g. a visit to the beach/park.
- Always allow the child to describe the image.
- It is important not to impose your own thoughts or suggestions on to the child's image. Guided imagery works better if it is rooted in the child's own experiences.
- The role of the professional is to guide and support the image through the use of descriptive questions, e.g. what can you see/smell/hear/feel?
- Discuss with the child where they would like their image to begin.
- Ascertain what position the child would like to be in prior to commencing, e.g. sitting/lying.
- Advise the child as to what will happen, whilst he or she is in the image/who will be in the room, etc.
- Explain all relevant information in simple age appropriate terms.
- Ascertain whether the child wishes to be told when the procedure is about to begin—some children do not want their image to be interrupted.
- Ensure both child and professional are clear about the journey the child wishes to take prior to commencement.
- Ensure that the child knows that they can open their eyes at any time.
- Reinforce and/or change the image when necessary. It is important that the child chooses a solid place to visit that can elicit lots of questions, e.g. where are you? What can you see/smell? Who is there?
- Always structure the image with a clear start, middle, and end.
- Count backwards 4, 3, 2, 1 at the end of the image to ensure the child is slowly brought back to the environment and surroundings.
- Discuss what went well and what could have been improved upon with the child/young person and carer/parent.
- Utilize relaxation techniques prior to beginning.
- Initial relaxation techniques, such as deep breathing and relaxation of muscles allow the child to commence the technique in a calm manner.
- Guided imagery can be practiced in any environment as long as the child has some where to sit comfortably.

Practice tips

- Guided imagery can be used to help a child cope with a variety of medical procedures, e.g. the taking of blood/insertion of long lines/removal of dressings/packing of wounds.
- Guided imagery is suitable for children from approximately 5yrs of age however children should be assessed developmentally to ensure they are capable of engaging in this technique.
- The child must have the ability to communicate effectively and use their imagination for the guided image to be successful.

Pitfalls

- The main difficulty arises when a child decides on a difficult image to expand upon; hence, the initial conversation is vital to the success of guided imagery.
- This coping strategy is not to be confused with hypnotherapy, which is entirely different and should only be carried out by a trained professional.
- Guided imagery is not meant as a substitute for pharmacological pain control.

Associated reading

Glasper A, Aylott M, Battrick, C. (eds) (2010). *Developing Practical Skills for Nursing Children and Young People.* Hodder Arnold (Publishers) Ltd, London, pp. 72–88.

Role of parents

Background

Parents/carers fulfill a vital role in all aspects of their child's care, including play. It is therefore extremely important to involve them in every way possible.

If the child is anxious about his/her treatment it may be necessary to initially work with the parents. Preparing parents/carers for their child's impending treatment can reduce anxiety levels and enable them to be positive and supportive throughout the procedure.

Equipment

- There is no specific equipment list. However, it is important to ensure that parents/carers are provided with the information necessary to help support their child through the use of play. The specific play equipment required would depend on the type of play being carried out.

Procedure

- Talk to the parents to ascertain the child's knowledge level regarding their admission/diagnosis.
- Ensure that parents are aware of what the procedure involves and what is likely to happen.
- Take advice from the parents in relation to their child's existing coping strategies.
- Take advice from parents in relation to the type of play activities their child enjoys.
- Ask parents to identify any situations/procedures that may pose particular difficulties for their child.
- Involve the parents in preparation for the procedure, e.g. a child due to undergo an ultrasound can put jelly on the parent and pretend to perform the scan.
- Ascertain whether parents are happy to accompany their child throughout the procedure. Some parents may suffer from anxieties that may make this difficult for them.
- Involve parents in the distraction process throughout the procedure, e.g. blowing bubbles while a dressing is being changed.
- Encourage parents to be involved with the child's care post-procedure. This could include supporting them to play with their child and taking on general caring again.

Practice tips

- Play is a great way to promote an element of normality for both the child and parent. This can reduce anxiety levels for both child and parent.

Pitfalls
- The hospitalization of a child can be extremely stressful for parents. Parental anxiety can be profound and can be transferred to their child. Any measures aimed at reducing this anxiety can be very beneficial.
- When in hospital parents are often worried about playing with their child especially if the child is connected to machines and monitors. It is important to advise and support parents through this.

Associated reading
Royal College of Nursing (2004). *Patient Information and the Role of the Carer*. [Online] Available at: ℘ http://www.rcn.org.uk/__data/assets/pdf_file/0010/78508/001375.pdf.

Multi-disciplinary approaches to play

Background

Play is a natural process that can be utilized to aid a child in their treatment and recovery. The focus of the NHS on multi-disciplinary care results in opportunities for play to be incorporated across a multitude of care disciplines.

Equipment

- Equipment will vary depending on the type of activity to be undertaken and its purpose (see 🕮 Practice tips, p. 160).

Procedure

- Often the play specialist will work alongside different disciplines in order to assist with treatment/procedures and facilitate continuity for the child and family.
- Play can be used to assist in a variety of ways. Specific suggestions are highlighted in the practice tips.

Practice tips

Here are a few examples of how play can be used as a tool by different professions.

Physiotherapy

- Children with respiratory conditions can be encouraged to perform breathing exercises by engaging in activities like blowing bubbles or using 'blow pens' as a craft activity (blowing paint across paper to make a picture). This can help improve lung function.
- Children who need to improve their mobility can be encouraged to take short walks/engage in small ball games.
- For children with restricted mobility kicking a ball from a sitting position encourages movement and can be a good starting point to work from.
- For those where exercise is a priority outdoor play and games like football can be encouraged.
- Children may not view this type of activity as a form of treatment. This can prove beneficial in terms of increased compliance.

Dieticians

- Within the hospital setting food can pose a significant issue for children. This may be due to a change in diet, a dislike of the food offered, or a reduced intake due to illness or surgery, particularly oral surgery.
- A child with severe reflux may become uninterested in food because they associate it with an increased risk of vomiting. In this situation it is useful to take the emphasis away from actually eating the food.
- Playing with food can make it seem less threatening, e.g. playing with yoghurt, mousse, ice cream on a tray. This is fun, messy, and there is a chance the child may taste the food through hand to mouth exploration.

- Role play with tea sets and plastic food can help to alleviate some of the fear associated with food.
- Some children may require a food supplement that may not taste nice. Play can allow experimentation:
  - Tasting the different supplements.
  - Deciding which is nicest.
  - Mixing them with flavoured syrups or others drinks.
  - Allocating them a score out of 10.
  - Parents/carers and health professionals can also take part in the tasting/scoring,

Psychology

- Often the clinical psychologist works closely with play specialists to help children deal with fear and anxiety prior to a procedure, e.g. needle phobia.
- The psychologist/child and play specialist can agree a coping strategy/ plan of action to assist the child in dealing with a potential procedure. (see 📖 Distraction, p. 150, 📖 Preparation and post-procedural play, p. 152, 📖 Directed and hospital role play, p. 154, and 📖 Guided imagery, p. 156).
- The play specialist can help implement this plan in order to reduce potential anxiety/trauma posed by the procedure.

These are just a few examples of how play can be used within the multi-disciplinary team. Many general play activities can be adapted to help support other professionals in their roles.

Associated reading

National Association of Hospital Play Staff. (2010). *NAHPS online*. Available at: ℜ http://www. nahps.org.uk/.

Developmental issues

Background

Monitoring a child's development is very important within the hospital setting. If a child is hospitalized for a long period, they may regress developmentally.

Play is important for children in hospital, as it aids normality and promotes development. Well children usually attend nursery or school, where they play and socialize, enabling them to learn new skills and reach developmental milestones. Depending on the child's condition, illness, or injury it may not be possible to carry out play in the same way. Developmental assessments may be carried out and a play programme devised for the child that will best suit their needs.

Equipment

- Developmental milestones checklists.
- Toys appropriate to those listed on the check list—see 📖 Practice tips, p. 162 for ideas.
- Appropriate environment.

Procedure

- Ensure that the developmental assessment is undertaken in an appropriate environment. This may depend on the areas of play to be focused upon (social, emotional, physical- fine/gross motor, cognitive, language, sensory).
- Ensure you have a range of developmental charts to hand as children will vary in terms of developmental ability, e.g. when assessing a child of 16 months ensure access to a checklist for 9–18 months and 18–24 months.
- Use toys to facilitate age appropriate activities (as identified on the checklist) to assess the child's developmental stage.
- Further assess the child's development through observation, e.g. watching them play and interact with family/siblings/others.

Practice tips

A suggested list of play activities that can be used within the medical setting to promote a child's development is given here. It is important that the activity is developmentally appropriate for the child, as well as being appropriate in relation to their condition/illness.

Social development

- Interaction with other children either in small or larger groups.
- Interaction with others during meal times/making meal times enjoyable.
- Going for walks outside.
- Facilitating realistic role play, such as homes, shops, hospital, and school.
- Singing/telling and listening to stories.

Emotional development
- Interaction with others.
- *Nursery/action rhymes:* these encourage interaction, and are fun which can lift the child's mood.
- Dolls.
- Role play.
- *Dressing up:* pretending to be a different character can afford the child an escape from the reality of being in hospital.

Physical development
- *Fine motor:* jigsaws, arts and crafts, building bricks, threading and lacing games.
- *Gross motor:* Rattles, baby gyms, walks, ball games, trikes and push along toys, mat play, rolling, sitting, crawling, walking.

Intellectual development
- Interaction with adults.
- Books.
- Walks to look at new environments (outdoors, shops, etc.).
- Drawing.
- Role play.
- Imaginative toys.

Language development
- Musical and interactive toys.
- Singing/music.
- Stories.
- Conversations.

This list is not exhaustive. It is important to involve the multi-professional team to ensure that activities carried out are those that will most benefit the individual's recovery, therefore, ultimately promoting development.

Pitfalls
- If developmentally appropriate toys and activities are not provided children will lose interest in the task.
- Assessing a child's development is important as children can regress to an earlier developmental stage post-treatment.
- In some cases developmental delay can be associated with the child's condition or illness.
- ❶ Chronically ill children are at particular risk.

Associated reading
Developmental checklists for children 0–5 years can be found at ℜ http://www.childrenstherapies. co.uk.

Sheridan M, Sharma A, Cockerill H. (2007). *From Birth to Five years: Children's Developmental Progress.* Routledge, Oxford.

Infection control[*]

* The majority of the topics in this chapter consist of revised material from a
previously published work, Chapter 4: Infection, authored by Jacqueline Randle,
Natalie Vaughan, and Mitch Clarke, from the *Oxford Handbook of Clinical Skills in Adult
Nursing*, edited by Jacqueline Randle, Frank Coffey, and Martyn Bradbury (OUP: 2009),
adapted with permission.

Standard precautions

Background

Standard precautions (formerly known as 'universal precautions') must be adopted at all times, to promote the safe practice of prevention and control of infection. Microorganisms can be transmitted through direct contact, indirect contact, and the air. The aim of standard precautions is to minimize the risk of infection to health care workers (HCWs), children/young people, their families/carers, and visitors.

Procedure

Standard precautions include the following:
- Effective hand hygiene.
- Appropriate covering of any cuts.
- Correct use of personal protective equipment (PPE).
- Safe handling and disposal of sharps.
- Safe handling and disposal of clinical waste and linen.
- Appropriate management of blood and other bodily fluids.
- Effective decontamination of equipment.
- Achieving and maintaining a clean clinical environment.
- Appropriate use of medical devices, including decontamination and servicing.
- Nursing children/young people in the correct environment.

Practice tips

- Prevention and control of infection is everyone's responsibility.
- Good prevention and control of infection must be an integral part of all clinical practice.
- A risk assessment should be conducted as part of the implementation of standard precautions, considering:
  - What is the source of infection?
  - How is the infection transmitted?
  - Are additional risk factors involved?
  - What are the individual patient risk factors?
  - Who are the individuals at risk?
  - What facilities are available or unavailable?
  - Is the staffing mix appropriate?
  - What are the contamination risks?
- On evaluation:
  - Is the patient still symptomatic?
  - Is the pathogen that caused the infection still present?
  - Has the pathogen spread to others or other clinical areas?
  - Do the special infection control precautions still need to be in place?
  - Should further advice, support, and guidance be obtained from the infection prevention and control team (IPCT)?

- HCW's must be familiar with and consistently apply local policies, procedures, and guidelines for prevention and control of infection. Any breach of practice must be reported according to the local reporting system.
- Effective communication between HCW's, patients, relatives, visitors, and the IPCT is vital. Documentation of procedures in place is essential.
- Ongoing training and education is required.

Pitfalls

- Standard precautions must be applied to all patients, regardless of age or whether they have a known infection or not.

Associated reading

British Medical Association (2006). *Health care associated infections: a guide for health care professionals*. British Medical Association, London.

Department of Health National Audit Office (2004). *Improving patient care by reducing the risk of hospital acquired infection: A progress report*. National Audit Office, London.

Department of Health (2007). *Saving lives: reducing infection, delivering clean safe care*. Department of Health, London.

Department of Health (2008). *Clean, safe care: reducing infections and saving lives*. DoH, London.

Pratt R, Pellow C, Loveday H, Robinson N, Smith G. (2001). The epic project: developing national evidence-based guidelines for preventing health care associated infections. *J Hosp Infect* **47**(Suppl.), S3–82.

Pratt R, Pellow C, Wilson J, et al. (2007). epic2: National evidence-based guidelines for preventing health care-associated infections in NHS hospitals in England. *J Hosp Infect* **65** (Suppl.), S1–64.

Wilson J. (2006). *Infection control in clinical practice*, 3rd edn. Baillière Tindall, London.

Hand hygiene

Background

Hands have microorganisms present, including some residual flora, as well as transient microorganisms that can lead to infection. Hand hygiene is the single most important factor in reducing the spread of health care-associated infection. Routine hand hygiene refers to the practices of both hand washing with soap and water and hand disinfection using products such as alcohol hand rubs. Both methods decrease the colonization of transient bacteria on the hands.

Equipment

• Hand basin, ideally with automatic mixer taps.
• Liquid soap.
• Alcohol gel.
• Paper towels.
• Foot-operated bin.

Procedure (see Fig 7.1)

• Remove all wrist jewellery (including wrist watches).
• Remove stoned rings.
• Turn on taps to a comfortable temperature, and wet hands and wrists.
• Apply enough soap to cover surfaces of the hands. Work up a lather.
• Vigorously rub hands together (palm to palm).
• Vigorously rub the back of each hand.
• Interlace and interlock fingers to cover all surfaces.
• Rotationally rub each thumb and wrist.
• Ensure that all of the soap is effectively rinsed off.
  • Routine or social hand washing should take 10–15s.
• Turn off the taps with disposable paper towels or elbows, to ensure hands are not re-contaminated.
• Dry all parts of the hands and wrists thoroughly using disposable paper towel, paying particular attention to the inter-digital surfaces of the fingers and thumbs. Thorough drying will decrease microbial growth and soreness.
• Dispose of the paper towel in a bin without re-contaminating hands.
• If decontaminating hands using alcohol hand rubs, follow this procedure using the alcohol hand rub in place of the soap, water, and paper towel. Allow to dry naturally for 30s.

Practice tips

• Hands must be decontaminated:
  • Immediately before/after every episode of direct patient contact.
  • After contact with the patient's immediate environment.
  • After contact with bodily fluids.
  • Before an aseptic technique.
  • After any activity or contact that potentially results in your hands becoming contaminated.

Associated reading

Royal College of Nursing (2012). *Essential practice for infection prevention and control. Guidance for nursing staff.* London.

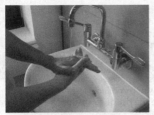

1. Palm to palm

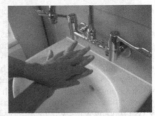

2. Right palm over left dorsum and left palm over right dorsum

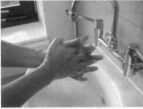

3. Palm to palm fingers interlaced

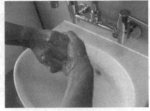

4. Backs of fingers to opposing palms with fingers interlocked

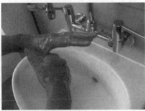

5. Rotational rubbing of right thumb clasped in left palm and vice versa

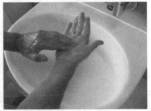

6. Rotational rubbing, backwards and forwards with clasped fingers of right hand in left palm and vice versa

Fig. 7.1 Hand-washing technique. Reproduced from Glasper et al., *Oxford Handbook of Children's and Young People's Nursing*, (Oxford: 2006) with permission from OUP.

- Hands that are visibly soiled or contaminated by dirt or organic material must be washed using liquid soap and water.
- When caring for a patient who has infective diarrhoea use soap and water between caring for patients, and between different care activities.
- An alcohol hand rub can be used between caring for patients or different care activities, if your hands are not soiled.
- Cover any cuts and abrasions with waterproof dressings.
- Avoid hot water as this can increase the risk of dermatitis.
- Use running water whenever possible.
- Nails must be kept short. Artificial nails and nail polish must not be worn.
- Emollient hand creams can be used to protect hands. If hand problems develop, seek advice from the occupational health department.

Pitfalls

- Gloves are often seen as a replacement for good hand hygiene. However, hands must still be washed with soap and water after the removal of gloves.
- Alcohol hand rub may not be easily accessible in all paediatric areas due to safety issues. In some instances, personal bottles of alcohol hand rub may be useful for ease of hand hygiene.

Personal protective equipment

Background
PPE is used to decrease the opportunity for microorganisms transmission, as well as offering protection to the person providing care.

Equipment
- Gloves:
  - Sterile.
  - Non-sterile.
- Aprons.
- Masks.
- Eye protection.

Procedure
The following may be utilized as personal protective methods. They are all single patient use:

Gloves
- Non-sterile may be used when there is a risk of contamination from bodily fluids, when special precautions are in place, when there is a risk of chemicals reacting with the skin, e.g. antibiotics.
- Sterile gloves should be used for surgical procedures, invasive aseptic procedures, preparation of sterile products.
- Non-latex gloves should always be made available.

Aprons
- Used when there is a risk of contamination from bodily fluids and when special precautions are in place.

Mask
- For procedures where blood splashes are a risk, for infectious or drug-resistant tuberculosis, and when there are special precautions in place.

Eye protection
- For procedures where blood splashes are a risk.

Practice tips
- PPE must be removed at the patient's bed space.
- Hands must be decontaminated after removing PPE.
- Adhere to local policies and guidance that designates a particular standard of face mask protection.

Pitfalls
- PPE should be removed after finishing the patient episode of care.
- Not having the required knowledge of the PPE necessary can lead to not wearing it correctly, resulting in an increased risk of infection.

Waste and linen management

Background

'Waste' refers to substances or objects that are no longer part of a cycle or chain. The disposal of waste is regulated by statutory regulations, and HCWs have legal and moral duties to dispose of waste properly. There should not be cross-contamination of different categories of hazardous waste, or between hazardous and non-hazardous waste. Linen refers to any bedding or hospital-supplied clothing worn by the patient.

Procedure

Underlying principles

- Household or domestic waste (e.g. packaging, paper towels, flowers, and other waste uncontaminated by potentially infectious substances) is disposed of in black plastic bags.
- Clear bags indicate recyclable municipal waste.
- Orange bags are for infected or potentially infectious waste.
- Yellow and black striped bags are for non-infectious healthcare waste.
- Medicine-contaminated waste is disposed of in yellow body, yellow lid sharps bins.
- Waste requiring incineration is disposed of in yellow plastic bags.
- Cytotoxic and cytostatic waste is disposed of in purple plastic bags or yellow and purple striped plastic bags, or if sharps in a purple lidded sharps container.
- Used or slightly soiled linen should be placed in a laundry bag and stored in a safe place prior to collection. When soiled, dispose of linen using aprons and gloves.
- Heavily soiled or infected linen should be placed in a soluble inner bag, then this placed in an outer bag and stored in a safe place away from the general public for collection.
- Change bags when three-quarters full.
- Ensure the correct disposal/storage of waste and linen, as it has consequences for patient safety, as well as cost implications. Always refer to local policy.

Practice tips

- In the community, the responsibility for waste disposal is the householder's, but clinical waste can be collected, on request, by the local authority.
- If the child/young person is treated by a HCW, the clinical waste produced as a result of the treatment is the responsibility of the HCW.
- Sharps bins are provided to patients who are required to use sharps as part of their treatment. Therefore, these must have arrangements in place for removal.
- Advise parents, children/young people and householders using sharps in the community not to dispose of sharps in soft drink cans, plastic bottles, or similar containers, because this can present serious hazards to staff disposing of domestic waste.

Pitfalls

- Do not forget about adhering to the correct disposal of confidential waste.

Associated reading

Royal College of Nursing (2012). *Essential practice for infection prevention and control. Guidance for nursing staff.* London.

Sharps management

Background

Sharps are any item that has the potential to cause a penetration injury.

Procedure

Underlying principles

- Avoid the use of sharps wherever possible.
- It is the responsibility of the sharps user to ensure that sharps are correctly used and disposed of.
- Dispose of sharps in the correct container immediately after use.
- Dispose of the entire needle and syringe; the needle should not be bent, broken, or disconnected.
- Do not re-sheath used needles under any circumstances.
- Do not re-sheath clean needles, unless there is safe means, e.g. a capping device.
- Ensure that sharps containers are available in close proximity to where the sharp is to be used.
- Sharps containers must conform to approved standards and be correctly assembled and labelled.
- Sharps containers should be emptied when three-quarters full or once week, securely closed, a label completed, and safely stored for removal.
- Containers must be removed by designated staff wearing appropriate PPE.

Action to be taken following a sharps injury

- Encourage the wound to bleed, but do not suck. Wash the wound under running water and apply a dry waterproof dressing.
- Report to line manager and complete an adverse incident form.
- If the injury is from a used sharp, medical advice should be sought to assess the potential risk of transmission of blood-borne viruses.
- Obtain advice from the occupational health or emergency departments, depending on local policy. Obtain further advice from the IPCT.
- Retain the sharp item and identify the source patient, if possible.
- Blood samples may be collected from the patient and HCWs if they consent.

Practice tips

- If undertaking a procedure where there is a risk of contact with blood or bodily fluids, always use appropriate PPE.
- Assess if the child/young person will be un-cooperative and consider if further protective precautions are required.

Pitfalls

- Do not re-sheath needles.
- Do not attempt to put sharps into nearly full containers.
- Sharps can be trapped in the entrance to the containers with flaps and injuring subsequent users.

Associated reading

Royal College of Nursing (2012). *Essential practice for infection prevention and control. Guidance for nursing staff.* London.

Aseptic non-touch technique

Background

The aim of the aseptic non-touch technique (ANTT) is to prevent micro-organisms on hands, surfaces, or equipment from being introduced to body sites, such as through surgical wounds or equipment, e.g. central venous lines. It is not always necessary to use sterile gloves and a sterile dressing pack for all procedures requiring ANTT, e.g. when changing an intravenous infusion bag, but the principles of ANTT should still be adhered to. The overall aim is to have no contact with key parts, and sterile and non-sterile parts should not touch.

Equipment

- Dressing trolley/suitable tray for procedure.
- Soap and water/detergent wipes.
- Yellow bin.
- Alcohol hand rub.
- Specific equipment for procedure, e.g. for a dressing change you will need a sterile dressing pack, sterile gauze, gallipot, 0.9% NaCl/normasol, sterile scissors, dressing.
- Alcohol swab.
- Sterile and non-sterile gloves. Sterile gloves to be used when avoidance of touching key parts is not possible.
- Apron.

Procedure

- Refer to the care plan or assessment so that the specific equipment can be prepared.
- Explain the procedure to both parent and child, and gain consent.
- Wash and dry your hands (see 📖 hand hygiene, p. 168).
- Put on a clean, disposable apron.
- Ensure the dressing trolley/tray is clean, using detergent and water or a detergent wipe (refer to local policy).
- Assemble equipment and put on it on the bottom shelf of the trolley.
- Check the expiry date and that sterile equipment packaging is intact.
- Open a sterile dressing pack on the top shelf if using a dressing trolley, touching only the corners of the paper and not touching the sterile inside of the packaging.
- Place any other sterile equipment onto the sterile field by gently dropping equipment onto the field, adhering to ANTT principles.
- If the procedure is a dressing change, remove the patients dressing.
- Change gloves before going to the patient.
- If sterile gloves are required, ensure that the first glove is placed on by only touching the inside of the glove, and the second by only touching the outside of the glove.

- Commence the ANTT using the following principles:
  - Only sterile items should come into contact with susceptible sites.
  - Sterile items should not come into contact with non-sterile items.
- Dispose of clinical waste and any sharps correctly.
- Wash hands with soap and water.
- Ensure the patient is comfortable.
- Clean the trolley using detergent and water/wipes (refer to local policy).
- Document the care episode.

Practice tips

- Effective hand decontamination is the most significant procedure in preventing microorganism transmission.
- Although it is possible to perform this technique independently, consideration should be given to having a second person wherever possible, so one person is 'sterile' and the other 'non-sterile'.
- Forceps can be used during an ANTT in preference to sterile gloves, but they could damage tissue.
- If appropriate, irrigation may be preferred when cleaning a wound. Whichever method is used, a light, delicate touch should be used.
- Consider administering analgesia before the procedure, if required.
- Consider the use of distraction, and a play specialist (see 📖 Distraction, p. 150).
- Prepare as much as possible in advance.

Pitfalls

- Taking 'short-cuts' can result in contamination.

Associated reading

Royal College of Nursing (2012). *Essential practice for infection prevention and control. Guidance for nursing staff.* London.

Peripheral intravenous cannula care

Background

Peripheral intravenous cannula (PICs) are plastic cannula inserted into a vein, and used to administer intravenous (IV) medication, fluids, blood products, and occasionally nutritional support.

Equipment

- Transparent dressing.
- Bandage.
- Splint.
- Syringe.
- Needle.
- 0.9% NaCl.
- Alcohol Wipe.
- Sharps Bin.
- Phlebitis Score.

Procedure

Underlying principles

- Explain the procedure and care of the PIC to the parent and child/young person.
- Decontaminate your hands before and after touching PICs and any PIC insertion site.
- Use ANTT when handling PICs (see 🕮 Aseptic non-touch technique, p. 174).
- Insertion and removal of PIC's should be documented clearly, with details of the site, size of the cannula used, date, time, and who inserted/removed it.
- Use a phlebitis grading scale to observe for signs such as pain, swelling, erythema, palpable venous cord, and pyrexia at the insertion site at least daily or more if necessary, and document your observations, taking action where necessary, e.g. alert medical staff, removal of PIC.
- As well as observation of the site using a phlebitis score, observe the surrounding tissue for infiltration and extravasation, the integrity of the device, and security of the connections should also be checked and documented at least daily, and every time the site is accessed or every hour if on a continuous infusion.
- PICs should be replaced every 72–96h, as per local policy. Any reason for not replacing the PIC must be documented:
  - Generally in paediatrics PICs are kept *in situ* as long as possible due to the difficulty of cannulation and lack of evidence indicating it causes an increase in acquired infection.
  - This requires nurses/doctors to be extremely vigilant in their assessment and care of a PIC.

- The PIC site should be covered with a transparent sterile semi-permeable dressing, and often protected with a splint and a bandage.
  - As well as for protection, many children/young people do not like the appearance of a PIC, and so a bandage can help with this.
- Replace the dressing using an ANTT when the dressing becomes damp, loosened, or soiled.
- A PIC should not get wet, and so assistance may be needed for the child to maintain hygiene.
- If a bionectar is *in situ*, it should be replaced every 72h.
- Remove the PIC at the earliest opportunity.
- If a PIC is removed, the reason for the removal and the condition of the site should be documented. If there are signs of infection, swab the site and send the canula tip off for culture.
- Patency should be established prior to administration of medication, between medication, after medication, and at regular intervals (at least daily) with 0.9% NaCl, usually 5–10mL. Flushing before, in-between and after medication administration also ensures that medications are not mixed.
- When accessing the PIC, a positive-pressure technique should be used.

Practice tips
- Avoid shaving at the insertion site because this causes micro-abrasions. This ↑ risk of bacterial colonization, which ↑ the risk of infection.
- Ensure that the insertion site can still be viewed easily.
- Regularly assess how secure the PIC is and the cleanliness of any dressings, e.g. children may get food on it, or pick at the bandage.
- If the child/young person is leaving the ward with the PIC *in situ*, ensure the PIC is secure, and consider further bandaging to ensure it will not become dislodged.
- Some PIC's can be positional; always document this so subsequent staff are aware.
- Even flushing of the PIC can be a traumatic experience for children so communication with the patient and parents/carers is important, as well as the use of distraction and of a play specialist (see 📖 Distraction, p. 150).

Pitfalls
- Poor documentation of PIC insertion sites.
- The patient may not understand the need for PIC and will try to remove it.

Associated reading
Royal College Nursing (2010). *Standards for infusion therapy.* RCN, London.

Specimen collection and storage

Background

The correct collection of specimens for investigations is essential to ensure accurate diagnosis. Specimens required will either be:

- *Bacterial:* cultured for up to 48h; informative for correct antibiotic treatment.
- *Viral:* as viruses do not survive long outside the human body, a transport medium is required for these samples.

Equipment

- Universal collection container for sample, e.g. sterile urine pot, microbial swab, and medium.
- PPE (see 📖 Personal protective equipment, p. 171).
- Bedpan.
- Sterile container.
- Urine bag.
- Alcohol swab.
- Syringe and needle.
- Tongue depressor.
- Laboratory request form.

Procedure

Underpinning principles

- Explain the reason for the procedure to both parent and child/young person, gain consent, and consider privacy and dignity.
- Decontaminate your hands before and after the procedure.
- PPE might be required following a risk assessment.
- Specimens should be collected at the appropriate time, using the correct technique and equipment.
- Ensure a sufficient sample is taken, and ideally taken before commencement of any causative treatment.
- Transport the specimens to the laboratory without delay or store them in a fridge or incubator as appropriate for the specimen.
- Different specimens require different medium and methods of sampling; if unsure, contact the receiving laboratory for advice before proceeding.
- Before taking a specimen, ensure any corresponding specimen documentation, request form, and container label is fully completed, including the patient's details, date and time specimen taken, the specimen taken, investigations required, relevant signs or symptoms, and any ongoing microbial drugs. Incorrect labelling may lead to the sample having to be re-taken.
- Document clearly when the sample is taken, sent, and ensure results are followed up.
- Do not contaminate specimens during transfer to the container.
- Inform both the parent and child when the results will be available.

Throat specimen collection

- Throat swabs are taken in order to isolate organisms known to cause upper respiratory tract infections.
- Explain to the patient that the procedure might cause a gagging, coughing, or sneezing.
- Put on non-sterile gloves.
- Obtain a good view of the throat before swabbing. A tongue depressor might be required.
- Gently, but firmly rotate the swab in any exudates from one or both anterior fauces.
- Avoid touching the lips, cheeks, tongue, or teeth.
- Place the swab in the appropriate transport medium.
- Remove gloves and decontaminate your hands.

Aural (ear) specimen collection

- Swabs are taken to see if infection is present in the ear canal.
- Put on non-sterile gloves.
- Direct a light into the patient's ear.
- Gently grasp the pinna of the ear, lifting it upwards and backwards.
- Gently rotate the swab into the external auditory canal. Do not push the swab beyond your visual path, as it may cause damage to the tympanic membrane.
- Place the swab in the appropriate transport medium.
- Remove gloves and decontaminate your hands.

Conjunctival (eye) specimen collection

- Put on non-sterile gloves.
- Ask the patient to sit down and tilt their head slightly backwards. Parents or another staff member may need to assist.
- Pull the lower lid down so that the conjunctiva is exposed and ask the patient to look upwards, if they are able.
- Run the swab firmly along the surface of the exposed conjunctiva, from the outer to the inner canthus.
- Twisting the swab will help ensure that epithelial cells are picked up.
- On completion, remove the swab from the lid and ask the patient to blink or close their eyes briefly, to help dispel any discomfort.
- Place the swab securely in the appropriate media and send it off to the laboratory.
- Remove gloves and decontaminate your hands.

Wound specimen collection

- Wound swabs should only be taken if there is clinical evidence of infection.
- Wearing gloves or using a dressing bag, remove the wound dressing.
- Rotate the swab in the wound, working from the middle outwards or zig-zag across to cover the full expanse of the wound:
  - Do not touch the surrounding skin.
  - For large wounds, swab the most contaminated area.
- Place the swab in the appropriate transport medium.
- If copious pus is present, aspirate a quantity using a sterile syringe and transfer into a sterile container.

- Remove gloves and decontaminate your hands.
- Swabs should be taken before wound cleaning, at which time the maximum number of bacteria is present.

Midstream urine

- Urine collection is common in paediatrics and is used to identify microorganisms that may be causing a urinary tract infection (UTI), as well as for other tests such as to indicate protein:creatinine ratios.
- Urine is sterile so the presence of bacteria is often indicative of an infection.
- Midstream urine (MSU) is used as the first stream of urine may be contaminated with bacteria from the skin.
- MSU can be difficult and time-consuming to obtain in children.
- Put on non-sterile gloves.
- If possible obtain the sample immediately after the patient has showered or bathed, or clean the area as follows:
  - *Female:* the vulva from front to back.
  - *Male:* the entire glans penis and behind prepuce.
- Ask the patient to void an initial stream into the toilet or bedpan. The MSU sample should then be collected in a sterile receiver, allowing the final stream into the toilet or bedpan:
  - 5–10mL of urine is sufficient for microbiological examination.
  - If the parent/carer is obtaining the sample, ensure they understand instructions and the importance of gaining a MSU.
- If the patient is unable to control the flow, or for infants, collect the whole specimen using a urine collection bag.
  - Using a urine collection bag can often result in a contaminated specimen if cleaning is not undertaken correctly.
- Place the specimen directly into a sterile container using a sterile syringe if necessary.
- Remove gloves and decontaminate your hands.

Catheter specimen of urine

- Urine samples may be obtained when an existing catheter is *in situ*.
- Samples are taken via a sampling port, and not from the drainage bag, as the sampling port will offer a less contaminated sample.
- Wash hands and apply PPE.
- Clamp the urinary drainage tube, if necessary, just below the sampling point and wait 15min.
- Wipe the sample point with an alcohol impregnated swab and allow to dry for 30s.
- Using ANTT aspirate the required amount of urine. This may be done using a sterile syringe, or a sterile needle and syringe.
- Release the clamp, if used.
- Transfer the urine to a sterile container and label as 'Catheter specimen of urine' (CSU).
- Remove gloves and decontaminate hands.

24-h urine specimen collection

- This measures the amount of urine produced in a day, so results found reflect any body chemistry changes.

- At the allocated time to start collection, ask the patient to empty their bladder into the toilet as this specimen must be discarded. If parents are monitoring collection, education regarding this is vital.
- Collect all subsequent voided urine using a bed pan, urinal, or urine collection bag, and add to the 24-h specimen container.
- At the start, ensure the container is labelled with the patient's details, start date and time.
- Discontinue collection after 24h and label the container.

Faecal specimen collection

- Many gastrointestinal (GI) disorders are due to intestinal parasites, which require laboratory investigation.
- Ask the patient to defecate in a bedpan or ensure parents know to keep nappies.
- Offer patient hand-cleaning facilities.
- Put on PPE.
- Observe the stool for colour, consistency, and volume.
- Using the spatula attached to the universal container lid, spoon a portion of faeces into the container. In the case of liquid faeces, a syringe might be required to obtain a specimen.
- Decontaminate your hands.
- Remove gloves and apron.
- Once a pathogen is isolated, no further samples are required, but if the sample results are negative yet diarrhoea continues take further samples. Repeat samples will also be required with certain micro-organisms such as *Salmonella*.

Practice tips

- If a request form is required from the medical team, ask for it to be completed in advance.
- For some samples distraction and/or a play specialist may be required.

Pitfalls

- Failing to document correct patient details on a specimen form will lead to repeated samples being required.
- Not sending the sample in a timely manner.
- Ensure the sample is stored correctly if it cannot be sent straight away.

Associated reading

Royal College of Nursing (2012). *Essential practice for infection prevention and control. Guidance for nursing staff.* London.

Care of the isolated patient

Background

There are two types of care of the isolated patient.

Source isolation

Aims to prevent the transmission of pathogenic organisms from spreading, either directly or indirectly. Reasons for source isolation may originate from:

- Enteric/faecal-oral route, e.g. diarrhoea and vomiting.
- Wound/skin, e.g. chicken pox, MRSA.
- Respiratory, e.g. bronchiolitis, whopping cough, meningitis.

Protective isolation

Aims to protect a susceptible patient from acquiring an infection, either directly or indirectly.

Procedure

Underlying principles

- Decontaminate your hands before and after any contact with the patient.
- When leaving the room, hands should be washed in the room, and alcohol rub used on leaving.
- Wear the correct PPE (see 📖 Personal protective equipment, p. 171). The choice of personal protective clothing should be determined by a risk assessment of the anticipated contact with the patient.
- Explain the need for isolation to both the parent and child/young person, and provide any necessary education.
- Consider the psychological, emotional, and developmental needs of the child/young person.
- Maintain confidentiality of a patient's diagnosis, while ensuring that staff and visitors are aware of the appropriate precautions for prevention and control of infection.
- Review the need for isolation regularly.
- The most appropriate type of isolation room should be selected:
  - For example, an en-suite facility for a patient with infectious diarrhoea.
  - In protective isolation the patient may need to be accommodated in a positive-pressure room.
- If isolation is not possible and if source isolation patients can be cohorted in a bay, with appropriate precautions for prevention and control of infection, e.g. bronchiolitis.
- Furniture and equipment should be kept to a minimum in an isolation room.
- Equipment should, where possible, be single-use only, designated for single-patient use or easily decontaminated.
- A trolley or dispenser for protective clothing must be allocated to an isolation room/cohorted bay, to provide equipment relevant to the type of special precautions for prevention and control of infection.

- The patient's documents and charts should not be kept in the room.
- Visitors should be encouraged to decontaminate their hands. They do not, generally, need to wear protective clothing, unless they are involved in the practical aspects of care.
- Avoid visits or transfers to other departments, where possible. Any receiving department should be notified in advance and the patient should be 'last on the list' if possible.
- Regularly and thoroughly clean both the equipment and the isolation room, complying with local guidance for cleaning and decontamination.
- Soiled linen and clinical waste must be bagged correctly and stored in a secure collection area.
- Spillages must be dealt with promptly, according to local policy.
- On discharge, ensure isolation cleaning of the room and ensure the curtains are changed.
- The room can only be occupied by another patient after thorough cleaning has taken place.
- In addition, when protective isolation is needed:
  - Before the patient is admitted, the room should be thoroughly cleaned using detergent and hot water, and the curtains changed.
  - Linen should be changed daily.
  - No-one with a cough, cold, or any other transmissible infection should enter the room, and there should be minimal visitors.
  - Hand hygiene is of the utmost importance for all those entering the room.

Practice tips

- Adhere to local guidance that designates specific responsibilities for cleaning the room and equipment.
- Staff should use the correct colour-coded cleaning equipment.
- Damp-dusting, normally using detergent and hot water, should be undertaken daily using a disposable cloth.
- The floor must be mopped daily.
- Alcohol hand rub alone is not effective against all enteric organisms, so hand-washing with soap and water followed by the use of alcohol hand rub should be used.

Pitfalls

- Consider the psychological needs of the patient to prevent feelings of isolation and vulnerability.
- HCW's not fully understanding the procedures and policies relating to isolation will place patients, HCW's, and visitors at risk.

Associated reading

Royal College of Nursing (2012). *Essential practice for infection prevention and control. Guidance for nursing staff.* London.

Chemotherapy handling precautions

Background

Cytotoxic drugs are used in treating childhood cancers (and sometimes inflammatory diseases). Cytotoxics may be genotoxic, oncogenic, mutagenic, and/or teratogenic, and exposure carries unknown long-term risks to handlers. Handling precautions are required, and pregnant staff should not be expected to handle them.

Procedure

- The handler must follow local and national guidelines, and only undertake those tasks for which they have been trained and authorized in their particular role.
- Incidents (such as spillage) and near misses must always be reported, according to local policies. These reports must be reviewed and actions taken to reduce future risk.
- Handlers must wear appropriate PPE:
  - Disposable nitrile or vinyl gloves and plastic apron for handling the drug, waste equipment, and the patient's body fluids.
  - A visor, face shield, goggles or safety spectacles if there is a risk of splashing.
  - Respiratory protective equipment to avoid inhalation of aerosols or powders.
  - Handlers must always wash hands after removal of PPE.
- Only staff who are suitably trained and experienced must prepare cytotoxics.
- Preparation should preferably take place in a designated area, within a central pharmacy or a pharmacy unit within an oncology clinic.
- On rare occasions, cytotoxics have to be prepared outside the pharmacy, e.g. if a drug has a very short half-life.
- A safety cabinet or pharmaceutical isolator should be used for preparation.
- Cytotoxics must be transported in clearly labelled leak-proof containers, which provide appropriate storage conditions for the medication during transit.
- Within clinical areas, cytotoxics should be stored in designated cupboards and fridges that are lockable, and are clearly labelled.
- Wherever possible, cytotoxics should be administered within normal working hours to ensure expert advice and assistance is readily available if required.
- The handler should wear disposable gloves and use a 'no touch' technique to avoid contaminating the patient and themselves.
- Disposal of cytotoxic waste must comply with the respective Health Board's/Health care Trust's Waste Policy.
- Suitable containers for cytotoxic waste should be available in all areas where cytotoxics are administered. These must be:
  - Purple coded bins clearly marked with the nature of the contents.
  - Made of puncture and leak-proof plastic with tightly fitting lockable lids.
  - Tagged with the department's coded tags so their source can be identified.

- Parents and other relatives should be advised to wear gloves when handling their child's vomit, urine, or faeces for up to 7 days after administration of cytotoxics.
- There are no known risks associated with a patient's excreta entering the public sewage system.

Practice tips

- If the patient is unable to take the drug in the form provided, contact the pharmacy department as they may be able to dispense a modified form.
- Doses of liquid preparations of oral cytotoxic drugs should be drawn up in an oral syringe over a plastic tray in case of spillage.
- At home, parents should be advised to wear gloves and to give medicines in the kitchen where the surfaces are most easily cleaned if any is spilt or spat out.
- For IV injection use luer lock syringes to reduce the risk of the spillage.
- For IV infusion prime the giving set with the same fluid as the drug is diluted in to reduce the risk of spillage and administrator contact.
- Young children who are being potty-trained should be put in nappies during and for a week after administration of chemotherapy.
- Scales (not jugs) should be used for measuring urine to avoid aerosolization.

Pitfalls

- All staff working in areas where cytotoxic medication is administered need to know where the cytotoxic spillage kit is located and how to use it.
- Contaminated hard surfaces, mattresses, furnishings, skin, and eyes should be washed thoroughly with copious amounts of cold water.
- In the event of spillage on clothing, the items should be removed as quickly as possible and washed separately from other clothing in the first instance.

Associated reading

Health and Safety Executive (2003). *Safe Handling of Cytotoxic Drugs.* Available at:
  ℜ http://www.hse.gov.uk/pubns/misc615.pdf.
Scottish Executive Health Department (2005). *Guidance for the Safe Use of Cytotoxic Chemotherapy.*
  [Issued under NHS HDL (2005) **29**, 4 July 2005]. Available at:
  ℜ http://www.sehd.scot.nhs.uk/mels/HDL2005_29.pdf.

Immunizations

Background

Babies are born with some immunity to infectious diseases and may receive passive immunity from mother to baby, e.g. via breastmilk. However, further active immunity is required; a vaccine is given that causes the body's immune system to make antibodies providing protection from a specific disease. Not only does the individual child/young person have protection, but by many having immunizations it offers 'herd protection'; decreasing the ability of the disease to spread (see Table 7.1).

Vaccines may be a 'live' version of the disease (causing a longer-lasting immunity), an inactivated form (this requires regular boosters) or may be an extract/detoxified exotoxin. If it is a live vaccine, then it should not be given to immunocompromised patients.

Table 7.1 General immunization programme

When	Immunization
2 months	Diptheria, tetanus, pertussis, polio, *Haemophilus* (known as DTaP/IPV/Hib, single jab)
	Pneumococcal
3 months	Diptheria, tetanus, pertussis, polio, *Haemophilus* (DTaP/IPV/Hib, 2nd dose)
	Meningitis C
4 months	Diptheria, tetanus, pertussis, polio, *Haemophilus* (DTaP/IPV/Hib, 3rd dose)
	Meningitis C (2nd dose)
	Pneumococcal (2nd dose)
12–13 months	Measles, mumps, rubella
	Meningitis C (3rd dose)
	Haemophilus (4th dose)
	(Hib and meningitis given as single jab)
	Pneumococcal (3rd dose)
3yrs and 4 months–5yrs	Diptheria, tetanus, pertussis, polio booster
	Measles, mumps, *Rubella* booster
12–13yrs	Cervical cancer (HPV) vaccine (girls only) 3 jabs given within 6 months
13–18yrs	Diptheria, tetanus, polio booster

Equipment

- Prescription.
- Cotton wool and tape.
- Vaccine required in syringe.
- Needle.
- Appropriate record for documentation, e.g. parent-held record and central recording system.
- Sharps bin.

Procedure

- Explain the procedure to the parent/carer and child/young person, discussing possible side effects and gain informed consent.
- Wash hands.
- Follow usual medicine safety guidelines/checks.
- Reconstitute and draw up the vaccine as per manufacturer instructions.
- Ensure the young person is comfortable and, if a child, ensure they are seated securely and comfortably on the parents lap if this is appropriate.
- Check parents/carers are happy to assist in holding them:
  - Expose the chosen site, removing any restraining clothing.
  - Administer the vaccine.
- Generally, immunizations are administered intramuscularly (IM) (see 📖 Intramuscular drug administration, p. 202), unless a child/young person has a bleeding disorder, when they may have it administered subcutaneously (SC), and a BCG is administered intra-dermally.
- Generally <1-yr-olds should receive vaccines via the anterolateral aspect of the thigh, older children/adults via the deltoid.[1]
  - Once immunization has been given wipe with a cotton wool ball.
  - Dispose of needle in the sharps bin and wash hands.
  - Record date, time, vaccine name, batch number, expiry date, site, dose.
  - Ask parent and child/young person to sit in the waiting area for 10min, as an adverse reaction is most likely to occur in this time.

Practice tips

- If there is a history of a reaction of the same vaccine do not administer.
- If the child has an acute illness, including fever, postpone the vaccine.
- If a child has a mild illness without fever the vaccine can still be given.
- For maximum protection, parents should be made aware that the full courses of vaccinations needs to be completed.
- If bleeding persists following vaccination a cotton wool ball can be secured to the site using tape, which should be removed at home.

Pitfalls
- If, for any reason, the vaccine is not given at the appropriate age due to illness or failed appointment, this will delay protection and further immunizations being administered.
- If a child is uncooperative this may cause anxiety for the parent and difficulty in administering the immunization; offer reassurance and the use of distraction, or other comforting techniques, with the child.
- If the child is not held securely there is a possibility the child may move and the nurse could sustain a needle stick injury.
- Adhere to correct storage of vaccinations.

Associated reading
℅ http://www.nhs.uk/Livewell/childhealth1-5/Pages/Childimmunization.aspx.

[1] *UK guidance on best practice in vaccine administration* (2001). Available at: ℅ http://www.rcn.org.uk/__data/assets/pdf_file/0010/78562/001981.pdf (accessed 24 February 2011).

Drug administration

Prescribing drugs

Background

Prescribing drugs may be undertaken by a number of health care professionals now. Doctors must have a full registration and hold a license to practice in order to prescribe. Nurse prescribers, or 'Independent non- medical prescribers', in the UK undertake a nurse independent prescribing course, which is an additional qualification then recorded with the Nursing and Midwifery Council (NMC). This allows nurse prescribers to prescribe any licensed medicine, for any medical condition that a nurse prescriber is competent to treat; including some controlled drugs. Additionally, as children's nurses, prescriptions can generally only be for children and young people up to the age of 19yrs. Where unlicensed medications are used, they may still be prescribed, but the prescriber takes responsibility (see 📖 Drug licensing, p. 217).

Prescribed drugs should be in an appropriate formulary, such as the British National Formulary for Children (BNFC),[1] and prescribers should be aware of clinical and cost-effective guidelines. The prescriber should always ensure an adequate patient history is taken, including:

- Any previous adverse reactions to medicines.
- Current medical conditions.
- Concurrent, or recent use of medicines.

Informed consent and negotiation with the child/young person/family should also be considered.

Equipment

- National formulary for children, current edition.
- Drug chart.
- Calculator.

Procedure

A prescription needs to be completed with:

- The patients surname, first name, date of birth, and full address.
- Weight/height and potentially surface area.
- The name of the prescribed item, quantity, and strength required.
- Frequency to be administered.
- Length of course of treatment.
- Route of administration.
- Any special instructions.
- Allergy status.
- Signature and date, and NMC registration number (if nurse prescriber).
- If there is unused space on a prescription pad, it should be blocked out by the use of a diagonal line.

Nurse prescribing

- A nurse prescriber can only prescribe for a patient he/she has personally assessed, or has access to sufficient information recorded in an easily accessible and comprehensive manner from a suitably qualified person. This ensures an awareness of any allergies and contraindications for the use of the drug.
- The prescription should only cover drugs for one calendar month of care; in hospital this is often only for 7–14days, as it is expected there will be a regular review of medications taking place.
- Most commonly, prescriptions will be on the hospital drug chart, however, on occasions, a prescribing pad may be used, e.g. outpatients clinics.

Practice tips

- Ensure there is access to patient's medical notes, any relevant charts, such as fluid balance and results.
- Try to ignore interruptions, as they can lead to prescribing errors.
- Do not be afraid to check calculations with another colleague.

Pitfalls

- Avoid use of decimal points when specifying strength, i.e. 3mg not 3.0mg.
- Quantities less than 1mg should be written, e.g. 500micrograms not 500mcg.
- Consider the possibility of pregnancy in female teenagers.
- Remember, when administering drugs, a registered nurse is accountable for actions and omissions.

Associated reading

Department of Health. (2006). *Medicines Matters—A Guide to Mechanisms for the Prescribing, Supply and Administration of Medicines*. DoH, London.
Nursing and Midwifery Council. (2010). *Standards for Medicines Management*. NMC, London.

[1] RCPCH Publications Ltd (2010). *British National Formulary (BNF) for Children*. BMJ Publishing Group Ltd, London.

Calculating drug dosages

Background

It is important that calculations for any drugs are done correctly, where children are concerned the need for correct calculation is vital for a number of reasons:

- Children differ physiologically, such as they have an increased metabolic rate and a less well developed physiological ability to deal with incorrect dosages. In addition, neonates have decreased drug clearance times.
- The range of dosages prescribed for children is much wider and may still be correct, e.g. 0.2mL and 2mL are both reasonable dosages to give to a child despite the large difference between them.
- The large range of sizes of children, from the smallest neonate to the largest adolescent means there is a wide variation in the dosages that are likely to be prescribed.

Equipment

- Appropriate formulary.
- Pen and paper.
- Calculator.
- Prescription.

Procedure

- There is some debate as to whether double checking reduces the number of errors made. Follow the policy of the organization you work for.
- If you do have two checkers, each should do their calculation individually and uninterrupted, i.e. independent, rather than double checking should occur.
- Calculations should be done without the use of calculators, although they can be useful to check the final answer.
- The most common formula used to calculate the correct drug dosage to give is, the amount of the drug you want, divided by amount of the drug in the formulation, multiplied by the amount it is in. This is often abbreviated to:

$$\frac{\text{what you want}}{\text{what you have got}} \times \text{what it's in}$$

e.g. paracetemol 90mg is prescribed for a child. The stock medicine supplied is 120mg in 5mL of solution.

$$\frac{90}{120} \times 5 = 3.75\text{mL}$$

Drug calculation exercises answers

- A child has been prescribed 25mg of prednisolone. The tablets that are available contain 5mg of prednisolone. How many tablets do you need to give?
  - 5 tablets.
- Rifampicin is prescribed at a dosage of 35mg. There is 100mg in each 5mL of syrup. How much will you need to give?
  - 1.75mL.
- Phenobarbital (phenobarbitone) 45mg is prescribed. It is available as a stock solution of 15mgs in 5mL. What volume will be required?
  - 15mL.
- A child has been prescribed 100mg of Gentamicin intravenously. It is available as 40mg in 1mL. What volume would be required?
  - 2.5mL.
- A child is ordered cephalexin suspension 80mg. It is available as a suspension containing 125mg/5mL. What volume would you administer?
  - 3.2mL.

General equipment
- Prescription chart.
- Children's formulary.
- Medication.
- Appropriate clean receptacle.

Associated reading

BNF. (2010). *British National Formulary for Children*. BMJ Group, London.
Kelsey J, McEwing G (eds) (2008). *Clinical Skills in Child Health Practice*. Elsevier Ltd, Philadelphia.
Nursing & Midwifery Council. (2010). *Standards for Medicines Management*. NMC, London.

Oral drug administration

Background
This is often the route of choice for many drugs if the child is conscious and able to swallow. A variety of formulations is available, e.g. tablets, capsules, syrups, and suspensions. It is convenient and simple, although it does not lead to the quickest absorption. Additionally, certain medications may be rendered inactive by gastric secretions and so other routes of administration are required.

Specific oral equipment
• Oral syringe. The smallest syringe for measuring a dose should be used.
• Medicine pot.

Oral administration principles
• Adhere to general principles (see 🕮 Drug administration, p. 196).
• If a sterile oral syringe is being used, it may be inserted into a syrup/suspension, however, if this is not the case the syrup/suspension should be poured into a medicine pot first.
• Tip the bottle away from the label when pouring into a medicine pot so if medicine spills it will not distort the medication label.
• If tablets are being given ensure that sufficient fluid is offered to wash them down with.
• On occasion, injection preparations are used orally. This should only be done with medical and pharmacy advice. Although the medication may be prepared with an IV syringe, it should be transferred to an oral syringe for administration to ensure a wrong route drug error does not occur.

Practice tips
• Offering the choice of a syringe or a spoon can be effective in encouraging children to take medicine.
• Where appropriate offer the choice of formula, e.g. liquid, capsule, or tablet.
• Consider use of age appropriate techniques, e.g. use of swaddling with infant, use of reward system with older child, encouraging independence with a young person.

Pitfalls
• Ensure suspensions are shaken prior to drawing up the medication.
• Where possible avoid dividing tablets. If the tablet is to be crushed ensure that it's suitable, e.g. not enteric-coated or sustained release. Crushed tablets may then be mixed with a small amount of food; if unsure, consult with pharmacy as there may be food interactions.
• It is not recommended that tablets or the content of capsules should be dissolved and a portion of the suspension administered.

Administration via enteral tube

Administration via enteral tube

Background

Medication should only be administered via an enteral tube where the child or young person is unable to take it orally. Drugs via this route are often unlicensed (see 📖 Drug licensing, p. 217).

Specific enteral equipment

- Enteral syringe.
  - For medication.
  - For aspirating nasogastric tube (NGT) must be >20mL syringe.
  - For flushing in between and at the end of medication.
  - If a 1mL syringe is used that is not enteral Luer then use an adapter.
- Water to flush. Consult local policy as to if this needs to be sterile; often sterile water is required for <1-yr-olds.
- pH paper.

Procedure

Adhere to general principles (see 📖 Drug administration, p. 196).

NGT

If it is a NGT, check the tube, by first visually ensuring that it has not changed position, and then testing the pH.

- Attach a 20 or 50mL enteral syringe to the end of the tube.
- Pull back to aspirate a sample of gastric contents.
- Test the contents on a pH strip.
- The Ph should be 5.5 or less.
- ❶ If you cannot aspirate or the pH is >5.5, do not administer the medication as the tube may not be in the stomach.
- If the tube is not testing, refer to your local policy for techniques to use such as re-positioning the child on the left side, re-aspirating, offering, or syringing a drink orally, and retesting (see 📖 Passing a nasogastric tube/nasogastric feeding, p. 416).

Gastrostomy

If it is a gastrostomy/PEG then visually check the patency and security of the tube.

- ❶ If there is any doubt concerning the correct position do not administer medication, but refer to local policy and seek medical/ specialist nurse advice.
- Attach an extension set if required.
- For further information on gastrostomy care and feeding see 📖 Gastrostomy care: cleaning, caring for, and changing, p. 424.

Nasogastric tube and gastrostomy
- Attach an enteral syringe and flush with (sterile) water to check patency, 5mL is sufficient.
- Attach the enteral syringe containing the medication.
- Administer the medication following your organizations policy, e.g. whether it can be given as a bolus or using gravity only. If a clamp is in situ on the extension set, remember to clamp/unclamp between medications.
- Flush the tube with a second enteral syringe of water in between and at the end of medication.
  - Consider if sterile water is necessary.
  - 5mL in between medication is sufficient.
  - 10mL at the end of medication is required, and 20mL if it is a percutaneous endoscopic gastrostomy (PEG).
- Re-attach the spigot to the end of the nasogastric tube, or detach an extension set where one has been used.
- The child should be observed at all times during the administration process. If any signs of distress are noted then it should be halted and appropriate help sought.

Practice tips
- Where possible, oral administration is preferred.

Pitfalls
- Some medications will affect the PH, this should be noted and documented where this is the case.
- Some medications should not be given via NGTs, such as enteric-coated tablets.

Intramuscular drug administration

Background

Intramuscular (IM) injections are generally avoided in children because of the pain and trauma involved. IM injections are used for where drugs cannot be delivered by any other method, e.g. immunizations. It offers a faster rate of absorption than the subcutaneous (SC) route, but less rapid than IV. Consideration should be given as to whether to use a local anaesthetic cream; and if to be used should be applied at the appropriate time in advance.

Specific intramuscular equipment

- Drug and, if required, diluent.
- Appropriate sized syringe (2mL or less).
- Hypodermic needle for drawing up medication (21G/23G).
- Appropriate sized hypodermic needle for administration (23G/25G).
- Sharps bin.
- Cotton wool.
- Gloves.

Procedure

- Adhere to general principles (see 🕮 Drug administration, p. 196).
- Wash hands.
- Reconstitute drug if required and withdraw correct amount of drug.
- Change the needle, disposing of used one in sharps container.
- Explain to child and family, and select an appropriate site:
  - Vastus lateralis in an infant.
  - Deltoid could be used in an older child.
  - The deltoid muscle can receive less volume and so should not be used when larger volumes of medication are required.
- The site should be socially clean. Cleansing with alcohol is not required.
- Pull the skin and SC tissue approximately 1 inch to the side (known as Z track technique).
- Insert the needle sharply at a 90° angle.
- Aspirate for blood, discarding syringe, and needle if blood is aspirated.
- Slowly inject solution (approximately 1mL in 10s).
- When it is complete withdraw the needle and apply gentle pressure for a few moments.
- Dispose of all the equipment appropriately.

Practice tips

- If repeated injections are to be given, rotate the site and record where it was given in the patients notes.

Pitfalls

- Avoid injecting large amounts of fluid into a small muscle mass as this may result in septic or sterile abscesses.
- Ensure you choose the correct site to avoid possible nerve complications.
- Dorsogluteal site is not recommended.

Subcutaneous drug administration

Background

Small quantities of drugs (<2mL) can be injected into the SC tissue. Drugs given in this way include anti-coagulants and insulin. Drugs are absorbed slower via this route compared to IM and IV.

Specific subcutaneous equipment

- Drug and, if required, dilutent.
- Appropriate sized syringe (1 or 2mL).
- Needle for drawing up medication (21G or 23G if drawing up from a glass ampoule).
- Appropriate sized needle for administration (25G).
- For insulin administration an insulin syringe or prefilled insulin pen should be used (see 📖 Insulin administration, p. 586).
- Some other SC drugs also come in pre-filled syringes.
- Sharps bin.
- Cotton wool.
- Gloves.

Procedure

- Adhere to general principles (see 📖 Drug administration, p. 196).
- Wash hands.
- Reconstitute drug if required.
- Withdraw correct amount of drug.
- Change the needle and dispose of the used one in an appropriate sharps container.
- Explain to child/young person and family, and select an appropriate site. The upper thigh, abdomen, upper arm, and buttocks may be used.
- The site should be socially clean; cleansing with alcohol is not required.
- Pinch the skin.
- Insert the needle at 45°. Some may be given at a 90° angle, such as when using an insulin pen. Utilize clinical judgement as to child's size, and refer to local policy.
- Slowly inject solution (approximately 1mL in 10s).
- When it is complete, withdraw the needle and apply gentle pressure for a few moments.
- Dispose of all the equipment appropriately.

Practice tips

- If repeated injections are to be given rotate the sites used and document this.
- Review the sites regularly for signs of bruising or fibrosis.
- For regular SC administration consider the insertion of a SC cannula.

Pitfalls

- Infection can be caused by poor technique.
- Ensure that you are aware of the unit of prescription, e.g. units in insulin or heparin, other medication may be millilitres.

Subcutaneous infusions

Background

SC infusions are the administration of medication or nutrients into the SC tissue usually over a prolonged period. The SC route can be used for several reasons:

- Where the treatment is not suitable for oral administration due to malabsorption, or inactivation by acids within the stomach, e.g. insulin.
- In preference to intravenous therapy as there is a reduction in the risk of infection, discomfort, or intravenous access is difficult.
- In preference to the intra-muscular route, e.g. due to the volumes required, and less risk of haematoma formation, or nerve damage.
- Families can be taught to self-administer treatment at home; therefore, minimizing hospital admissions.
- Many differing treatments can be administered via SC infusion including:
  - Isotonic fluid replacement.
  - Immunoglobulin replacement.
  - Insulin.
  - Somatostatin analogues.
  - Opioids, e.g. morphine.
  - Anti-emetics.

In theory, as subcutaneous tissue is found all over the body, any site can be used. However, the site chosen for the infusion is dependent upon the volume, rate of absorption and whenever possible the patient should be involved in the choice of site. When regular treatment is given, the site should be rotated. The most frequently used sites include:

- The abdomen, avoiding the umbilical area.
- The upper lateral aspects of the thighs.
- The upper outer quadrant of the buttocks.
- The lateral aspects of the upper arms.

Equipment

- Medication.
- Luer lock syringe.
- SC needle/cannula for the infusion.
- Syringe driver and SC giving set.
- Sterile adhesive dressings or clean paper tape.
- A sharps bin.

Procedure

- Following local policy, check the medication and prescription.
- Using a clean technique, avoiding touching the key parts; prepare and draw up the medication and diluents as prescribed.
  - Attach the syringe/giving set to the needle/cannula and prime.
  - Set up the infusion pump as per prescription, local guidelines and manufacturer's instructions.
  - Place the child in a position that is comfortable for them.

- If the child is immunocompromised cleanse the skin for at least 30s using a 70% isopropyl alcohol swab and leave to dry for 30s. In all other cases, ensure the skin is visibly clean.
- Lift a skin fold (ensuring that only SC tissue and not muscle is lifted) and insert the needle. The angle of insertion will depend upon the type of needle, its length and the amount of SC tissue the child has.
- Secure the needle/cannula.
- Commence the infusion.

During the infusion
- Check the insertion site for any leaking. If this occurs the rate of infusion may need to be reduced.
- Undertake regular observations to detect any adverse reactions to the medication.
- Observe the insertion site for signs of phlebitis.
- Check and document the infusion rate and volume infused according to local policy.

On completion of the infusion
- Remove the tape/dressing that is securing the needle/cannula.
- Remove the needle/cannula; disposing of them according to local policy.
- Hold cotton wool or gauze on the site and apply a plaster if required.

Practice tips
- Anaesthetic cream can be used prior to the needle insertion.
- The abdomen is frequently chosen as the insertion site as it generally provides greater absorption of larger volumes and more freedom of movement during infusions.
- Erythema or blanching and swelling at the site of infusion may be seen, however, this should quickly diminish as the drug is absorbed and usually disappear completely within 2–4h of the infusion being completed.
- For continuous infusions, a Teflon cannula may reduce the risk of phlebitis and prolong the life of the infusion site. For intermittent infusions the needle is removed after the infusion is completed; therefore, a metal needle or butterfly needle may be more appropriate. IV cannulae may also be used.

Pitfalls
- Due to the nature of subcutaneous tissue, blood may enter the giving set; if this occurs the infusion device will need re-siting to prevent IV administration.

Associated reading
Mills W, Fiske K. (2009). *Subcutaneous Access (Infusions and Injections)*. Available at: ℘ http://www.ich.ucl.ac.uk/clinical_information/clinical_guidelines/cpg_guideline_00154.

Intraosseous administration

Background
The intraosseous (IO) route has become the route of choice when a child has no other central access already *in situ* in a clinical emergency.

This is an ideal site when urgent vascular access is needed as the medullary cavity (bone marrow) does not collapse when a patient is hypovolaemic or in circulatory failure. Medications delivered via this route begin to act almost as quickly as those delivered via a central vein and quicker than those delivered via a peripheral vein.

❶ As this is a vascular route, medications should only be administered by healthcare personnel who have undergone recognized training and been deemed as competent. Check and adhere to local policy.

Site selection
Optimum sites are:
- Tibia (2–3cm below tibial tuberosity).
- Femur (3cm above lateral condyle).

These sites avoid epiphyseal plates and joint spaces, which is advised. Other sites can be used, but infected skin or wounds should be avoided, as should fracture sites.

Equipment
Single use IO needles. Assess size required individually.

General guide to needle size
- 0–6 months—18G.
- 6–18 months—16G.
- >18 months—14G.
- Sterile gloves.
- Apron.
- Alcohol wipe/skin preparation.
- Syringes.
- Needles for injection.
- NaCl 0.9% for injection.
- Sterile 3-way tap and extension tubing.
- Specimen bottles (if and as required).
- Local anaesthetic agent.
- IV fluid administration set (if required).
- Adhesive tape.
- Child's medication chart.
- Medication and/or fluids.

Procedure
- Wash hands.
- Check expiry date and remove IO needle from packaging.
- Check needle to ensure it has no cracks in hub or cannula.
- Check trocar can be unscrewed and withdrawn easily.
- Screw trocar into cannula until tip protrudes from the end of cannula.

- Prime 3-way tap and extension tubing and turn 3-way tap to 'off'.
- Explain process as appropriate to child and family.
- Determine and identify entry site.
- Position child safely (with support to maintain position as needed).
- Clean insertion site area and allow to dry.
- Immobilize limb.
- Wash hands and apply gloves and apron.
- Position cannula at an angle of 90° to skin.
- Using a screwing action, apply pressure to needle hub until there is an obvious loss of resistance (almost like a 'pinging' sensation!).
- Ensure cannula is stable in upright position.
- Remove trocar and attempt aspiration of bone marrow with 5mL syringe (in clinical emergency omit bone marrow aspiration).
- If no marrow can be aspirated, use clinical judgement to endorse correct placement of cannula.
- If fluid is aspirated from the marrow, the laboratory needs to be advised it is not blood.
- Flush cannula with 0.9% NaCl from pre-primed extension set with 3-way tap.
- Administer medications and fluids as prescribed.
- Observe site and associated limb for signs of extravasation, leakage, compartment syndrome.
- Discontinue administration if these complications arise and seek medical assistance.
- Secure needle and/or extension tubing as required to maintain stability.
- Dispose of all equipment/waste according to local policy.
- Record procedure and administration of medications/fluids in health record.
- Continue to observe site frequently (at least hourly) while cannula is *in situ*.

Practice tips

- Bone marrow or spinal needles can be used if IO needles not available.
- Avoid 'rocking' motion as cannula is inserted, which could splinter bone.
- Bone marrow may be difficult to aspirate as it is highly viscous and the lumen of the cannula is relatively narrow.
- Securing of cannula can be achieved by taping a clean gallipot over it.

Pitfalls

There are risks associated with this form of administration, amongst them namely:

- Infection.
- Extravasation.
- Embolism.
- Compartment syndrome.
- Tissue necrosis.

Associated reading

Advanced Life Support Group. 2005. *Advanced Paediatric Life Support: The Practical Approach*. 4th edn BMJ, London.

Intrathecal administration

Background

This method of delivery involves the injection of medication into the sheath surrounding the spinal cord, and requires the process of lumbar puncture.

Principles

- Medication may be delivered via a single dose or a continuous dose administered through an intrathecal pump which will be surgically implanted just below the skin of the stomach with a tube connected to the base of the spine.
- Medications given via this route currently are:
  - Some analgesics.
  - Some chemotherapy agents.
  - Baclofen.
- ❶ Administration of intrathecal medication is limited to suitably trained medical personnel.
- For care of a child who is undergoing lumbar puncture, see 📖 Assisting with lumbar puncture, p. 398.

Administration via eye

Background
Only locally acting medication is instilled into the eye. Whilst not painful it can be uncomfortable and may cause short-term blurring of vision.

Specific equipment for eye
- Medication including appropriate dropper.
- Swab.
- Tissue.

Procedure
- Adhere to general principles (see ⊞ Drug administration, p. 196).
- A baby should be swaddled in a towel/blanket.
- Ensure the child/young person is either lying down, or their head is slightly extended backwards.
- Draw the lower eyelid down.
- The drops should be applied to the inner aspect of the eye (whether it is open or shut), i.e. nearest the nose.
- When it has disappeared, a further drop can be applied if prescribed.
- The dropper should not come into direct contact with the patient.
- If ointment has been prescribed the lower lid should be gently pulled down to allow it to be instilled, and administered in a line across the lower lid.
- Any excess can be gently wiped off with a clean tissue, whilst the eye is closed.
- If both drops and ointment are prescribed, leave 5min between the applications of these.

Practice tips
- Eye medication should be sterile.
- If both eyes require medication then separate containers should be used for each eye.
- Remove medication from the refrigerator some minutes prior to instillation.

Pitfalls
- Instillation of medication to the eye can be problematic especially in babies and toddlers. Preparation and distraction is essential.

Administration via ear

Background
Only locally acting drugs are instilled in the ear. There are specialized preparations. While it is not painful it can be uncomfortable.

Specific equipment for ear
- Medication: generally with dropper already attached.
- Tissue.

Procedure
- Adhere to general principles (see ▢ Drug administration, p. 196).
- Ask the child to lie on their side with the effected ear uppermost.
- After washing your hands, draw up medication into the dropper, making sure that it is at room temperature.
- Gently pull the pinna up and back before applying the prescribed drops directly into the ear canal. If the child is <3yrs, pull the pinna down and back.
- If at all possible the child should then stay in this position for 3–5min, so preparation for age appropriate distraction is a good idea.

Practice tips
- Gentle rubbing of the area immediately in front of the ear may help the medication travel and relax the child.

Pitfalls
- The practice of inserting small cotton wool plugs should be avoided as it may cause complications.

Administration via nose

Background

The lining of the nose is very vascular which allows fast systemic absorption. Drugs with local action, e.g. decongestants may also be instilled in the nose.

Specific nasal equipment

In addition to the general equipment required for medication administration, paper tissues can be useful.

Procedure

- Adhere to general principles (see 📖 Drug administration, p. 196).
- Clear secretions. If the child is able to (aged 2yrs or above) ask them to blow their nose.
- After washing your hands, draw up the medication in the dropper.
- The child should lie on the bed with their head extended slightly over its end.
- They should then turn slightly towards the side on which the drops are to be instilled.
- Taking care not to touch the nose (or anything else) with the dropper instill the prescribed number of drops.
- Discard any medication left in the dropper.
- The child should remain in that position for 30–45s.
- Repeat the process if medication is required in the other nostril.
- If medication is to be administered via a nasal spray then secretions should be cleared as described.
- The child/young person's head should be upright.
- One nostril should be gently pushed closed, whilst the spray is applied to the other.
- If the child is able they should breathe in gently through their nose during the administration.
- If needed the procedure should be repeated with the other nostril.

Practice tips

- Nasal medication can leak into the throat and leave an unpleasant taste, so have a drink to hand.

Pitfalls

- Bacterial contamination may occur if nasal dispensers come into contact with the nose or if the drugs are not stored correctly.

Per rectum administration

Background
Per rectum (PR) administration of medication may be used where it is not possible to give orally, e.g. if the child is vomiting or where local action is required. Often this is in the form of a suppository, which is in solid form and dissolves once inserted, or an enema that is usually liquid and inserted using a nozzle.

Specific per rectum equipment
- Disposable gloves.
- Lubricating jelly.
- Tissues.
- Disposable sheet or similar.
- Commode.

Procedure
- Adhere to general principles (see 🕮 Drug administration, p. 196).
- Ask the child to empty their bladder.
- Ensure the child/young person's privacy.
- Place an incontinence sheet on the bed/chair if necessary.
- Ensure a commode or toilet is nearby.
- Ask the child to lie on their left side, legs flexed with the topmost one higher, if possible.
- If using a suppository, lubricate it.
- Gently introduce the lubricated suppository or nozzle of the enema and administer the dose. Insert rounded end first if it is a suppository.
- In younger children it may assist retention if you gently hold the buttocks together for a short while after administration.

Practice tips
- Consider if there should be two practitioners present for the procedure.
- Consideration of privacy and dignity issues is vital.
- Ensure enema is at least at room temperature.

Pitfalls
- If poor technique is used rectal administration can cause physical pain, discomfort, and embarrassment, as well as distrust of the nurse.

Topical drug administration

Background
Topical medication is applied directly to the skin. Most usually it is intended to have a local action, rather than being absorbed systemically. Types include creams, lotions, ointments, emollients, gels, and pastes.

Specific topical equipment
• Gloves.
• Dressings/bandages if required.

Topical administration principles
• Adhere to general principles (see 🕮 Drug administration, p. 196).
• Wear gloves when applying topical medication to prevent absorption of the medication.
• Follow instructions given with the specific product/care plan.
• Avoid applying to surrounding skin.
• Time hygiene care/bath/shower around topical administration.

Practice tips
• Remember that skin thickness varies both with age and site. The face has the thinnest skin, whilst the thickest is on the soles of the feet and palms.
• All topical drugs are for single patient use only.
• Use of distraction may be important with this administration as the child may be reluctant for cream to be applied, and may try to scratch cream off immediately after application.

Pitfalls
• Drugs can be absorbed systemically even when intended for local use; this is particularly true of neonates and infants.
• With multiple topical administration medicines, there may be specific sites and orders to administer them in; follow the prescription, and care plan carefully, referring to specialist advice as required.

Cytotoxic medication

Background

Only appropriately trained staff should handle and administer cytotoxic medicines.

Principles

- Where possible the medicines should be reconstituted in specially adapted pharmacy areas.
- Appropriate protective clothing should be warn, e.g. gloves, gowns, and goggles.
- Prior to the administration of cytotoxic medication the child's blood counts should be checked to ensure that it is safe to go ahead.
- Any required supportive treatment, e.g. anti-emetics or hydration should be administered prior to the cytotoxic medication.
- The nurse should be aware of the treatment protocol and the side effects of the drug.

Practice tips and pitfalls

- If cytotoxic medicines are to be administered intravenously then an extravasation kit should be available.
- Intrathecal chemotherapy will be dispensed in Luer slip syringes, rather than a standard syringe to prevent accidental administration of inappropriate medicines by this route.
- Care must be taken dispose of patient waste safely as it will contain cytotoxic material.

Associated reading

Department of Health (DoH). 2008. *Updated National Guidance on the Safe Administration of Intrathecal Chemotherapy*. DoH, London.

Covert administration of drugs

Background

Where ever possible covert administration of drugs should be avoided, especially where the child is of an appropriate age to withhold consent.

Principles

If it is unavoidable and in the best interests of the patient the following steps should be taken in addition to the general steps when administering medication:

- Advice should be sought from a pharmacist about the most suitable carriage for the drug.
- Inform the parent/carer and gain consent.
- Where it is at all possible tablets should not be crushed (especially those with special coatings) nor capsules opened.
- Where it is necessary medicines should be mixed with a small amount of food or liquid rather than in a whole drink or portion of food.
- The patient should be observed until the entire carrier has been consumed.
- All details should be recorded in the child's records.

Administration of medication by the young person, parent, or carer

Background
Self-medication has been shown to be beneficial in a number of cases, especially where the child or young person suffers from a chronic condition requiring on-going medication, e.g. asthma, diabetes, or cystic fibrosis. If self or carer medication administration is to be utilized, an education programme should be undertaken, ensuring they understand all stages of the administration process. Only when they have been deemed competent should they be allowed to take the medication without direct supervision. Whilst in hospital any medication should still be recorded on the child's/young person's prescription chart; the nurse is still responsible for ensuring the medication has been taken. A key may be given to the patient/carer for medication storage and removed from them on discharge.

Equipment
There should be documentation for the parent/carer, young person, and staff detailing medication being self-administered.

Principles
- Prior to a young person, their parents, or carers giving or taking medication, an assessment must be made of their ability to do so.
- Ensure that for each medication they are aware of:
  - The drug effects and side effects.
  - Contraindications.
  - How and when to administer the medication.
  - What to do in the case of an error.
- This should be documented within the patient's notes.

Drug licensing

Background

Not all medicines used in children are licensed for use. This does not mean that they are not tested; however, because of the ethical and practical difficulties of running large scale randomized controlled trials in children and young people companies often do not apply for the licences in these groups.

Medication that is licensed, but used outside its licensed indications is commonly known as 'off-label'.

Equipment

Refer to Children's formulary such as the BNFC for details on unlicensed drugs.

Principles

- If these drugs are used in children and young people the prescriber takes responsibility, rather than the pharmaceutical company.
- Parents/carers and, if appropriate, the child or young person, should be informed that the drug is unlicensed.
- Extra support may be needed to reassure in this instance.

Patient group directions

Background

A patient group direction (PGD) allows specific registered healthcare professionals to supply and/or administer a medicine to a patient without the patient seeing a prescriber.[1] In children's nursing, a PGD can only be used by qualified children's nurses who have undergone specific training in the supply and administration of the drug listed in the 'PGD'.

Equipment

- Copy of patient group direction.
- Drug chart.
- BNFC.

Procedure

- A PGD includes the following criteria:[2]
  - A written instruction for the supply of a licensed medicine in an identified clinical situation.
  - The patient may not be individually identified before presenting for treatment.
  - Drawn up locally by doctors, pharmacists, and other health professionals.
  - Must meet legal criteria.
  - Signed by, e.g. a doctor, chief pharmacist, and approved by an NHS Hospital Trust Board.
  - Must improve patient care and not be to the detriment of patient safety.
- The patient is to have an identified clinical condition.
- There must be a list of individuals who are named as competent to supply/administer each PGD, and a register kept of their names.
- An annual assessment of knowledge is taken regarding each specific PGD, as part of the nurse's personal development plan update.
- When supplying PGD's, it can include a flexible dose range. This is important in children's nursing, when doses are often related to age or weight.
- Drugs that are frequently administered by PGD include:
  - Salbutamol inhalers via spacers.
  - Diarolyte-rehydration solution given orally.
  - Ametop® (tetracaine gel) and EMLA® (lidocaine cream); both are used for topical local anaesthesia.
  - Oxygen; should be treated as a drug and prescribed prior to delivery, as administration of inappropriate concentrations may have serious or fatal consequences.[3]

Practice tips

- Clearly identify the patient's condition and check for any contraindications against using the drug; using for example a Children's National Formulary for this.
- Ensure a complete set of clinical observations have been taken and you have considered implications of any abnormal findings.

Pitfalls

- Ensure local PGD policy, and local medicines code is adhered to at all times.

Associated reading

[1] National Prescribing Centre. (2009). *Patient Group Directions. 'A Practical Guide and Framework of Competencies for All Professionals Using Patient Group Directions'*. Available at: http://www.npc.co.uk/non_medical/resources/patient_group_directions.pdf (accessed 24 February 2011).

[2] Department of Health. (2006). *Medicines Matters—A Guide to Current Mechanisms for the Prescribing, Supply and Administration of Medicines*. DoH, London.

[3] BNF. (2010). *British National Formulary for Children*. BMJ Publishing Co., London.

Controlled medication

Background

The misuse of drugs act 1971 (with regulations in 1985 and 2001) lists drugs in 5 schedules. Nursing is concerned with schedules 2 and 3. All of the drugs listed are regulated in relation to prescription, requisition, storage, administration, disposal, and recording. Drugs that are controlled include morphine based drugs and some anti-convulsants. Additional statutory measures for the management of controlled drugs are laid down in the Health Act 2006 and its associated regulations. CD's should always be stored in a locked cupboard within a locked cupboard.

Equipment

In addition to the standard equipment, controlled drugs (CD) have a separate record book in which a running tally is maintained and is double signed.

Principles

In addition to the usual steps the following actions should be taken when administering controlled drugs:

- Specific prescription requirements for controlled medication exist and should be adhered to.
- As well as the patients prescription chart the ward controlled medicines record book should be used. All controlled medication stationary should be securely stored.
- Controlled medicines must be checked by two people, one of whom must be a registered nurse.
  - Refer to local policy.
  - In the community a second competent person (which may be the carer) may witness the administration and balance.[1]
- The total number of tablets or ampoules should be checked against the number recorded in the book.
- The number required should be removed and the rest returned to the locked cupboard, and the controlled medicines book be amended accordingly.
- If the entire ampoule is not used the remaining medicine must be disposed of and this documented.
- If irregularities are found between amounts present and those recorded, re-check CD medication against records. If irregularities are definite then this is a clinical incident and should be reported as such. A senior nurse in charge of the area should be alerted as well as pharmacy. Follow local policy.
- The medication should then be administered in the usual way.
- It may be that the young person and parents/carers require additional reassurance because of the view that many controlled dugs are addictive.

Associated reading

[1] Nursing & Midwifery Council. (2010). *Standards for Medicines Management.* NMC, London.

Intravenous access and care

Venepuncture

Background

Venepuncture is the introduction of a needle into vein to obtain a representative blood sample for haematological, biochemical or bacteriological analysis.[1]

Venepuncture or phlebotomy is one of the most common invasive procedures performed in clinical practice today. For the nurse who is performing venepuncture, it is their responsibility to be familiar with blood tests commonly undertaken, the requirements for each test (fasting, pre drug administration, etc.) and know the normal blood component values.

Principles of practice

- The smallest gauge needle should be utilized to minimize damage to the vein.
- The vacuum system is likely to cause small veins to collapse so is not recommended for small children.
- If the child is receiving intravenous (IV) fluids, ideally another limb should be utilized, but if this is not possible then a vein below the level of the cannula should be utilized with the IV infusion stopped for 5–10min prior to venepuncture.
- Avoid areas with a pulse present as an artery could be punctured.
- Avoid areas where the skin is broken or where rashes are present.

❶ Preparation is essential. This should include:
- Use of local anaesthetic topical agents.
- Distraction therapy.
- Good clear explanation to the child and parents.
- Positioning of the child and parent.
- Good infection control measures.
- Knowledge of the child's previous experiences.

Selection of a vein

- Selecting the right vein is the most crucial aspect of venepuncture apart from gaining the child's cooperation.
- The superficial veins of the arm are usually the site of choice, namely branches of the basilic, cephalic, median cephalic, and median cubital vein. Care must be taken to avoid the brachial artery; this should be done by palpation and then avoiding it. The vein should feel soft and bouncy, be straight, and free from valves. In the infant, it may be difficult to palpate a vein so transillumination may be used.
- In the infant, the superficial veins in the dorsum of the hand, the dorsal venous arch or the metacarpal veins may be more accessible.
- Children who have blood taken on a regular basis will usually instruct you on which vein to use.
- It is rare to have to use the veins in the lower limbs for routine venepuncture and this should be avoided if at all possible as the risk of thromboembolisim has been identified.

Equipment

- Butterfly needle or needle-appropriate gauge for child's size.
- Syringe/s.
- Vacuum system may be used in an older child.
- Disposable tourniquet.
- Alcohol swab.
- Appropriate collection tubes.
- Specimen request form.
- Low linting swab.
- Hypoallergenic plaster.
- Apron.
- Non-sterile gloves.
- Sharps bin.

Procedure

- Confirm the identity of the child.
- Explain procedure appropriately and gain consent.
- *Assemble team:* nurse to hold limb, play therapist to distract child.
- Ensure privacy for the child.
- Check all equipment is ready and prepared.
- If child's skin is visibly dirty, wash with soapy water and dry.
- Wash and dry hands thoroughly.
- Apply non-sterile gloves and apron.
- Remove local anaesthetic cream.
- Bring the prepared equipment to the child.
- Assess veins and identify suitable vein/veins by palpation.
- Support limb with a pillow and ask parent/carer to hold child securely, ensuring that they are comfortable doing this and that child will be safe during procedure. The child may wish to lie down.
- Apply tourniquet or ask staff to squeeze the limb being utilized gently. The older child could be asked to make a fist. The vein may be gently tapped or stroked in order to increase its prominence.
- Release the tourniquet.
- Wash and dry hands thoroughly.
- Apply non-sterile gloves and apron.
- Reapply the tourniquet.
- Clean skin with an alcohol-based solution and allow to dry.
- Apply ethyl chloride spray if indicated, following manufacturer's instructions.
- Remove the cover from the needle and inspect.
- Stabilize skin with the thumb, stretching skin downwards. The vein can be stretched using the forefinger and thumb of the non-dominant hand. This applies traction to the vein thus anchoring it and preventing it rolling.
- Insert the needle at a 30° angle.
- Reduce the angle of descent when a flashback is seen. This will be in the tubing if using a butterfly device or in the hub of the needle if using a syringe. If using a syringe, pull back on the plunger of the syringe before commencing so as blood will flow into the syringe once the vein has been punctured.

- Slightly advance the needle into vein.
- Using very gentle pressure, withdraw the required amount of blood into the syringe. If using a needle, allow the blood to drip into the appropriate sample bottles without exerting any pressure on the needle.
- Loosen and remove tourniquet or relax pressure on limb.
- Remove needle from vein.
- Apply gentle digital pressure with the low lint swab over the puncture site for approximately 1min.
- Transfer the blood to the appropriate sample tubes in the correct order as soon as possible. Gently invert the tubes at least six times.
- Label all samples immediately.
- Inspect puncture site and apply sterile hypoallergenic plaster checking their allergic status to plasters first.
- Ascertain comfort status of child.
- Dispose of all waste appropriately.
- Wash and dry hands.
- Follow local procedure for transportation of samples to laboratory.
- Document venepuncture in child's care records.

Practice tips

- If it is difficult to palpate a vein or if the child's hands are cold then remove the tourniquet, and apply moist warm heat either in the form of a warm compress or place child's hands in a bowl of warm water.
- When inserting the needle and an arterial puncture occurs, remove the needle at once and apply pressure until the bleeding stops. Document in the child's care records.
- If a nerve is touched, remove needle at once and apply pressure. Document in the child's care records.
- Avoid having the tourniquet on for too long as this will cause haemo-concentration due to venous stasis and will also be very uncomfortable for the child.
- If a blood sample is required for calcium levels, release the tourniquet before drawing the sample or an inaccurate reading may result.
- Do not exert excessive pressure on the syringe—insert the blood gently into the sample tubes and invert (do not shake).
- If a haematoma occurs at the venepuncture site, remove the needle, apply pressure until bleeding stops. Use an ice pack if necessary and elevate the affected limb. Document in the child's care records.
- Good positioning and excellent distraction of the child is essential to reduce fear and trauma for the child.

Associated reading

[1] Lavery I, Ingham P. (2005). Venepuncture: best practice *Nursing Standard* **19**(49), 55–65.

Inserting and securing a peripheral intravenous line

Background
Peripheral intravenous cannulae are increasingly being inserted by nurses. A flexible plastic tube is inserted into a vein thus providing direct access to the circulatory system for the purpose of administration of intravenous fluids and medication.

Indications for use
- Short term therapy of 3–5 days.
- Bolus injections or short, intermittent infusions.

Choice of device
The principle of using the smallest, shortest gauge cannula in any given situation should be adhered to (see Table 9.1).

Table 9.1 Choice of cannula size

Cannula gauge	Age of child
26 gauge	Neonate and infant
24 gauge	Child
22 gauge	Older child
18 gauge	Older child in an emergency situation

Insertion site
- This will depend on the age of the child, clinical condition, indication for use, type and duration of therapy, and condition of the child's veins.
- Previous history of infusion devices should be considered.
- The antecubital fossas (median vein), dorsum of hands (dorsal venous network) wrists are common sites for insertion of a cannula in a child.
- The scalp and long saphenous vein of the lower limb may also be used in infants if none of the other areas are suitable.
- In an older child, the basilica vein or cephalic vein may also be used.
- Where possible areas of flexion should be avoided and the child should be given a choice about the site utilized.
- Areas where skin is broken or inflamed should also be avoided.

Choosing a vein
The vein to be cannulated should be easy to palpate, feel bouncy, refill when depressed, and be straight and free from valves. Valves may be felt as small lumps, and the presence of valves will make it difficult to advance the cannula and to get backflow of blood.

Preparation for procedure

Prior to insertion of the cannula, the following points should be considered:

- Obtain consent from the child and/or parents.
- Check the child's identity and review treatment plan.
- Organize distraction therapy.
- Use appropriate local anaesthetic topical agents
- Use of sucrose for the young infant.
- Familiarization with correct holding technique for procedure.
- Assess veins for suitability.
- Follow local NHS Trusts policy for insertion of cannula.
- Competence in aseptic non-touch technique (ANTT).

Equipment

- *Cannulae:* use appropriate gauge.
- Tissues to remove local anaesthetic cream.
- Skin cleansing solution.
- Extension set.
- Needle-free valve.
- 0.9% normal saline drawn up into 10-mL syringe.
- Ethyl chloride spray.
- Entonox (if to be used).
- Specimen bottles, if sample to be collected at same time.
- Non-sterile gloves.
- Cotton wool ball.
- Tourniquet-disposable,
- Sterile dressing. Splint.
- Kling bandage.
- Non-sterile tape.
- Portable light.

Procedure

- Give appropriate information and gain consent.
- *Assemble members:* nurse to hold limb, play therapist/nurse to distract child.
- Ensure privacy for the child.
- Check all the equipment is ready.
- Wash and dry hands thoroughly.
- If child's skin is visibly dirty, then this should be washed with soapy water and dried.
- Remove local anaesthetic cream.
- Assess veins and identify suitable vein/veins by palpation.
- Wash and dry hands thoroughly again.
- Apply non-sterile gloves and apron.
- Support limb with a pillow and ask parent/carer to hold child securely, ensuring that they are comfortable doing this and that child will be safe during procedure.
- Apply tourniquet or ask staff to squeeze the limb being utilized gently.
- Clean skin with an alcohol-based solution for 30–60s and allow it to dry.

- Apply ethyl chloride spray if indicated as per manufacturer's instructions.
- Remove needle guard and check the cannula.
- Stabilize the skin with the thumb, stretching the skin downwards, or the vein can be stretched using the forefinger and thumb of the non-dominant hand. This will apply traction to the vein, thus anchoring it and preventing it rolling.
- Hold cannula with bevelled end up, enter skin at 10–45% angle[1] and using a steady motion, advance cannula until a 'flashback' of blood is seen in the chamber of the cannula.
- Decrease angle of cannula so as to prevent puncture of the posterior vein wall and gently advance the cannula off the stylet. Continue to insert the plastic cannula into the vein, while keeping the skin taut until the hub of the cannula is touching the skin.
- Never re-introduce the stylet into the plastic cannula once you have removed it.
- Loosen and remove tourniquet or relax pressure on limb.
- Apply pressure with one finger to the vein above the insertion site and fully remove the stylet.
- Secure cannula with an appropriate transparent sterile dressing such as Tegaderm™ IV dressing.
- If blood samples are to be obtained, do so now before flushing the cannula. Attach an extension set to the cannula with a 10-mL syringe, withdraw the required amount of blood. Gentle squeezing pressure or tourniquet may need to be utilized again at this stage.
- Attach the extension tubing (should be luer lock) with the needle-free valve in situ and using a 10-mL syringe primed with 0.9% normal saline, flush the cannula using a pulsatile flush ending with positive pressure and close the clamp.
- Inspect the site for signs of leakage or swelling, and clean away any blood from area.
- Apply the correct size disposable splint and cover with a bandage.
- Ensure child and parent/carer are comfortable and pain free. Explain altered care needs, i.e. restriction in movement now that cannula is inserted.
- Remove gloves, wash hands, and dispose of all waste correctly, following universal precautions.
- Document insertion in care records and place intravenous cannula care bundle in child's care records.

Associated reading

Department of Health (2007). *Saving Lives: reducing infection, delivering clean and safe care*. DoH, London.

Royal College of Nursing (2003). *Restraining, holding still and containing children and young people: guidance for nursing staff*. RCN, London.

---

[1] Dougherty L, Lister S. (2008). *The Royal Marsden Hospital Manual of Clinical Nursing Procedures*, 7th edn. Wiley-Blackwell, Oxford.

Maintenance of peripheral intravenous sites and systems

Background

Once *in situ*, the peripheral cannula and intravenous systems present a risk of infection, phlebitis, extravasation, and embolus for the child. Use of ANTT (see ⌨ Aseptic non-touch technique, p. 174) helps to reduce these risks of contamination by the patient's skin flora at the time of insertion or by the introduction of organism into any part of IV system can occur. It is a requirement that all NHS Trusts audit key policies and procedures for infection prevention under The Health Act 2006.[1] A care bundle and local trust policy should be followed to enable this process to be monitored.

Equipment

- Sterile dressing.
- Visual phlebitis score.
- Normal saline to flush.
- Splint.
- Bandage.
- 10-mL luer lock syringe to flush.
- Alcoholic chlorhexidine gluconate bp 2% and isopropyl alcohol 70%.
- Wipes.

Procedure

- *Hand hygiene*: follow correct hand hygiene procedure before and after each cannula inspection (see ⌨ Hand hygiene, p. 168).
- Site inspection should be carried out daily using the Phlebitis Score. (see Table 9.2).

Practice tips

- *Dressing*: transparent, semi permeable, sterile dressing should be *in situ* and intact. If soiled or non-adherent then it should be replaced.
- *Accessing the cannula:*
  - Should be via an 'add on device' such as a Smartsite® or Bionector®.
  - If an extension set with a three-way tap is being used then it should be luer lock and must be used in accordance with the manufacturer's instructions.
  - ANTT and the correct cleansing solution, which should be allowed to dry before use should be utilized in accordance with local policy.
- *Flushing:*
  - Ensures patency, using 0.9% normal saline utilize a pulsatile action and end with a positive pressure.
  - 0.9% normal saline should be prescribed or follow a patient group direction.
  - Patency of the cannula should be checked before the administration of any fluids or medication.

Table 9.2 The Phlebitis score

Grade	Clinical criteria	Action
0	No symptoms-site appears healthy	Continue to observe cannula
1	Erythema at site with or without pain	Possible signs of phlebitis Close observation of cannula
2	Pain with erythema and/or oedema at IV site	Early stage of phlebitis Re-site cannula immediately
3	Erythema and/or oedema with streak formation. Palpable venous cord <2.5cm	Medium stage phlebitis Re-site cannula Consider treatment
4	Pain at IV site with erythema streak formation, induration, palpable venous cord >2.5cm	Advanced stage of phlebitis or the start of thrombophlebitis Re-site cannula Commence treatment
5	Pain along path of cannula, erythema, induration, palpable venous cord, pyrexia, possible purulent discharge	Advanced stage thrombophlebitis Commence treatment Re-site cannula

- *When flushing the cannula:*
  - Initially aspirate the device to check for blood return.
  - If no blood is returning, attempt to gently flush the cannula.
  - If resistance is met, stop, and remove device.
  - Flush volume of should be at least double volume of the cannula and 'add on devices'.

Administration sets
- Should be changed no more frequently than after 96h when used for continuous infusion, but at least every 7 days. ❶ Local policy may vary—check! Where possible, system should remain 'closed'. Fluid type will also determine when it should be changed.
- Change the needleless components at least as frequently as the administration set. There is no benefit to changing these more frequently than every 72h.
- *Blood or blood products set*: should be discarded as soon as the transfusion is completed, maximum two units.
- *Intermittent infusion sets*: should be changed every 24h if they remain connected to the device, but discard immediately if disconnected.

Replacement

- Replace peripheral catheters in children only when clinically indicated.
- If cannula inserted in an emergency situation and aseptic technique has been compromised, it should be replaced within 24h or as soon as possible.
- *Securing:* once secured with a primary dressing a splint may be utilized Take care to position the splint so as circulation will not be impaired. Splint should be correct type for the site and is single use only. A bandage may then be applied and changed as required.

All peripheral IV cannula care should be documented in the child's care record or on the care bundle.

Pitfalls

- Securing the cannula is essential to avoid dislodgment.
- Complaints of pain at the site it should not be ignored.
- Inadequate flushing will lead to occlusion of cannula.
- Failure to recognize phlebitis and infiltration will lead to patient morbidity.

Associated reading

Ayliffe GAJ, Lowbury EJL, Geddes AM, Williams JD. (2000). *Control of Hospital Infection*, 4th edn. Arnold, London.

CDC (2011). *Guidelines for the prevention of intravascular catheter related infections* CDC, New York.

Department of Health (2007). *High Impact Intervention No 2. Peripheral intravenous cannula care bundle.* HMSO, London.

Jackson A. (1998). Infection control: a battle in vein infusion phlebitis. *Nurs Times* **94**(4), 68–71.

---

[1] Department of Health (2006). *The Health Act (2006) Code of Practice for the Prevention and Control of Healthcare Associated Infection*. HMSO, London.

Changing infusion bags and lines

Changing infusion bags and lines

Background
The changing of the intravenous fluid bag and administration sets must be undertaken using ANTT (see 📖 Aseptic non-touch technique, p. 174) and as per local policy. Incorrect procedure places the child at risk of sepsis or possible air embolus. Any fluids or drugs that are to be added to the intravenous fluids must be compatible.

Equipment
- Prescription chart.
- Administration set.
- Intravenous fluid.
- Sterile field.
- Alcoholic chlorhexidine gluconate bp 2% and isopropyl alcohol 70%.
- Wipes.
- Gloves.
- Apron.

Procedure
- Assemble equipment.
- Wash and dry hands thoroughly.
- Apply sterile gloves and apron.
- Check intravenous fluid as per local policy against the prescription chart.
- Observe the outer wrapper and discard bag if not intact.
- Check the fluid expiry date, colour, clarity, and for the presence of any particles.
- Check the outer wrapper of the administration set to make sure it is intact and that it has not expired.
- Open administration set and close the roller clamp.
- Open the intravenous fluid bag and expose the port by removing the protective cover.
- Remove the protective cover on the administration set spike and using ANTT, insert into the intravenous fluid bag.
- Hang the intravenous fluid bag on a drip stand.
- Squeeze the drip chamber of the administration set until it is half full.
- Slowly open the roller clamp and prime the administration set until the fluid reaches the end of the line following the manufacturer's instructions. This should expel the air from the line—also visually inspect the line for the presence of any air. If air is present, then open the roller clamp to allow more fluid through the line expelling any remaining air.
- Close the roller clamp.
- If using a burette, then fill approximately 30mL of fluids into the burette and close the fluid fill clamp before opening the roller clamp to prime the line.
- Label the line with the date and time that it has been first used.
- Insert the administration set into the appropriate infusion pump.
- Check patient identity.

- When using a needleless device, e.g. Smartsite® decontaminate as per local policy.
- Ensure patency of intravenous cannula prior to connecting intravenous infusion by flushing with 0.9% normal saline as prescribed.
- Connect administration set to intravenous cannula via needleless device.
- Secure administration set as required.
- Set the infusion rate and other parameters as prescribed.
- Open roller clamp and commence infusion.
- Document all required details, batch number, expiry date, time infusion commenced, name of first and second checker on prescription chart.
- Document date and time of that the administration set was changed in child's care records along with the serial number of the pump being used.
- Remove apron and gloves and dispose of all waste.
- Commence/maintain fluid balance chart.
- Wash and dry hands thoroughly.

Practice tips

- Always allow IV fluid to flow slowly through the line, so as to avoid 'air bubbles' from occurring.
- Place the roller clamp near the intravenous fluid bag so the nurse can have easy access to this in the event of pump malfunction.

Associated reading

Doughty L, Lamb J. (2008). *Intravenous Therapy in Nursing Practice*, 2nd edn. Blackwell Publishing, Oxford.

Use of intravenous infusion devices

Background

Infusion devices are designed to accurately measure the amount of fluid or drugs delivered via the intravenous route over a prescribed period of time, thus achieving an effective therapeutic response, whilst maintaining patient safety. The infusion of fluids or medication into children is classified as high risk and accuracy is essential. When administering intravenous fluids there are many considerations for the children's nurse who is required to be competent in the calculation of drug doses, maintenance of accurate fluid balance, the use of specific paediatric infusion devices and be able to manage any complications as they occur. Any infusion device should be used in accordance with the Medicines and Healthcare Products Regulatory Agency (MHRA) risk classification system.

❶ Ensure you are trained, competent and (where necessary) have been assessed as such before using any infusion device. If in doubt, check!

Types of intravenous controllers, pumps, and infusion devices

Manual flow control devices/gravity devices

They are rarely used in the clinical area now due to the risk associated with their use. They are entirely dependent on gravity to deliver the infusion. The system consists of an administration set with a roller clamp that controls the flow rate of the fluid. They are available with a variable drop size. Their use is dependent on many variables, such as fluctuations in venous pressure, viscosity of the fluid, and position of the patient. They may be used with gravity drip rate controllers, but while the drop rate is controlled by a battery or mains powered occlusion valve they have no pumping mechanism.

Electronic infusion pumps

These include:
- Volumetric pumps.
- Syringe pumps.
- Specialist pumps: patient-controlled analgesia (PCA) pumps, ambulatory infusion devices.

Volumetric infusion pumps

This type of pump works by calculating the volume delivered. The pump measures the volume displaced in the reservoir in the administration set for every pump cycle. The pump calculates every fill and empty cycle the reservoir delivers as a given amount of fluid; hence, the term volumetric. Volumetric pumps may be accurate to within 5%. The benefits of using volumetric infusion devices are:
- Can detect air in the administration set.
- Variable pressure measurement.
- Range of alarms, e.g. end of infusion, high venous pressure.
- Secondary infusion facility.
- Multichannel and dual channel facility.
- Programmed to deliver set volumes.

It is essential that the correct administration set is utilized for the type of volumetric pump being used. Neonatal/paediatric volumetric pumps should be available in all children's clinical areas.

Syringe pumps

Syringe pumps are highly accurate, low volume devices that are generally used to deliver small volumes of highly concentrated medication to the child. The plunger of the syringe is driven forward at a controlled rate to deliver the medication to the child.

The syringe size is usually 60mL so the volume for infusion is limited to this, but other size syringes may be used. The syringe is attached to an extension/administration set, which is then connected to the peripheral intravenous cannula.

The volume delivered is usually in millilitres per hour. Anti-siphonage valve administration sets should be used to prevent free flow. It is essential that the correct syringe is used so as to reduce the risk of infusion error. The children's' nurse must be competent in all aspects of the use of the syringe pump.

Patient controlled analgesia pump

See 📖 Patient-controlled analgesia, p. 124.

Battery operated syringe drivers

This is a portable battery-operated device that is used to deliver drugs either the parenteral or subcutaneous route. They are used in palliative care or for long-term management of certain conditions, such as for the administration of dechelating agents. They either deliver as an hourly rate or as a daily rate. They are calculated as millimetres per hour or millimetres per day. It is essential that the user is aware of which pump they are using so as to avoid error from occurring.

Practice tips

- Read the infusion device instructions.
- Check the service date of the infusion device.
- Is the device in good working order, clean, battery charged?
- Be able to set up the infusion device with the correct administration set.
- Be familiar with the alarm system and be able to recognize pump failure.
- Know what you need to monitor during the infusion.
- Know where to document information and where to report adverse incidents.
- Keep equipment clean and plugged in when not in use.

Associated reading

🔗 http://www.mhra.gov.uk.

Perucca R. (2001). Types of infusion therapy equipment. In: Hankins J (ed.), *Infusion Therapy in Clinical Practice*, 2nd edn. WB Saunders, Philadelphia.

Assisting with venous cutdowns

Background

Cutdowns are used when venous access in a sick child is difficult due to poor circulation. With the increased use of intraosseous needles it is not a commonly performed procedure, but one you may be asked to assist with.

Equipment

- 1% lidoocaine for injection (used if the child is still responsive to pain).
- Size 15 scalpel blade.
- Curved haemostats.
- Fine pointed scissors.
- Strong ligatures ×2.
- IV cannula (gauge will depend on the size of the child).
- 10-mL syringe with 0.9% saline.
- Bionector® or other access device.
- Sterile dressing.
- Sterile gloves.
- Sterile field.
- Antiseptic agent according to local policies.
- Suture.
- Sharps bin.

Procedure

- Performing a venous cutdown is a high risk procedure. The decision to undertake it will be made by a senior medic. The procedure should be explained and consent obtained from the adult with parental responsibility if at all possible.
- Gather and prepare appropriate equipment.
- Monitor the child's vital signs throughout the procedure.
- Position chosen limb in a position as directed by the medic.

The doctor will:
- *Select the appropriate vein:* this will usually be the brachial or saphenous vein.
- Prepare the skin.
- Place sterile field in appropriate position.
- If child conscious locally anaesthetize the skin with 1% lidoocaine.
- Undertake procedure aiming to insert an intravenous catheter directly into a visible vein.

The nurse will:
- Wash hands and don personal protection equipment (PPE).
- Prime access device and syringe with 0.9% saline ready for attachment to cannula.
- Secure the limb chosen by the medic.
- Cover insertion site with a sterile transparent dressing.
- Observe site for any bleeding.
- Ensure the documentation is complete according to local policies.

Practice tips

- When immobilizing the limb, ensure you keep your hands well out of the way. You may want to help support the limb by rolling up a pillow case and placing under the limb selected.
- If the child is not conscious and the family is present, suggest they look away or leave the room if appropriate, if you feel it will add to their distress.
- If the child is conscious, distraction tactics maybe helpful.
- A splinted limb may make the site more secure so this could be considered.

Pitfalls

- Contraindicated in trauma to the limb.
- Difficult procedure to undertake that is not common practice.
- Sometimes performed in stressful situations so many medics not familiar with it.
- Invasive so increased risk of infection, haematoma, phlebitis, and nerve damage.
- Scarring common.

Associated reading

Chappell S, Vilke GM, Chan TC, et al. (2006). Peripheral venous cutdown. *J Emerg Med* **31**(4), 411–16.

Managing central venous catheters

Background

A central venous catheter (CVC, often referred to as a central line) is a silicone, polyurethane, PVC, or Teflon® tube whose distal tip ends in one of the major central veins, most often the superior vena cava. Insertion sites may vary.

There are two main purposes:

- To deliver drugs (especially irritant or vesicant drugs), fluids or parenteral nutrition (PN) directly into the fast-flowing central circulation.
- To enable regular blood sampling.

The decision to site a CVC is a multidisciplinary one. Accessing central lines is a skilled nursing procedure, and should only be undertaken by competent and confident practitioners.

The main goals of care are maintenance of patency, prevention of infection, and preservation of the catheter's integrity. Regardless of the type of CVC, these principles are the same.

Equipment

- 10-mL luer lock syringes (or larger).
- Needles.
- Sterile/non-sterile gloves (according to local protocol).
- 0.9% sodium chloride (saline) for flushing.
- Heparinized 0.9% NaCl (heparin) solution for final flush.
- Clean working surface (e.g. rigid, deep-sided plastic tray).
- 2% Chlorhexidine/ 70% isopropyl alcohol swabs for cleaning ports and hubs.

Procedure

- Ensure catheter is clamped before any procedure is commenced to minimize risk of introducing air into the circulation.
- Use strict ANTT according to local protocol. Effective hand washing and the use of appropriate gloves is crucial.
- Establish type, size, material, and location of line (see Table 9.3). Details should be in the child's notes; the size (French gauge (FG)) is often printed on the side of the line itself.
- Establish patency and correct placement of the catheter *before* continuing procedure. Aspirate ('bleed back') the line with an empty 10-mL syringe or one filled with 0.9% NaCl.

❶ A strong, brisk 'flashback' of blood should be *clearly visible* in the syringe on aspiration.

- *Continue with procedure:* withdrawal of blood (using a new syringe) for sampling or a fresh saline flush prior to the dose of drugs or fluids.
- Use a brisk push-pause technique when flushing to create turbulence in the line and clear any debris.
- Use an infusion pump for fluids and drug infusions. IV administration sets in continuous use (i.e. without disconnection) can safely be changed every 72h. Exceptions are the administration of blood (12h) or PN (24h) due to enhanced potential for microbial growth.

Table 9.3 Types of CVCs and indications for use

Length of dwell	Short- and medium-term (e.g. PICC lines)	Long-term (e.g. Hickman® lines, implanted ports)	
	Often temporary lines for use in hospital environment in acutely sick children	Enables treatment or blood sampling in children with long-term conditions, e.g. cancer, cystic fibrosis	Non-tunnelled
	Sometimes inserted in the clinical area under local anaesthetic or sedation. Often by nurses	Surgically-inserted in theatre under general anaesthetic	Skin is punctured and the line inserted directly into the blood vessel, either peripherally or centrally
Type of catheter	Tunnelled	Implanted port	
	Percutaneously inserted via skin incision and fed along a large vein until the tip reaches the SVC. The line is tunnelled under the skin from the entry site to the chest wall where it exits the skin	Also a surgically inserted, tunnelled line. Attached to an internal reservoir sited under the skin which is accessed via a special non-coring needle	
		Designed for intermittent use and for children with long-term conditions	
	Sutured in place, often has an integral cuff which anchors the line in the tunnel by encouraging tissue growth around it	Needle removed at the end of a course of treatment or when vascular access not needed	
Distal end	Open-ended	Valved	
	External clamp attached to the line to close it off to the air when accessed	No clamp needed due to a valve at the distal end which opens and closes when line is used	
Lumens	Single lumen	Double or multi-lumen	
	Most often used for TPN. Should not be routinely used for blood sampling	For regular blood sampling, simultaneous administration of incompatible drugs, fluids and blood, and sometimes pressure monitoring. Each lumen can be used independently	

- At the end of the procedure, always flush the line with 0.9% NaCl to clear the line of infusate and maintain patency. Heparinized 0.9% NaCl may also be required depending on type of line and local protocol, although evidence for its effectiveness in preventing occlusion is inconclusive.
- Re-dress and flush long-term lines *weekly* (usually 5mL 10IU/mL heparinized 0.9% NaCl) and implanted ports *monthly* (5mL 100IU/mL heparinized 0.9% NaCl). NB. Heparin flushes are not usually needed for lines with a valve at the distal end.

Troubleshooting

If good blood return is difficult to obtain:
- Check for external kinks and unseen clamps, and change the non-injectable bung before more advanced troubleshooting.
- Try aspirating with a syringe smaller than 10mL, due to the lower force required to withdraw fluid without creating a vacuum.
- Repositioning is often all that is needed to encourage blood return. Ask the child or young person to:
  - Raise his/her arms.
  - Roll onto one side.
  - Cough.
  - Sit up from a lying position or vice versa.
- Flush the catheter with 10–20mL 0.9% NaCl and try aspirating again. This is safe, providing the saline can be instilled without *any* signs of pain, discomfort, or swelling.
- If the line is an implanted port, try re-accessing with a new non-coring needle if tolerated.
- *Do not* proceed if no blood can be aspirated or blood return continues to be only minimal. Seek specialist advice.
- Maintain positive pressure on flushing when the syringe is removed or clamp applied in order to prevent backflow of blood.
- A smaller bore catheter is more likely to block than a larger one and may need flushing more frequently to maintain patency. Larger lumens of a multilumen line are best used for sampling and administering blood due to its higher viscosity than other fluids.

Practice tips

- Check if the child uses a name for their line—'wiggly', 'worm', etc.
- Loop the line into an S or C shape under an appropriate dressing to avoid it pulling. Younger children may need the ends of their lines tucked away in a small bag or pouch.
- Always discard first few millilitres of blood obtained (unless needed for blood cultures) before taking other samples. This is to avoid distorting blood results by contaminating or diluting the sample with fluids already in the line. Reassure parents that discarding this blood will not harm the child.
- Multilumen lines are intended to be used as such. Blood, and drugs or fluids can be infused simultaneously.
- Intermittent flushing with heparinized NaCl is used to prevent blockage. Heparin is *not* a thrombolytic agent and cannot therefore be used to treat occlusions.

- The more often a CVC is accessed or manipulated, the higher the risk of contamination. Be organized, group accesses together where possible (e.g. taking blood samples at the time when drug doses are due).
- Change injectable bungs and dressings weekly, using strict ANTT. Perform both procedures when the weekly heparin flush is due; this will help reduce both stress for the child and the risk of introducing infection.
- Always use a luer lock syringe that screws onto the bung.
- Use the time spent accessing the catheter to inspect the site—this should be done at least daily in hospital.
- Alternate lumens used for each access in multilumen CVCs so they are all flushed equally regularly. Note lumen used each time on the child's drug or fluid chart.
- Periodically, measure the length of catheter extending from the skin to check the line has not migrated. In a Hickman® line, look for protrusion of the cuff.
- Have a set of plastic clamps close at hand at all times in case of sudden damage to or disconnection of the line.

Pitfalls

- Take care with femoral lines due to the risk of contamination with faeces and urine.
- Children should be encouraged to shower, rather than bathe with a CVC *in situ* to minimize risk of infection. Swimming *must* be avoided.
- Some lines may not 'bleed back' well enough for regular blood sampling due to their small bore or not being designed for this purpose. Check manufacturer's instructions.
- ❶ *Never* use undue force when attempting to flush any CVC; this can rupture it. ❶ Remember: the smaller the syringe, the greater the pressure exerted inside the line. This is reversed when aspirating.
- Avoid three-way taps on CVCs due to increased risk of contamination.
- Any splits, perishing, leaks, or visible cuffs are suggestive of damage and increase risk of complications. ❶ *Never* use a damaged catheter—seek specialist advice immediately. CVCs can be repaired, but only by those trained and competent to do so.

Associated reading

Department of Health (2007). *High Impact Intervention No 1 Central venous catheter care bundle.* Available at: ℘ http://www.clean-safe-care.nhs.uk/index.php?pid=4.

Pratt RJ, Pellowe CM, Wilson JA, et al. (2007). National evidence-based guidelines for preventing healthcare-associated infections in NHS hospitals in England. *J Hosp Infect* **65**, S1–S64.

Royal College of Nursing (2005). *Standards for infusion therapy*, 2nd edn. RCN, London.

Parenteral nutrition

Background
A nutrient solution comprised of dextrose, amino acids fat, electrolytes, vitamins, micronutrients, and water. Administered intravenously when the intestine cannot be used, or cannot absorb or digest adequate amounts of nutrition. PN can be temporary or permanent. It can be given for 24h a day or overnight in long-term patients, as this gives them more freedom during the day. PN can be given in conjunction with other feeding methods or administered as total parenteral nutrition (TPN) when no food or feed is given by other routes.

For dextrose and amino acid concentrations of under10% a peripheral line maybe used, but a central line, such as a Hickman® or peripherally-inserted central catheter (PICC) line must be used for concentrations of 20–30% as extravasation may cause vein sclerosis or burns.

Storage
PN is prepared on daily basis and stored in a temperature-controlled fridge. Electrolytes are tailored to the patients need, but if being administered long-term in stable patients, their nutritional alterations will be minimal. The PN should be removed from fridge 30min before administering.

Complications
Sepsis
The dextrose and lipid content of PN makes it a potential harbour for microorganisms. The child will be vulnerable to infection so vital signs should be monitored. Temperature over 38°C should be reported, blood cultures taken, and local protocol followed.

Hyper-/hypoglycaemia
• Due to glucose content of the fluid.
• Abnormal liver function may result from long-term therapy.

Prerenal azotemia
If PN formula contains excessive amino acids, and insufficient glucose and lipids the body will turn to protein for energy-causing fluid retention.

Occlusion of line
Lipids are viscous in nature, and can cause gradual or sudden occlusion.

Equipment
• Infusion pump.
• Sterile drapes/dressing pack.
• Sterile gloves.
• Cleaning agent—as per local policy.

Procedure

- Explain procedure to patient/carer and gain consent.
- Wash and dry hands.
- Open dressing pack/drape and place all equipment on sterile area.
- 2 nurses should check PN solution as per local policy against the prescription. The infusion should also be checked for any signs of leakage, clarity, particles, turbidity, and expiry.
- Put on gloves, prime set, maintaining sepsis.
- Clean patient's line as per local policy.
- Attach administration set and attach to pump.
- Commence infusion.

Care during infusion

- Monitor fluid balance.
- Check vital signs 4-hourly, report any pyrexia above 38°C.
- Monitor blood glucose 4–6 hourly.
- Monitor weight, biochemistry.
- Patient may require mouth care, if nil by mouth.
- Check that line remains safely connected to child and that infusion is running as prescribed at least hourly.
- Ensure full documentation of procedure and type and amount of all PN and fluids administered.

Practice tips

- Never add anything to the infusion.
- Use a dedicated line wherever possible for the PN.
- Use strict aseptic technique.
- Protect infusion from sunlight.
- Discard any unused solution.
- If line is broken during infusion do not reconnect the PN.

Associated reading

Coyne I, Neill F, Timmins F. (eds) (2010). *Clinical Skills in Children's Nursing.* Oxford University Press, Oxford.

Kelsey J, McEwing G. (2008). *Clinical Skills in Child Health Practice.* Elsevier, Oxford.

Care of the perioperative patient

Pre-operative care

Background

Approximately 450,000 children aged between 0–16yrs undergo a surgical procedure in England every year and as such require both physical and psychological preparation.[1] This tends to be an anxiety provoking time for both child and parent; thus it is important that they are engaged in the preparation process and fully involved in their care pre and post operatively. This chapter considers the immediate pre-operative care required by a child and their family.

Equipment

- Identification band.
- Allergy band if appropriate.
- Stethoscope.
- Thermometer.
- Blood pressure (BP) monitor.
- Weighing scales.
- Operation gown or child's own pyjamas.
- Age appropriate preparation aids (see Chapter 6).
- Pre-operative checklist.
- Pre-operative medications if required.

Procedure

- On admission orientate the child and family to the environment.
- Use age appropriate communication skills and language.
- Consider the use of a play specialist to assist in preparing the child.
- Complete and sign all admission paperwork.
- Apply an identification band.
- Apply an allergy band if appropriate.
- Weigh the child as per policy and document on the prescription chart.
- Perform and document a full set of baseline observations reporting any concerns to the surgical team: temperature, pulse, respiratory rate (RR), oxygen saturations/BP.
- Ensure that the child is clerked and reviewed by appropriate medical personnel.
- Ensure that the child and family understand the procedure.
- Provide time for the child and family to ask questions.
- Ensure the issue of who bears parental responsibility is confirmed.
- Ensure that all necessary consent forms are signed, dated, have the correct procedure identified, and include an appropriate signature (see 📖 Seeking consent, p. 20).
- Ensure that the child has been reviewed by an appropriate anaesthetist and assessed for any potential complications prior to leaving the ward for theatre.
- Ensure that the child has adhered to appropriate fasting protocols (see 📖 Fasting times and principles, p. 248).
- Conduct all checks identified on the theatre checklist and document clearly (see 📖 Theatre checklist: how to prepare patients, p. 252).

- Ensure the child has a shower as close to the time of surgery as practical to minimize the risk of post-operative infection.[1]
- Encourage the child to empty their bladder prior to surgery. For young children ensure a new nappy is applied (see 📖 Practice tips, p. 247).
- Ensure that the child has changed into their own pyjamas or a hospital gown (dependent on local policy) in a timely fashion prior to surgery.
- Apply topical local anaesthetic cream to an appropriate site 60min before insertion of an IV cannula. (Refer to manufacturer's instructions as recommended timings may vary dependent on the product used.)
- Administer any prescribed pre-operative medication as per hospital policy at the correct time in order to achieve the desired effect. (Timings may need to be altered in consultation with the anaesthetist depending on the progression of the list.)
- If appropriate, check that the operation site has been correctly marked and that this is still visible.
- Ensure all patient notes are complete.
- Ensure all pertinent scans, X-rays, reports accompany the child to theatre.
- Once contacted by theatre ensure the child is safely transferred as per local policy.
- Dependent on hospital policy accompany the child/parent into the anaesthetic room, and provide appropriate distraction to assist the child and family cope with the anaesthetic process.
- Once the child is anaesthetized escort the parent from the anaesthetic room and provide appropriate support.

Practice tips

- Both parent and child may become anxious, distressed, or agitated if the progress of the list is slower than expected. Clear communication on progress can help to alleviate this.
- Encouraging a child to empty their bladder prior to surgery is beneficial, as they may receive substantial amounts of intravenous fluid in theatre. ❶ A full bladder is more prone to damage during abdominal surgery.[1]
- Play is a very effective way of preparing a child and their family for upcoming procedures.

Pitfalls

- Parental anxiety can be easily transferred to the child. Where appropriate, parents should be given the option of accompanying their child into the anaesthetic room. This should be a choice, rather than an expectation and appropriate support must be provided.
- Emergency admissions may not allow much time for preparation. In such cases it may be important to engage the child in post-procedural play (PPP); see 📖 Preparation and post-procedural play, p. 152.

Associated reading

[1] Glasper A, Aylott M, Battrick C. (eds). (2010). *Developing Practical Skills for Nursing Children and Young People.* Hodder Arnold (Publishers) Ltd, London.

Fasting times and principles

Background

General anaesthetic agents can reduce the body's normal reflexes that would usually stop regurgitated gastric fluid reaching the lungs.

❶ Inhalation of gastric juices can be fatal. Fasting prior to general anaesthesia (GA) aims to reduce both the acidity and volume of stomach contents so reducing the risk of regurgitation and subsequent aspiration. Fasting policy varies from Trust to Trust. Prolonged periods of fasting may not only lead to dehydration and hypoglycaemia, but can also be distressing for the child and their family. Current research has identified that there is no need for an excessive fasting period in paediatric patients prior to surgery.[1]

Procedure

The following advice is based on current Royal College of Nursing (RCN) guidelines:

Pre-operatively for healthy children undergoing elective surgery

- The '2–4–6 rule' may be applied:
  - 2 = Water or clear fluids may be given up to 2h prior to induction.
  - 4 = Breast milk may be given up to 4h prior to induction.
  - 6 = Solids/cow's milk/formula milk may be given up to 6h prior to induction.
- Chewing gum should not be allowed on the day of surgery as studies have shown that chewing gum can lead to an ↑ in gastric fluid volume.
- Sweets are classified as solid foods so should not be consumed within 6h prior to induction (this includes boiled sweets and lollipops).
- Regular oral medication can be continued pre-operatively unless contraindicated or advised otherwise by the relevant medical team.
- 0.5mL/kg (up to 30mL) of water may be given orally to help children take their medication.[2]

Pre-operatively for high risk children undergoing elective surgery

- Some children are considered more likely to regurgitate under anaesthetic, these include:
  - Obese children.
  - Diabetic children.
  - Children with stomach disorders, e.g. oesophageal reflux.
- Higher risk children may follow the same regime as healthy children unless contraindicated.[2]
- Guidance should be sought from the anaesthetic team as to whether fasting times should be increased for individual high risk children.

Emergency surgery

- Children admitted in an emergency situation should be treated as having a full stomach unless it is possible to ascertain a reliable estimate of the last time they ate or drank.
- If possible the child should follow the normal fasting protocol.[2]
- Medical, surgical, and anaesthetic review will be required, and a decision taken on the urgency of the treatment required.

Post-operative guidance in healthy children

- Once the patient is alert and fully orientated, and providing there are no complications or contraindications oral fluids can be offered.
- It is advisable to start with clear fluids or breast milk.
- The child should be observed for any signs of post-operative nausea or vomiting. If evident appropriate action should be taken (see 📖 Managing nausea and vomiting, p. 408).
- Once oral fluids are being tolerated the child may commence solid foods.
- ❶ Advice must be sought regarding a post-operative regime for children who have existing gastrointestinal (GI) conditions; or who have undergone abdominal or GI surgery.

Practice tips

- Many children take medicine in liquid, rather than tablet form. If regular medication is required close to induction and constitutes a fluid volume of ↑ 30mL seek advice from the anaesthetic team.
- If an elective operation is delayed a decision should be sought from the anaesthetic team as to whether to give the child a drink of clear fluid.
- Clear fluids can be defined as 'those through which newsprint can be read'.[2]

Pitfalls

- Carbonated drinks are not usually accepted as constituting clear fluids; however, more research is required into this area.
- Care must be taken to ensure that the child and the family fully understand the fasting instructions and adhere strictly to them as otherwise surgery may be delayed or cancelled.
- It can be useful to remind the child and family of the '2–4–6' timings as they get close, subsequently reinforcing what must no longer be eaten or drunk once the time period has elapsed.
- It may be necessary to remove all drinks and food from the child's bedside, and parents should be encouraged to eat and drink away from their children so as not to cause further distress.

[1] Brady M, Kinn SO, Rourke K, et al. (2008). *Preoperative fasting for preventing preoperative complications in children*. Available at: ℘ http://www.thecochranelibrary.com (Accessed 29 September 2010).

[2] Royal College of Nursing. (2005). *Perioperative Fasting in Adults and Children: An RCN Guideline for the Multidisciplinary Team*. Available at ℘ http://www.rcn.org.uk (Accessed 29 September 2010).

Sedation

Background

When admitted to hospital, a child may be required to undergo tests and procedures that can be both painful and unpleasant. This can induce high levels of stress and anxiety for both the child and family. Procedural sedation is the practice of administering sedative drugs to a child or young person in order to help them cope with these procedures. The main aims of sedation are: to relieve stress and anxiety, assist in pain relief, keep the child still to allow the procedure to be managed safely, induce appropriate sleep.

NB. This section relates only to light sedation (conscious sedation where the child is able to respond purposefully to verbal commands either alone or in response to light tactile stimulation. ❶ Reflex withdrawal from a painful stimulus is not a purposeful response). Deep sedation and anaesthesia should only be undertaken in conjunction with an appropriately trained anaesthetist.

Equipment

- Working oxygen and suction.
- Appropriately sized oxygen mask and suction catheters.
- Rebreath bag and mask (all sizes).
- Airways (all sizes).
- IO needles (16G, 18G).
- Completed prescription chart.
- Sedation drugs.
- Reversal drugs.
- O_2 saturation monitor and probe.
- Sedation checklist (local policy).
- Observation chart.
- Written signed consent.

Procedure

- Appropriately trained medical personnel should establish the child's suitability for sedation by assessing:
  - The child's current medical condition.
  - Past medical problems (including previous problems associated with sedation or anaesthesia).
  - Any known allergies.
  - Current medication to identify potential drug interactions.
  - Airway status.
  - Weight.
  - Developmental or psychological status.[1]
  - ❶ Further specialist advice should be sought if there is concern relating to potential airway or breathing problems.
- Explain the procedure to the child and family in age appropriate terms and gain valid consent.
- Recheck the child's allergy status.
- Check all equipment is in working order and easily accessible including full resuscitation equipment.

- Perform and record a full set of baseline observations (see 📖 Vital signs/examination, p. 6).
- Obtain accurate weight in kg to ensure the correct dose of sedation.
- Complete pre-sedation checklist (refer to local policy).
- Ensure appropriate fasting times have been adhered to. (See 📖 Fasting times and principles, p. 248).
- If able ensure that the child goes to the toilet pre-sedation to ensure that the child does not need to urinate during the procedure.
- Administer sedation as prescribed. Follow local policy and best practice in relation to administration of medicines (see Chapter 8).
- Once sedation has been administered keep the child calm and encourage them to relax and go to sleep.
- Attach a saturation monitor and set alarm limits as recommended by the medical team (to continuously monitor saturation levels and help detect any respiratory depression).
- In addition, if the child is <1yr attach an apnoea monitor.
- Monitor the child continuously for changes in: RR, oxygen saturations, heart rate, depth of sedation, coping, pain, distress, nausea, or vomiting, and take appropriate action if required.
- Document pulse, RR, and oxygen saturations at least every 10min throughout the procedure.
- Post-procedure continue observations until the following have returned to normal:
  - Vital signs.
  - Responsiveness and orientation level.
  - Pain and nausea have been adequately controlled.
  - There is no risk of further ↓ in consciousness.
- Document the effectiveness of the sedation.

Practice tips

- If an apnoea alarm is *in situ* this needs to be removed during an MRI Scan as the monitor is not compatible with the scan machine.[1]
- ❶ Drugs used for sedation are potent and can lead to airway obstruction, apnoea, and hypotension; thus the nurse administering sedation must observe closely for signs and be skilled in managing airway obstruction.

Pitfalls

- When administering the sedation if a child vomits or does not take the full dose, discuss with the appropriate medical team to ascertain whether further sedation is required.
- ❶ Sedation is generally contraindicated in children with existing airway problems, raised intracranial pressure, difficult behavioural problems.

Associated reading

[1] NICE. (2010). *Sedation in Children and Young People: Full Guideline* (Draft) May 2010. Available at: 🕾 http://www.nice.org.uk/nicemedia/live/11967/48518/48518.pdf (accessed 27 September 2010).

Theatre checklist: how to prepare patients

Background

On the day of surgery it is important that the nurse reinforces all of the physical and emotional preparation previously received by the child and family whilst also ensuring and maximizing the child's safety in preparation for their pending surgery. Pre-operative theatre checklists are one method of facilitating this.

Equipment

Relevant theatre checklist.

Procedure

The content identified on theatre checklists may vary from Trust to Trust. The following provides a guide only—please refer to the appropriate policy for your relevant Trust.

- A pre-operative theatre checklist should be completed directly prior to the child going to theatre to ensure it is as up to date as possible.[1]
- The nurse should work through the list and perform all required checks clearly recording them on the pre-operative documentation.

Common checks include ensuring that:
- An identification band is *in situ*—ensure it is:
  - Clear.
  - Legible.
  - Contains the patient's correct name, date of birth, hospital number.
  - Corresponds to all documentation.
- Baseline observations are documented and are within normal acceptable limits.
- The child's weight has been recorded in kg on the prescription chart and pre-operative checklist. (Weights should be checked by two health professionals, and initialed by both).
- Any allergies have been clearly identified on both the pre-operative check list, and the prescription chart and an appropriate allergy band is *in situ*.
- A moving and handling assessment has been completed and enclosed.
- A pressure sore risk assessment has been undertaken and clearly documented, including any required action plan to reduce risk.
- The consent form has been completed and all sections appropriately signed.
- All prescribed pre-operative medication has been given in accordance with local policy.
- Fasting protocol has been adhered to (see 📖 Fasting times and principles, p. 248).
- If appropriate the time that topical local anaesthetic cream was applied has been recorded.
- All case notes, drug cards, X-rays, and scans are available, and ready to be sent to theatre with the patient.

- Any loose, capped, or crowned teeth have been clearly identified and any unfixed braces, dentures, and plates have been removed to reduce the risk of accidental ingestion, inhalation, or damage.
- Any external prosthesis has been removed—this includes items like hearing aids, spectacles, contact lenses (see 📖 Practice tips, p. 253).
- All jewellery, hairpins, etc., have been removed or covered appropriately (see 📖 Pitfalls, p. 253).
- All makeup and nail varnish has been removed to ensure that the anaesthetist is able to examine for signs of hypoxia.
- The patient/parent/carer has signed to verify that the correct site has been marked. Ensure this corresponds with the notes.

The following should also be documented on the pre-operative checklist:
- Any areas of broken skin/rashes/sores.
- Any known infection that the patient may be suffering from in particular any infections such as methicillin resistant *Staphylococcus aureus* (MRSA; follow local policy).
- Any medications that have been given prior to surgery other than prescribed premeds, e.g. analgesia, inhalers, should be clearly identified.

Practice tips
- Hearing aids, spectacles, contact lenses may be removed in the anaesthetic room in order to ensure appropriate communication is possible up until the last moment.[1]
- For older children and young people remember to check for any body piercings.
- Some children and young people like to take a familiar object down to theatre with them, e.g. a favourite toy. All personal items should be clearly labelled and identified on the pre-operative documentation.

Pitfalls
- It is important to either remove or cover jewellery as metal and other materials can be a risk factor for burns from cautery equipment used during surgery. In addition they can contribute to pressure sore development during prolonged surgery.[1]

[1] Glasper A, Aylott M, Battrick C. (eds). (2010). *Developing Practical Skills for Nursing Children and Young People.* Hodder Arnold(Publishers) Ltd, London.

Recovery from anaesthesia: immediate care

Background

During recovery from anaesthesia the patient is at risk of adverse events related to the airway, breathing and circulation. Staff must be competent to provide safe, effective care and there must be at least two appropriately trained staff present until the child/young person meets the discharge criteria. Care should be delivered on a one to one basis until the patient is safe for discharge to the ward.

Equipment

- Piped oxygen.
- A selection of oxygen masks.
- Wall mounted suction.
- Monitoring appropriate to age, clinical need, and surgical procedure.
- Selection of oropharyngeal airways.
- Anaesthetic breathing system appropriate to weight of child.
- Thermometer.
- Vomit bowls.
- Full paediatric resuscitation equipment.

Procedure

On arrival to the recovery room

- Ensure the recovery environment is stocked and safe.
- A comprehensive handover should be given by the anaesthetist and scrub staff, including any post-operative instructions.

Initial assessment

Recovery from anaesthesia algorithm (see Fig. 10.1).

Perform a rapid assessment of:

- ABCDE (please refer 📖 Vital signs/examination, p. 6).
- Attach monitoring.
- Provide supplemental oxygen as prescribed.

Airway

- Is the airway clear? Use gentle suction if necessary.
- Is the patient maintaining their own airway?
  - A head tilt, chin lift, or jaw thrust manoeuvre must be performed immediately if the patient is not maintaining their own airway.
  - Place the patient onto their side or elevate the bed head up to relieve partial obstruction.
  - Any patient with an airway adjunct *in situ* must always receive supplemental oxygen.
- Continuous monitoring and reassessment is crucial until the patient is fully able to maintain their own airway.

Breathing
- Oxygenation will only be achieved once the airway is patent.
- A 'look, listen, and feel' assessment must be undertaken.
- If there are no breaths or ineffective respiration, intervention must be taken in accordance with the algorithm in Figure 10.1.
- The recovery practitioner must be aware of the management of common airway difficulties in particular:
  - Laryngospasm.
  - Bronchospasm.
  - Residual neuromuscular blockade.
  - Malignant hyperthermia.
  - Chest pain.
  - Tension pneumothorax.

Circulation and vital sign monitoring
- Visual observation must be used in conjunction with monitoring. The frequency will depend on the stage of recovery, surgery, and clinical condition of the patient. However, the following must be assessed and documented every 5min until the patient is fully awake:
  - Heart rate, rhythm, and pulse amplitude.
  - Oxygen saturation levels and administration.
  - Level of consciousness.
  - Skin colour, perfusion, and capillary refill time.
  - Respiration rate, pattern, and effort.
  - Pain intensity at rest and on movement.
- The following must also be recorded:
  - Temperature.
  - BP.
  - Urine output.
- When appropriate the following may also be required:
  - Central venous pressure (CVP).
  - Arterial BP.
  - End tidal carbon dioxide levels.

Practice tips
- ❶ An unconscious patient must never be left unattended.
- The anaesthetist should not return to theatre until satisfied that the patient is in a stable condition.
- Care must always be delivered in a systematic ABCDE approach.

Pitfalls
- ❶ Remember that chest movement does not mean a clear airway.
- A patient with a laryngeal mask airway should be left completely undisturbed until the patient is able to open their mouth on command.
- Oropharyngeal airways must be removed once the patient begins to regain consciousness to prevent coughing, vomiting, or laryngospasm.
- Do not make a child or young person assume a position that they do not want to. It will increase anxiety, the effort of breathing, and oxygen consumption.

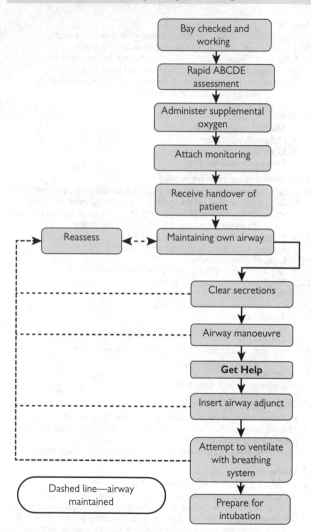

Fig. 10.1 Recovery from anaesthesia algorithm.

Associated reading

Association for Perioperative Practice. (2007). *Standards and Recommendations for Safe Perioperative Practice*. AFPP. Harrogate.

Collecting patients following surgery

Background

A thorough and comprehensive handover between theatre recovery staff and ward staff prior to transfer of the post-operative child is essential. This will ensure adequate risk assessment and aid the selection of appropriate transfer equipment and personnel to enable safe transfer back to the ward.

Equipment

Equipment required may vary depending on the condition of the patient, their surgery, and underlying medical conditions.

Essential equipment is:
- Oxygen cylinder, a well-fitting mask, and tubing.
- Portable suction equipment.
- Vomit bowl.
- Tissues.
- Pocket mask.

Additional items which may be required:
- Portable monitoring equipment.
- Selection of airway adjuncts.
- Bag-valve-mask.

Procedure

The parents or carers of the child should have been called to the recovery area prior to discharge. However, if this has not been possible, ensure parental presence when collecting a child post-operatively.

Handover of care

A comprehensive handover of clinical details and care must be given to the receiving ward nurse, this must include:
- The surgical procedure undertaken.
- Intraoperative complications (if any).
- Drains, dressings, and sutures *in situ*.
- Fluid balance, noting blood loss, drainage, intravenous fluids, or any oral intake.
- Anaesthetic drugs given.
- Details of any untoward incidents in recovery/action taken.
- Details of intravenous or intra-arterial access.
- Any drugs given, e.g. analgesia, antibiotics, and anti-emetics.
- Any post-operative instructions including analgesia plan, wound care, and discharge date (if recorded).

Joint assessment

The following must be checked jointly at handover, allowing any discrepancies or concerns to be addressed prior to discharge from the recovery area:
- A full set of vital signs as documented.
- Sedation score must be acceptable. The child must be responsive to voice, and have displayed signs of normal behaviour.
- Wound site must be assessed—any unexpected bleeding, swelling, or altered neurovascular observations must have received a surgical review and have an action plan documented.

- Surgical drains must be connected and working, drainage must be within expected limits, and documented.
- Intravenous (IV) fluids or drug infusions must match the prescription, the rates, and doses must be correct for the child's weight.
- Pain assessment.
- Epidural block level (when appropriate).
- Care needs arising from any regional anaesthetic blocks.
- Neurological observations (when appropriate).

Documentation

The receiving ward nurse must ensure that all documentation is present and completed including:

- Operation notes.
- Anaesthetic record.
- Analgesia prescription chart if appropriate.
- Drug chart.
- Fluid prescription.
- Post-operative instructions.

Transfer

- The patient must be transferred by an appropriately trained, competent registered practitioner.
- Prior to transfer it is important to ensure that the patient is comfortable and that their dignity is maintained.
- Temperature should be checked at the point of discharge and steps taken to conserve warmth.

Practice tips

- Where the patient is unstable or requires transfer to an intensive care area, an anaesthetist should be present for the transfer and medical handover.
- Transfer risk assessments may be used to guide choice of equipment and personnel required for transfer.
- When assessing sedation score a familiar voice should be used; children may ignore a stranger's voice, but will be more likely to respond to a parent or carer.
- Parents and carers are integral in assessing normal behaviour and must be utilized in the assessment.

Pitfalls

- Remember to take a vomit bowl on transfer even if the patient denies nausea. The motion of the bed or elevator may trigger nausea.

Associated reading

Glasper A, Aylott M, Battrick C. (eds) (2010). *Developing Practical skills for Nursing Children and Young People.* Hodder Arnold (Publishers) Ltd, London.

Post-operative care

Background
A swift and comprehensive assessment of the post-operative patient will ensure a smooth and timely discharge to home, and minimize potential complications.

Equipment
Prior to collecting the child from theatre, ensure that the child's bed space has working:
- Piped oxygen.
- Wall mounted suction.

Ensure that monitoring equipment appropriate to assess the child's medical condition following the surgical procedure is available including:
- Saturation monitoring.
- Apnoea monitoring.
- BP monitoring.
- Stethoscope.
- Pen torch.

Procedure
- Prior to collecting the child from theatre, ensure that the bed space is clear from obstructions and personal items, and that all equipment is in clean, working condition.
- The care area should be calm, quiet, and allow for continuous observation of the patient as appropriate.
- Following handover of the patient complete an immediate assessment of airway/breathing/circulation (ABC).

Assess and document vital signs including:
- Heart rate and pulse amplitude.
- Respiratory rate, depth, and rhythm.
- Oxygen saturation levels and fraction of inspired oxygen (FiO_2).
- Sedation score (AVPU).
- The frequency of observations will vary depending on the clinical need of the patient and the surgical procedure.
- Complete an extensive pain assessment, at rest, and on movement (when awake) utilizing a pain assessment tool appropriate to the child's age and level of development. Parents must be involved in the pain assessment process in order to allow accurate assessment:
  - A referral to the pain service may be required if there are likely to be ongoing pain problems.
  - Regular multimodal analgesia should be administered in accordance with prescribed regime and pain guidelines.
  - The child should be positioned in such a way as to maximize comfort and post-operative safety.

Additionally the following must be assessed and documented.
- *Wound site specific to surgery:* observe for bleeding, or swelling at, or around the wound site, excessive swallowing following oral surgery, abnormal neurovascular observations in limbs, or digits distal to the surgical site, abdominal distention, epidural insertion site.

- *Dressings:* if any wound fluid leaks out onto a dressing (strike through) the dressing should either be changed or have a further dressing placed over the top as once 'strike through' is evident the dressing no longer provides an effective barrier to the entry of pathogens.
- *Drainage:* drains to be secured and working (suction to be applied if required). The amount of fluid in the drain should be observed and recorded as per post-operative instructions.
- All observations of wounds, dressings, and drains must be specific and measurable to allow early identification of deterioration and complications to be treated. Surgical review must be sought with any concerns.
- *Fluid balance:* including blood loss.
- *Urine output:* to monitor renal function as part of the circulatory assessment; it is also important to chart when a patient is able to pass urine post-surgery.
- *Nausea and vomiting:* utilize pharmacological and non-pharmacological methods of anti-emesis.
- Skin integrity and pressure areas.
- Neurological observations (where appropriate).
- The frequency of ongoing observations will be determined by the clinical condition of the patient/specific surgical or anaesthetic requirements, but would normally be taken at 5–15min intervals initially.
- Encourage oral fluids and light diet promptly, and as tolerated unless contraindicated. Any specific surgical instructions must be followed where appropriate and tolerated.

Practice tips

- Prior to accepting a patient post-operatively, ensure that the discharge and transfer criteria are met (refer to 📖 Recovery from anaesthesia: immediate care, p. 254 and 📖 Collecting patients following surgery, p. 258).
- Maintain open and honest communication with the child/young person, and their family. It may be useful to utilize the play team in education and post-operative advice.
- A range of non-pharmacological methods of pain management should also be considered.

Pitfalls

- Do not forget to ensure appropriate measures are in place for those at risk of developing pressure sores or the breakdown of skin integrity.
- Embarrassment or lack of understanding often discourages staff from using non-pharmacological methods of pain management, e.g. guided imagery, resulting in under-utilization.
- Do not assume that oral fluids will be detrimental in the nauseated patient. Often a dry mouth and hunger are triggers and easily rectified with a sip of water or an ice pop.

Associated reading

Glasper A, Aylott M, Battrick C. (eds) (2010). *Developing Practical Skills for Nursing Children and Young People.* Hodder Arnold (Publishers) Ltd., London.

Emergency and high dependency care

Airway obstruction

Background
Airway obstruction can be described as partial or complete. The onset may be progressive in a sick child or sudden in a well child, depending on its cause. In either case, respiratory distress will often be noted, which may quickly progress to a loss of consciousness and a life-threatening event. Early recognition is therefore vital.

The obstruction may occur at any level of:
- Pharyngeal airway.
- Tracheal airway.
- Laryngeal airway.

❶ *Children* may be more susceptible to airway obstruction due to their anatomical differences:
- Young children have a large head and a short neck.
- The face and mandible are small, and the tongue is comparatively large.
- Teeth may be loose.
- The base of the mouth is easily compressible.
- Infants <6 months are obligate nasal breathers.
- 3–8-yr-olds often have adenotonsillar hypertrophy.

Causes
- Viral or bacterial infections.
- Croup.
- Epiglottitis.
- *Abscess:* peritonsillar or retropharyngeal.
- Foreign body.
- *Burns:* chemical or thermal.
- *Allergic reaction:* e.g. nuts, antibiotics, drug therapy, bee stings.
- Trauma.

Observe for:
- *Infection:* coryza, cough, temperature, wheeze, stridor, cyanosis, respiratory distress, difficulty in swallowing, drooling, pain, and facial swelling.
- *Allergic/burns:* hives, itching, swelling, nausea, vomiting, rash, blisters, burns.
- *Foreign body:* sudden onset difficulty in breathing, persistent cough, grasping of throat.
- *Trauma:* obvious penetrating injury, tracheal deviation, bruising, or swelling.

Procedure
- Nurse 'high risk' children where they can be easily observed, with working oxygen, suction, and resuscitation equipment to hand.
- ❶ Do not examine a child with a partially occluded airway unless an appropriate medical/anaesthetic team is available.
- Keep the child comfortable and quiet.
- Oxygen and medications/interventions should be withheld until a medical and anaesthetic team is fully assembled if you feel the child will not tolerate them.

❶ A partially occluded airway may quickly become fully obstructed with poor management!

Practice tips

- Simple techniques, such as head tilt–chin lift can maintain an open airway in an unconscious child, with added adjuncts, such as oropharyngeal/nasopharyngeal airways if required.
- If such adjuncts are used, reassessment of the airway following insertion should be undertaken.
- The use of any adjunct does not guarantee a patent airway.

Associated reading

Cleaver K and Webb J. (eds). (2007). *Emergency care of children and young people*. Blackwell Publishing: Oxford.

Barry P, Morris K, and Ali T. (eds). (2010). *Paediatric intensive care*. Oxford University Press: Oxford.

Airway opening manoeuvres

Background

Airway obstruction can be one of the primary causes of respiratory arrest in children. In some cases, a prompt, simple manual airway opening manoeuvre can correct the obstruction and prevent respiratory arrest.

Children have a number of anatomical differences that will affect positioning required in airway opening manoeuvres:

- In younger children a large head combined with a short neck, means that excessive neck flexion will narrow the airway.
- A short and soft trachea means over-extension, as well as flexion of the neck will cause tracheal compression.
- The floor of the mouth is easily compressible, requiring careful positioning of fingers when holding the jaw for airway positioning.

As a child's airway anatomy changes with age, different age groups will require specific airway opening manoeuvres. For the purpose of this chapter, we will use three different age groups.

- Neonates/Infants (birth to 1yr).
- Children (between 1yr and puberty).
- Adult (puberty and older).

The basic manoeuvres that will assist and maintain an airway are;

- Head tilt/chin lift.
- Jaw thrust.

The ideal position for the rescuer when managing an airway is at the patient's head, ensuring you are comfortable (think about back position and reducing bending) and are free of danger/obstruction.

If there is any obvious debris visible in the mouth that can be safely removed then remove them.

▶ A blind finger sweep is contraindicated in children as it can damage the soft palate and push a foreign body further into the airway.

Neonates/infants (birth to 1yr)

Head tilt/chin lift

In an infant the desirable position for airway opening is described as neutral. As the infant has a large occiput they naturally adopt a sniffing position, therefore further extending the neck may obstruct the airway.

The rescuer places one hand on the forehead holding it in a neutral position, the fingers of the other hand should then be placed on the hard part of the chin, and the chin should be lifted upward (see Fig. 11.1).

Care must be taken not to grip too hard as this may damage the soft tissue.

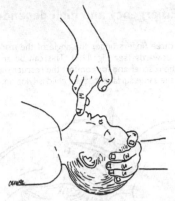

Fig. 11.1 Chin lift in infants. Reproduced with kind permission of Wiley-Blackwell Publishing from Advanced Life Support group (2005). *Advanced Paediatric Life Support. The Practical Approach.* 4th edition. BMJ Books, London.

Children (1yr to puberty)

As a child's head is now smaller in proportion, when using a chin lift manoeuvre the rescuer should use the sniffing position, with the head slightly tilted (see Fig. 11.2). As with infants careful positioning of the fingers is required to avoid damage to the soft tissue.

> ► If there is a suspected trauma, always consider the possibility of a cervical injury. If a cervical injury is suspected then a head tilt–chin lift manoeuvre could worsen a c-spine injury. Therefore, the safest airway opening manoeuvre in this situation is the jaw thrust.

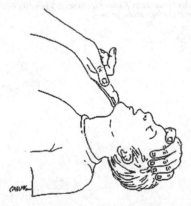

Fig. 11.2 Sniffing position; airway opening manoeuvre in children. Reproduced with kind permission of Wiley-Blackwell Publishing from Advanced Life Support group (2005). *Advanced Paediatric Life Support. The Practical Approach.* 4th edition. BMJ Books, London.

Place two or three fingers under the angle of the mandible bilaterally and lift the jaw upwards (see Fig. 11.3). This can be an uncomfortable manoeuvre for the rescuer and for comfort the rescuer should ideally rest their elbows on the same surface that the child is lying on.

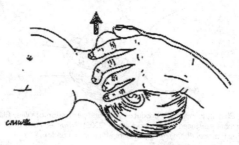

Fig. 11.3 Jaw thrust manoeuvre. Reproduced with kind permission of Wiley-Blackwell Publishing from Advanced Life Support group (2005). *Advanced Paediatric Life Support. The Practical Approach.* 4th edition. BMJ Books, London.

▶▶ There are rare occasions in trauma where a jaw thrust may be difficult to maintain the airway. If there is more than one rescuer, the second rescuer should apply c-spine immobilization.

If jaw thrust is not sufficient to maintain the airway, and there is only one rescuer, the airway should always take priority and the rescuer should consider a gradual head tilt.

Associated reading

Advanced Life Support Group (2005). *Advanced Paediatric Life Support: The Practical Approach*, 4th edn, Blackwell Publishing, London, pp. 24–5.

Performing suctioning

Background

Performed to remove excessive or retained secretions from the respiratory tract, or obtain specimens for laboratory examination, following a respiratory assessment. It may be performed as a single procedure by experienced and competent nursing and medical staff (or by suitably trained parents/carers), or may be incorporated into a chest physiotherapy regime. The frequency of suctioning is determined by the child's clinical condition; however, the principles are the same for suction via the pharynx or via an artificial airway, e.g. tracheal tube or tracheostomy.

Equipment

- Suction unit (piped vacuum system or a portable unit) and tubing.
- Suction catheters of appropriate size and type:
  - Rounded tip.
  - 2 or 3 (but no more than 3) lateral holes that should be smaller than the distal hole.
  - Integrated vacuum control.
  - Catheters should not exceed 50% of the airway's internal diameter (other than when a Yankauer sucker may be used to clear thicker matter from the mouth).
  - If suctioning via a tracheostomy or endotracheal tube (ETT), the suction catheter can be measured by doubling the size of the internal diameter, e.g. 3.0mm diameter, use a 6 French gauge (FG) suction catheter.
- Approximate guide to catheter selection for a natural airway are:
  - Infant 5–6 FG.
  - Child <5yrs 6–8 FG.
  - Child >5yrs 8–10 FG.
  - Each child should be individually assessed.
- Irrigant (if deemed appropriate/necessary).
- Non-sterile gloves.
- Apron.
- Bowl of clean tap water.
- Tissues.
- Disposal bag.
- Labelled specimen container (if required).
- Blanket (for holding child if necessary).
- Oxygen.

Preparation of child and family

- Explanations to both child/young person and family should be given appropriate to age and condition.
- Explanations should include:
  - Reason for suction and what it will entail.
  - Potential risks.
  - Duration.
  - Expected outcome.

- Child and family should be told that appropriate holding may be necessary.
- Individual requirements of child should be addressed, e.g. nebulized medication, pre-oxygenation:
  - Pre-oxygenation may be deemed necessary for some children.
  - Adequate hydration of the child should be ensured and/or humidification of inspired gases.
  - Hyperinflation may be required for some ventilated children. This must only be performed in consultation with medical staff and by a suitably experienced nurse or physiotherapist.

Procedure

- Check all equipment to ensure fully operational.
- The negative pressure of the unit must be checked and altered if necessary prior to attaching the catheter.
- Recommended pressures (subject to individually assessed needs) are:
  - Infant 6–9kPa (60–80mmHg).
  - Child 9–11kPa (80–100mmHg).
  - Older child 11–15kPa (max. 120mmHg).
- Ensure resuscitation equipment is readily available.
- Place child on their side (if possible):
  - Two people may be required, one to perform the procedure and the other to hold the child.
  - If not appropriate to place on side, the child/young person can be placed with their face up, and neck slightly extended.
- Perform clinical handwash.
- Pre-oxgenate child if required.
- Put gloves on. The catheter should only have contact with the child's airway and the practitioner's glove.
- Remove suction catheter from packaging and attach to suction tubing.
- Turn on suction at appropriate pressure.
- Ensuring that no negative pressure is being applied (i.e. maintaining integral vacuum control) introduce catheter gently into airway:
  - For natural nasal airway suction, the distance from the level of central incisors to the angle of the lower jaw is determined—the catheter should be inserted just beyond this point.
  - For artificial airway suction, the length of the airway should be measured and recorded, and the catheter inserted just beyond this point.
  - Medical staff may instruct a different insertion distance, e.g. post-tracheal surgery.
  - If suctioning with a Yankauer, then it should be inserted via a convex angle along the roof of the pharynx, with no 'blind' suctioning.
- Apply negative pressure as individually assessed by occluding the port.
- Withdraw catheter from airway, avoiding any rotation.
- The maximum duration of each suction attempt should be determined by child's response, but should be no more than 10s.
- Removal of viscous secretions may be aided by use of an irrigant—but these should not be used routinely—only on medical advice. Sodium chloride may be instilled, or saline nebulizers administered.

- Monitor child continuously throughout procedure:
  - Respiratory rate and quality.
  - Colour.
  - Heart rate.
  - Oxygen saturation of arterial blood (SaO_2).
  - Quantity, colour, and viscosity of secretions.
- Take immediate appropriate action if condition deteriorates.
- Catheters are designed for single use only; catheter and glove should be changed on each pass, unless in an emergency.
- No more than 3 suction passes are recommended. Always allow recovery of the child between each pass. Seek medical advice if suctioning is not effective after 3 attempts.
- If the child is receiving oxygen therapy, recommence oxygen delivery as soon as procedure is completed.
- Clean child's nose/mouth as required and ensure that they are comfortable.
- Give reassurance and information as appropriate to both young person/child and family.
- Suction tubing and flow controls should be flushed with clean water.
- Discard personal protection equipment (PPE) according to local policy.
- Perform clinical handwash.
- Record procedure in health record, including details of aspirate obtained and any clinical reactions. Inform medical and nursing personnel as appropriate.
- Suction tubing and jars should be regularly emptied and washed or changed as per local policy.

Practice tips

- Catheters should not be kinked prior to insertion as a method of vacuum control.
- When removing glove, wrap the used catheter around the gloved hand, pull glove back over soiled catheter and discard safely.
- When a child requires regular suctioning, keep spare gloves and an ample supply of the correct-sized suction catheters at the bedside.

Pitfalls

- Airway suctioning can lead to tracheobronchial trauma, hypoxia, pneumothorax, cardiovascular changes, intracranial pressure alterations, bacterial infection, and other complications.
- ❶ There may be specific complications when there is a head injury.
- Use of irrigants should only be considered on the advice of medical staff—not all the solution is recovered on suctioning, there is a risk of inhalation and it is frightening and uncomfortable for the child.
- Yankauers should not be used for nasal suctioning.
- Physiotherapists may utilize airways, and deep suctioning techniques; these should not be used unless the person is appropriately trained and understands the further risks.

Associated reading

Moore T. (2003). Suctioning techniques for the removal of respiratory secretions. *Nurs Stand* **18**(9), 47–53.

Insertion of oropharyngeal airway

Background
The oropharyngeal airway (OPA), oral airway, or Guedal airway is an airway adjunct, which is used to maintain a patent airway. Its presence in the airway should prevent the tongue from falling back over the epiglottis in the unconscious child.

The OPA should only be used for an unconscious individual as its presence in the airway of a semi-conscious or conscious person is likely to stimulate the gag reflex and may lead to airway obstruction.

Equipment
• Correct-sized OPA, chosen by measuring from mouth corner to ear tip. This should be the approximate length of airway selected.
• Tongue depressor.
• Lubricating gel.

Procedure
• Wash hands.
• Consider lightly lubricating airway.
• *Insert airway:*
  • In infant and child up to 8yrs, depress tongue and insert airway with tip pointing down into throat.
  • In child above 8yrs and adult, insert airway with tip pointing upwards and then when contact is made with the back of the throat turn the airway by 180°, so that it is pointing down into the throat.
• Observe child closely while airway *in situ*. If conscious state is achieved then gag reflex may lead to obstruction.
• To remove the airway, simply pull out gently.
• Dispose of used airway as per local infection control policy.

Practice tips
• Use of an OPA may greatly assist in maintaining open airway during resuscitation procedures.

Pitfalls
• Trauma and bleeding in the airway can be caused by inaccurate sizing of airway.

Associated reading
Cleaver K and Webb J. (eds). (2007). *Emergency care of children and young people.* Blackwell Publishing: Oxford.
Barry P, Morris K, and Ali T. (eds). (2010). *Paediatric intensive care.* Oxford University Press: Oxford.

Insertion of nasopharyngeal airway

Background

Equipment

Procedure

Insertion of nasopharyngeal airway

Background

A nasopharyngeal airway (NPA) is a shortened endotracheal tube used to relieve upper airway obstruction. The tip of the tube will usually be placed to sit just above the epiglottis, and may remain in place (with weekly changes) for weeks or months as may be required in some conditions.
❶ The decision to insert a nasopharyngeal airway will be undertaken by senior medical personnel. Insertion should only be undertaken by an appropriately trained and experienced health professional.

NPA insertion is contra-indicated in cases of severe head injury or facial surgery.

Equipment

- Oxygen and suction.
- Saturation monitor.
- Suction catheters.
- Lubricating gel, e.g. KY jelly®.
- Zinc oxide tape or non-latex alternative cushioned hypoallergenic adhesive dressing, e.g. Duoderm®.
- Non-sterile gloves.

Procedure

- Assess child's respiratory function.
- Observe respiratory rate, depth and effort, heart rate, temperature, and oxygen saturation.
- *Assess respiratory distress:* increased effort, chest recession, nasal flaring, head bobbing, sweating, poor colour, tachycardia, or bradycardia, restlessness, confusion.
- Record all observations to provide appropriate baseline.
- Provide full and appropriate explanations, and gain consent.
- Prepare child as appropriate for their age and cognitive level, considering the involvement of play specialist.
- In advance of the airway insertion, the airway will need to be individually fashioned for the child. For this you will need:
  - *0–2 months:* 2.5–3.0mm ETT.
  - *6 months:* 3.5–4.0mm ETT.
- ETT.
- Portex™ tracheal tube holder (0.5mm smaller than ETT size).
- Sutures.
- Measure the child's length from crown of head to heel, review neck X-ray and consider individual assessment to determine approximate tube length.
- Ensure the child is held appropriately to avoid pulling at insertion.
- Ensure the child's nostrils are clear.
- Ensure oxygen and suction are available at the bedside.
- Perform a clinical hand wash.
- Prepare equipment.
- Put on non-sterile gloves.
- Apply lubricant to catheter.
- Insert nasopharyngeal airway gently into the nostril.
- If there is any difficulty putting the airway in place, pass a suction catheter through the airway and into the nostril as an introducer.

- Pass the tape through the loops of the tracheal tube holder and then onto the face.
- Secure the NPA.
- Perform suction on the NPA to ensure patency.
- Clear away equipment as per local guidelines.
- Wash hands.
- Throughout the procedure you should observe:
  - Oxygen saturation.
  - Respiratory rate.
  - Heart rate.
  - Vomiting, retching, and coughing.
- A lateral neck X-ray will be needed to confirm correct airway position.
- Record details of NPA insertion in child's health record, including length and diameter of airway.

After insertion

- Monitor oxygen saturation, respiratory rate, heart rate, oxygen requirements 2–4-hourly as condition indicates.
- Consider apnoea monitoring for those <1yr of age.
- Suction is likely to be required:
  - Before feeds.
  - After feeds.
  - 2–4-hourly if a child is on continuous feeds.
  - As clinically indicated.
- If secretions yielded are thick or discoloured:
  - Send a specimen for microbiological analysis.
  - Consider delivering humidification via headbox or mask.
  - Consider injecting 0.5mL of 0.9% NaCl into the airway prior to suctioning—only do this as directed by medical staff.
- Change airway weekly and/or whenever it becomes blocked.
- Alternate between different nostrils when changing.
- Change tape daily, taking care when removing not to debride skin.
- Keep nostrils clean and observe surrounding skin for soreness, giving appropriate skin care as required.
- ❶ Replace airway immediately if it is blocked or falls out.
- Keep a spare set of prepared airway and tapes (and a set of the next size down) with child at all times.
- Oxygen, suction and resuscitation equipment should be available at all times. Portable equipment should accompany the child if they move away from piped systems.

Pitfalls

- It may be difficult to pass the NPA. Consider the following:
  - Make sure NPA diameter is not too wide.
  - Ensure enough lubricant is being used.

Associated reading

Cleaver K and Webb J. (eds). (2007). *Emergency care of children and young people*. Blackwell Publishing: Oxford.

Barry P, Morris K, and Ali T. (eds). (2010). *Paediatric intensive care*. Oxford University Press: Oxford.

Assisting intubation

Background

❶ This procedure should only be undertaken by a suitably trained and competent practitioner—usually a medic. Communication during intubation is key—the practitioner is unable to see anything except for the vocal cords once the procedure has commenced so cannot see what is being passed or assess the patient's observations.

Equipment

- Monitoring (electrocardiogram (ECG) and oxygen saturations).
- Intravenous (IV) access.
- Bag and mask and/or Ambubag™ and mask.
- Guedel airway.
- Scissors.
- Elastoplast®.
- Drugs including flush.
- Laryngoscopes.
- Suction—Yankauer and suction catheters.
- ETT × 3.
- Lubricating gel.
- Stethoscope.
- Magill's forceps.

Preparation

Prepare drugs as per local policy but commonly remembered using the acronym AIMS:

A = atropine.
I = induction agent.
M = muscle relaxant.
S = sedative.

Prepare ETT, consider the need for a cuffed or uncuffed tube, and estimate size and length using the following equations:

For a child aged 2–12yrs

Size of ETT = age/4 + 4.
- Length of oral ETT = age/2 + 12}
- Length of nasal ETT = age/2 +15}
- Check local policy as ETTs are now often uncut. Have an ETT of the estimate size, and one a size above and one a size below. Keep the ETT clean in the packet and apply a little lubricating gel to the end.

Prepare Elastoplast® tape or preferred method for securing the ETT. Position child appropriately so head is clearly accessible (remove head of bed or cot), and adjust height of the bed, cot or trolley where possible.

Procedure

- Wash hands and prepare equipment.
- Ensure IV access is patent.
- Attach monitoring and maintain close observation of the child.
- Position child.
- Aspirate nasogastric (NG) tube if *in situ*.
- Child will need pre-oxygenating with a bag-valve-mask device.

- Ensure drugs are administered and flushed.
- Check monitoring and position so it is visible and possibly audible.
- Pass appropriate laryngoscope into the practitioner's left hand, ensuring the light is bright.
- Suction as requested using the Yankauer, to improve visibility.
- Once the vocal cords have been visualized, pass the ETT into the practitioner's right hand.
- Apply cricoid pressure if requested.
- Remove mask from bagging device, but keep mask close to hand.
- Attach a suction catheter to suction tubing, but keep Yankauer close to hand.
- Once ETT is in position pass bagging device and check for equal bilateral chest movement and good oxygen saturations, listen for air entry with a stethoscope.
- If positioned correctly, tape the ETT into position. Record length and size of ETT and perform a chest X-ray (CXR).
- If positioned incorrectly remove ETT, reattach mask to bagging device and pre-oxygenate then repeat procedure, repeat drugs as required.
- Suction ETT as appropriate.
- Consider ongoing ventilation, sedation, and analgesic needs.
- Explain to family.

Practice tips

- Observe the child and their vital signs. Remember the practitioner intubating can't see them.
- Bradycardia can be caused by both hypoxia and vagal nerve stimulation so have atropine to hand.
- Pass a nasogastric tube (NGT) as soon as possible to remove air from the stomach caused during bagging, then leave on free drainage during ventilation until feeding is commenced.
- Consider placing a roll under the child's shoulders for positioning.
- Keep spare laryngoscopes to hand (both straight and curved blades) as batteries can fail unexpectedly.
- Magill's forceps are required for nasal intubations and a bougie should be available in case of difficult intubation, a Guedel airway may assist bagging during pre-oxygenation.
- If intubation and ventilation continue, aim to change the tapes daily if the child is adequately sedated, and carefully move the ETT to the alternate corner of the mouth to reduce pressure and facilitate mouth care. This is to be carried out by two nurses once deemed safe and appropriate by medical staff. The tapes should also be renewed if they become loose or heavily soiled.

Pitfalls

- If no chest movement is seen on the left side pull back the ETT slightly as it may be too long and have gone down the right main bronchus.
- If ETT unable to be passed despite trying with a smaller size, use a bag-valve-mask device and get more senior help.

Associated reading

Cleaver K and Webb J. (eds). (2007). *Emergency care of children and young people*. Blackwell Publishing: Oxford.

Barry P, Morris K, and Ali T. (eds). (2010). *Paediatric intensive care*. Oxford University Press: Oxford.

Assisting with cricothyrotomy

Background

This procedure is carried out when normal intubations nasal, oral or endotracheal are not possible. For example, in cases of oedema of the throat a cricothyrotomy is usually an emergency procedure. This procedure does not require manipulation of the cervical spine.

In cricothyrotomy, the incision or puncture is made through the cricothyroid membrane in between the thyroid cartilage and the cricoid cartilage.

❶ Performing a cricothyrotomy is a high risk procedure. The decision to undertake it should be made by senior medical personnel only.

Equipment

- Sterile towels.
- Bag valve mask with tracheotomy tube adaptor.
- Tracheal hook.
- Trousseau introducer.
- Or 3-way venous cannula tap with up to 6L of oxygen via oxygen tubing.
- Large bore IV cannula.
- Sterile gloves.
- Antiseptic agent and cleaning agents.
- Scalpel.
- Suitable distraction aids, e.g. story book, tape, etc.

Procedure

- Undertake comprehensive nursing and medical assessment.
- Explain procedure to patient if able to understand and parents. Written and verbal consent should be obtained if possible.
- Consider local anaesthetic.
- Gather and prepare all equipment (see Table 11.1).
- Monitor all sedated or seriously ill children with continuous pulse oximetry.
- Position child in the supine position and if no cervical spinal injury place a pillow under their shoulders to slightly lift the head back exposing the neck.

Table 11.1 Equipment needed

Age	Device
0–1	Wide bore IV cannulation device
1–10	Wide bore IV cannulation device or quick trac 1.5mm
10–14	6 or 7mm internal diameter tracheotomy tube or paediatric quick trac 2.0–3mm
14 plus	Mini trac 4.mm

Doctor will:
- Prepare skin.
- Towel up sterile field.
- Clean area using local infection control measures.
- Undertake procedure by locating the thyroid and the cricoids membrane.
- Stabilize the cricothyroid membrane with one hand and insert local anaesthetic via syringe and needle.
- Either:
  - Pierce with a large-bore cannula attached to a syringe aiming at 45° to the skin, caudally in the sagittal plain.
  - Aspirate as introduced.
  - Confirm position by withdrawal of air, then slide the cannula over needle into airway; or
  - Using the scalpel make a transverse incision (about an inch long) directly over the cricothyroid membrane.
  - Cut through the cricothyroid membrane (hear a popping sound).
  - Withdraw scalpel and enlarge hole with tracheal hook.
  - Insert a trousseau introducer followed by a mini trac or an ETT.
- Provide ventilation either with:
  - An IV cannula with a 3-way tap attached to regulated oxygen flow, or:
  - With a tracheal tube adapter and a bag-valve device with the highest available concentration of oxygen pushing high flow oxygen gently into the airway.
- Determine if ventilation was successful by auscultation and observing chest rise and fall.

Practice tips
- An additional member of staff to undertake distraction will be invaluable.
- There are many kits available on the market for this procedure.
- Cricothyrotomy is considered at best a temporary solution and replacement by other methods must be considered as soon as possible especially in children.

Pitfalls
- Haemorrhage caused by insertion.
- Insertion into right main bronchus if ET tube is used.
- Injury to larynx and vocal cords.

Associated reading
Cleaver K and Webb J. (eds). (2007). *Emergency care of children and young people*. Blackwell Publishing: Oxford.
Barry P, Morris K, and Ali T. (eds). (2010). *Paediatric intensive care*. Oxford University Press: Oxford.

Haemodynamic monitoring

Background
There are four factors that directly affect a patients' haemodynamic status:
- *Chronotropy:* heart rate.
- *Intravascular volume:* circulating volume of fluid in the intravascular space.
- *Vasoactivity:* changes in the internal diameter of blood vessels.
- *Inotropy:* strength of myocardial contractions.

Therefore, to ensure accurate and safe management of children and young people with cardiovascular instability (potential or actual) it is fundamental to continuously observe their haemodyanmic status.

Continuous haemodynamic monitoring
- Gives an indication of the patients' cardiovascular status and allows for trends, compromise, and deterioration to be identified.
- Assists practitioners in understanding efficacy of interventions (such as administration of fluids and vasoactive drugs).
- Includes heart rate, central venous pressure (CVP), and invasive blood pressure monitoring.

Heart rate
A patients' heart rate should be initially assessed on admission, at the beginning of each shift, or if their condition changes by palpating an appropriate pulse:
- *Infant:* brachial or femoral pulse.
- *Child/adolescent:* radial or carotid pulse.
- Counting rate for 60s.

This will allow the collection and interpretation of information relating to pulse:
- Rate.
- Rhythm.
- Strength.

However, for continuous heart rate monitoring the use of 3- or 5-lead ECG and/or pulse oximetry is required (in high dependency/critical care both is necessary).

Equipment
- Appropriate monitor (3- or 5-lead ECG +/– pulse oximetry).
- 3- or 5-lead ECG leads.
- Pulse oximetry leads and appropriately-sized probe.
- ECG dots.

Procedure
Pulse oximetry
- Explain procedure to patient and family.
- Attach leads to monitor and the pulse oximetry probe to the lead.
- Attach probe to desired site (patients' finger/toe/hand (infant)/bridge of nose/ear lobe) following manufacturer guidelines.
- Turn on monitor.

- Ensure probe is picking up a good trace (shown in Fig. 11.5).
- Set appropriate limits.
- Document findings.
- Inform medical team if reading outside of normal range.

3/5 lead ECG

- Explain procedure to patient and family.
- Ensure privacy is maintained by drawing curtains around patient.
- Remove patients top to allow access to chest area.
- Attach leads to monitor.
- Turn on monitor.
- Apply ECG dots/stickers to the patient and attach the ECG leads as shown in Fig. 11.4.
- Ensure leads are picking up a good trace (shown in Fig. 11.5).
- Set appropriate limits.
- Document findings.
- Inform medical team if reading outside of normal range (see Fig. 11.5).

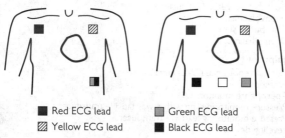

■ Red ECG lead   ■ Green ECG lead
▨ Yellow ECG lead   ■ Black ECG lead

Fig. 11.4 Attachment of ECG leads.

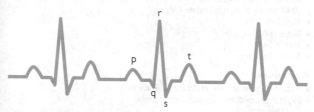

Fig. 11.5 A normal ECG trace (sinus rhythm): p wave - atrial depolarization through the right atrium to the left atrium; qrs complex - rapid depolarization of the right and left ventricles; t wave - repolarization of the ventricles.

Central venous pressure monitoring

The pressure of the returning blood that flows from the systemic veins to the right atrium is called central venous pressure. CVP is determined by the function of the right heart and the pressure of venous blood in the vena cava.

CVP monitoring is indicated in patients:
- With continuing hypovolaemia secondary to major fluid shifts or loss.
- Requiring infusions of inotropes.
- With hypotension who do not respond to initial management.

Factors that increase CVP include:
- Fluid overload.
- Forced exhalation.
- Mechanical ventilation.
- Tension pneumothorax.
- Heart failure.
- Pleural effusion.
- Decreased cardiac output.
- Cardiac tamponade.

Factors that decrease CVP include:
- Hypovolaemia.
- Distributive shock.
- Deep inhalation.

Equipment
- Central venous line (CVL) *in situ*.
- Prescription.
- Appropriate monitor.
- Pressure monitoring line with 3-way tap +/– transducer.
- Pressure monitoring lead +/– transducer.
- Leveling device.
- Inflatable pressure bag.
- Universal PPE (in line with local policy).
- 500mL bag normal saline (IV).
- 10ml ampoule normal saline (IV).
- 10-mL syringe.
- Green IV needle.
- Sterile field.
- Alcohol wipe.

Procedure
- Assess patient for the need for CVP monitoring.
- Explain procedure to patient and family.
- Turn on monitor.
- Attach pressure monitoring lead +/– transducer to monitor.
- Using an ANTT, attach the pressure monitoring line to the 500mL bag of normal saline and prime the line.
- Assemble green needle to 10-mL syringe and draw up 10mL normal saline.
- Access the patients CVL using the ANTT.
- Flush the lumen with 10mL normal saline to ensure line is not blocked.
- Attach pressure monitoring line.

- Insert 500mL bag of normal saline into pressure bag and inflate to appropriate pressure, in line with local policy (e.g. infant 100mmHg = 1mL/h; child/adolescent 150mmHg = 1.5mL/h; adult 300mmHg = 3mL/h).
- Place pressure monitoring line into transducer/attach to lead.
- Ensure transducer is at the level of the patients' right atrium, approximately the mid-axillary line in the 4th intercostal space using the leveling device.
- Zero the monitoring line by:
  - Turn 3-way tap off to patient and open to bung.
  - Open bung to the air.
  - Select 'zero CVP' on monitor.
  - Ensure reading on monitor is '0'.
  - Replace bung onto 3-way tap.
  - Turn 3-way tap off to the bung and open to the patient.
- Ensure transducer is picking up a good trace (shown in Fig. 11.6).
- Set appropriate limits.
- Document findings.
- Inform medical team if reading outside of normal range.

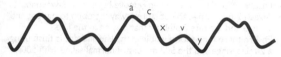

Fig. 11.6 CVP trace: a wave - atrial contraction; c wave - closure of tricuspid valve; x descent - atrial relaxation; v wave - ventricular contraction with tricuspid valve closure; y descent - tricuspid valve opens.

Invasive blood pressure monitoring

Continuous invasive blood pressure monitoring is achieved by transducing an intra-arterial line and is indicated in patients:
- Receiving a continuous infusion of vasoactive drugs (e.g. inotropes).
- With haemodynamic instability.
- Receiving anaesthetic/sedative agents.
- Requiring critical care transportation/transfer.
- Requiring intracranial pressure monitoring (ICP).

Equipment

- Arterial line *in situ*.
- Prescription.
- Appropriate monitor.
- Pressure monitoring line with 3-way tap +/− transducer.
- Pressure monitoring lead +/− transducer.
- Leveling device.
- Inflatable pressure bag.
- Universal PPE (in line with local policy).
- 500 ml bag Normal Saline (IV) with 500IU heparin.
- 2 × 2-mL syringes.
- Alcohol wipe.

Procedure

- Assess patient for the need for invasive blood pressure (BP) monitoring.
- Explain procedure to patient and family.
- Turn on monitor.
- Wash hands, apply alcohol gel and apply PPE.
- Attach pressure monitoring lead +/– transducer to monitor.
- Attach the pressure monitoring line to the 500-mL bag of normal saline with 500IU heparin, and prime the line and 3-way tap.
- Cleanse arterial line hub with alcohol wipe.
- Attach 3-way tap and pressure monitoring line to arterial line.
- Insert 500-mL bag of normal saline with 500IU heparin into pressure bag and inflate to appropriate pressure, in line with local policy (e.g. infant 100mmHg = 1mL/h; child/adolescent 150mmHg = 1.5mL/h; adult 300mmHg = 3mL/h).
- Place pressure monitoring line into transducer/attach to lead.
- Ensure transducer is at the level of the patients' right atrium, approximately the mid-axillary line in the 4th intercostal space using the leveling device.
- Zero the monitoring line by:
  - Ensure arterial line is clamped remove bung from 3-way tap.
  - Attach 2-mL syringe to hub, turn 3-way tap open to patient and syringe and aspirate 0.5mL air that may be in the line.
  - Ensure there is no blood visible in the line, if there is flush using a 2-mL syringe and the 500-mL bag of normal saline with 500IU heparin.
  - Remove syringe, turn 3-way tap off to patient and open to air.
  - Select 'zero art line' on monitor.
  - Ensure reading on monitor is '0'.
  - Replace bung onto 3-way tap.
  - Turn 3-way tap off to the bung and open to the patient.
- Ensure transducer is picking up a good trace (shown in Fig. 11.7).
- Set appropriate limits.
- Document findings.
- Inform medical team if reading outside of normal range.

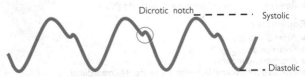

Fig. 11.7 Invasive blood pressure trace.

Practice tips
- Remember the ECG monitor only measures electrical activity through the cardiac muscle and not cardiac output so if there are any changes in the patient's condition it is important to palpate a pulse (e.g. Pulseless Electrical Activity (PEA)).
- There may be some difficulties in keeping ECG dots attached (especially if the patient is sweaty). As long as the skin is intact, try wiping the site with an alcohol wipe and allow to dry, then apply the ECG dots.
- Ensure the pulse oximetry probe site is changed at a minimum of 4-hourly as the infra-red light emitted can damage skin (especially in neonates) and pressure sores can form.
- The pulse oximetry trace and reading can be effected by a reduction in peripheral blood flow caused by:
  - Hypovolaemia.
  - Cardiac failure.
  - Hypotension.
  - Cold.
  - Vasoconstricting inotropic drugs.
- The pulse oximeter trace may also be affected by:
  - Bright overhead lights.
  - Shivering and vigorous movement.
  - Nail varnish.
- Normal CVP values in a spontaneously breathing patient is 2–8mmHg, rising by 4–6mmHg during mechanical ventilation due to the increase in intrathoracic pressure.
- The CVP measurement may still be in the normal range even with hypovolaemia due to vasoconstriction.
- Ensure that the CVP or invasive BP line is zeroed at a minimum of 4-hourly or whenever the patient/transducer moves.
- Obtain 4-hourly non-invasive blood pressure readings to ensure reliability of invasive blood pressure reading.

Setting up a fluid warmer and infusion system

Background

A child's body is made up of ~70–80% water. Hormones and the renal system control the normal distribution of fluid in the intra- and extracellular spaces in the body by maintaining varying pressures and osmotic gradients.

Illness or injury can disrupt these controls allowing fluid shift or loss resulting in the need for rapid infusion of warm fluids. In these cases, the fluid used should be crystalloid (Hartmann's or 0.9% saline). Blood may also be used to replace significant blood loss. In resuscitation the initial fluid requirement will be 20mL/kg for illness and 10mL/kg for trauma.

Equipment

- Gloves.
- Apron.
- Crystalloid fluid/blood.
- IV fluid giving set appropriate for the fluid to be administered.
- Fluid warmer such as a 'hot line' mounted on a drip stand.
- Suitable giving set for the fluid warmer used.
- Wide bore extension set.
- 3-way tap.
- 50-mL syringe.

Procedure

- Collect all equipment required.
- Wash hands.
- Connect the appropriate fluid and giving set together.
- Hang the fluid on the drip stand.
- Connect the first giving set to the giving set appropriate for the fluid warmer to be used.
- Connect a wide bore extension set.
- Add a 3-way tap to the end of the wide bore extension set.
- Run the fluid through the completed system.
- Ensure the giving set for the fluid warmer is inserted in to the warmer and switch on the fluid warmer.
- Connect the completed system to the cannula inserted in the patient.
- Connect a 50-mL syringe to the 3-way tap ensuring the tap is off to the patient.
- Release all the clamps on the circuit.
- Open the 3-way tap to the fluid and draw back the appropriate amount of fluid to maximum of 50mL in to the syringe.
- Turn the 3-way tap ensuring it is closed to the system, but open to the patient.
- Push the fluid quickly in to the patient from the 50-mL syringe.
- The 3-way tap should then be closed to the patient and the steps repeated as appropriate.

Practice tips

- If unsure of the method of fluid administration as long as the initial giving set is appropriate to the pump available this system can be set up as previously stated and used without the 50-mL syringe.
- If a pump is used the rate of infusion will be far slower than the fluid being pushed in via the 50-mL syringe.
- By using wide bore giving sets and extension sets this allows a faster drawing up of fluid or blood speeding up the administration of the fluid to the patient.
- An assistant can be useful in operating the 3-way tap and keeping count of the amount of fluid administered.
- This system is suitable for use with a cannula, as well as an intraosseous needle.
- Ensure the insertion site of the cannula or intraosseous needle is observed during administration of the fluid looking for signs of extravasation. If this occurs administration of the fluid should be stopped immediately.
- Normal saline can be kept in an incubator in preparation. Advice should be sought from the hospital pharmacy on the temperature and the time that this may remain in the incubator.
- Where blood is to be administered ensure a giving set with a filter is used.

Pitfalls

- Care should be taken to ensure that the system does not pull or drag the cannula out of the patient due to its weight. The giving sets can be secured to the bed and the patient to prevent this from occurring.

Associated reading

Hazinski MF. (2008). *Nursing care of the critically ill child.* 2nd ed. Elsevier Mosby: Missouri.
Stack CG. (2004). *Essentials of paediatric intensive care.* Cambridge University Press: Cambridge.

Care of intra-arterial line blood pressure (BP)

Background

An intra-arterial line can provide accurate continuous monitoring of systemic arterial BP. Generally, arterial lines are cared for in theatres or high-dependency areas and rarely on general children's wards due to the significant risk to the perfusion distal to the cannulated artery.

An intra-arterial line must not be used for drug administration

Common sites for insertion of an arterial line are the brachial, radial, femoral, and dorsalis pedis arteries.

Potential complications from insertion of an intra-arterial line;

- Blanching/cyanosis of the limb, due to interruption to peripheral circulation.
- Thrombosis/embolism.
- Infection—cellulitis.
- Haemorrhage—from site or loose connection anywhere in giving set.
- False reading—check against non-invasive BP reading.
- Iatrogenic anaemia.

Procedure

At start of each shift check;

- Infusion fluid, usually saline or heparinized saline, and the expiry date. The fluid should be changed every 48 h.
- The position of the transducer and recalibrate.
- The flush rate and the waveform on the monitor.
- The alarm limits on the monitor and that the alarm is on.
- Ensure site is clearly labelled as arterial.
- The site must always be exposed—the colour and warmth of the limb distal to the intra-arterial line should be closely observed.

If there are any indications that the blood supply to the limb is affected, i.e. cool, mottled, or discoloured, the line may need to be removed.

Hourly checks

The following checks should be carried out at least hourly, so giving early indication of any disruption to the circulation, or displacement of intra-arterial catheter:

- Check site for bleeding, redness, and swelling.
- Check connections, taps, etc., on giving set, for leakage and backflow.
- Check flush rate/pressure bag (100mm/Hg = 1mL/h. 200mm/Hg =2mL/h).
- Observe waveform continuously for damping.
- Check limb for warmth and perfusion.

Practice tips
Arterial waveform in relation to ECG
Normal arterial pressure can be represented by a waveform that reflects systole, valve closure, and diastole (see Fig. 11.8).

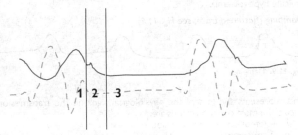

Fig. 11.8 Arterial waveform in relation to ECG.

1. The systolic pressure is the peak of the initial upstroke of the waveform, which occurs just after the QRS complex of the ECG. Systolic pressure reflects the peak pressure recorded when the heart contracts and forces blood into the arterial system.
2. The dicrotic notch is thought to represent the closure of the aortic valve.
3. The downstroke after the dicrotic notch represents ventricular diastole.
4. The diastolic BP is pressure recorded when the heart relaxes, and represents resting arterial tone.

Associated reading
Cook K and Langton H. (eds). (2009). *Cardiothoracic care for children and young people: a mulitdisciplinary approach*. Wiley-Blackwell: Oxford.
Davies JH and Hassell LL. (2007). *Children in intensive care: a survival guide*, 2nd ed. Churchill Livingstone Elsevier: Oxford.
Stach CG. (2004). *Essentials of paediatric intensive care*. Cambridge University Press: Cambridge.

Factors affecting blood pressure monitoring

If arterial pressure waveform 'swings' markedly with ventilation, this may indicate hypovolaemia.

Damping (flattened trace; see Fig. 11.9)

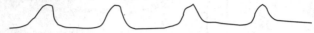

Fig. 11.9. Damping.

This represents the loss of the physiological signal in the transmission circuit, the most common causes are:
- Occlusion of catheter tip by a clot.
- Loose connection.
- Inadequate irrigation rate.
- Catheter tip positioned incorrectly.
- Clots or air bubbles in the tubing or transducer (see 📖 Trouble shooting, p. 291).

Catheter fling (see Fig. 11.10)

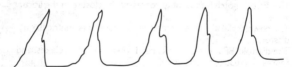

Fig. 11.10. Catheter fling.

- The motion of the catheter tip within the vessel accelerates fluid movement in the catheter. Can lead to 10–20mmHg being superimposed on the pressure wave. Ensure catheter is correctly positioned and is well secured.
- *Positioning*: abnormally high or low readings can occur as a result of improper levelling. The transducer should be level with the atria. Calibration should occur at the beginning of the shift after each position change.
- *Temperature*: the transducer is affected by changes in environmental temperature and therefore requires calibration at least once per shift.
- Ensure intra-arterial catheter and connections including transducer are visible at all times.
- Record arterial BP on the chart in red pen and record a non-invasive BP at least every 4h in black pen.
- Use clear labelling to indicate it is an intra-arterial line. Red lines, caps and labels are commonly used.
- Intra-arterial lines should only be accessed as per unit policy, but this is generally an extended role for nurses.

Pitfalls

Trouble shooting

No reading
- Check 3-way taps are in the correct position.
- Check line is not kinked or occluded.
- Catheter may be occluded, try to aspirate any clot and flush, but not if no clot aspirated as clot may be flushed into circulation. Remove line.
- Transducer may not be connected to monitor.

Inaccurate readings
- May be due to damage to the dome—change set.
- May be due to air bubbles—see 📖 Pressure signal damped by trapped air bubbles, p. 291.
- May be due to blood in the dome—may be able to flush out, but may continue to read inaccurately and may require a new set.
- Monitor and line may need recalibrating.
- May be leaks in the system—check.
- Transducer may not be level with midline of the chest.
- Abnormally high or low readings may be due to catheter fling—ensure catheter is well secured and correctly positioned.

Pressure signal damped by trapped air bubbles
- Close tap to patient.
- Hold 'dome' upwards so that air can rise.
- Open tap to air (remaining closed to patient).
- Flush slowly so that air is flushed out.
- Ensure that all connections are secure and not loose.
- If this fails the entire flush system may need changing.

Blood backing up in the line
Often due to reduced pressure in the system.
- Check pressure bag is 'pumped up', use clamps to prevent deflation.
- Check and tighten all connections.
- Check 3-way taps are in correct positions.

Bleeding at the puncture site
May be due to migration or dislodgement of the catheter, or enlarged puncture site due to movement of the catheter within the artery. It could also indicate clotting problems.
- Apply firm pressure to the site for 5–15min.
- Check stability of catheter, check pulse and capillary refill distal to the site to ensure adequate peripheral perfusion.
- Retape securely.
- Check clotting.

Compromise to the circulation distal to the catheter site
Decreased pulse volume, blanching, pallor, cyanosis, cool skin (may be due to blockage of catheter (clot) or spasm of the artery).
- Observe very closely.
- Vigorous flushing may cause arterial spasm, if not quickly resolved the cannula should be removed.
- If circulatory integrity is in doubt it may be necessary to remove the cannula.

Mechanical ventilation

Background

Mechanical ventilation comprises any form of mechanical device used to assist or replace the work normally undertaken by the respiratory muscles. This can be achieved by generating:

- A positive pressure that forces gases into the respiratory tract
  - Modes include: pressure controlled ventilation (e.g. bi-level positive airway pressure (BiPAP), pressure support (PS), continuous positive airway pressure (CPAP), assisted spontaneous breathing (ASB), volume controlled ventilation (e.g. controlled mechanical ventilation (CMV), synchronized intermittent mandatory ventilation (SIMV)).
  - Can be delivered non-invasively via a tight fitting face mask or invasively via an ETT or tracheostomy.
- A negative pressure around the thoracic cavity that sucks gases into the respiratory tract:
  - Can be delivered by an iron lung or cuirass jacket.
  - Requires a patent airway.

Possible indications for mechanical ventilation include:

- Routine anaesthesia for surgery, clinical investigations, and procedures.
- Impaired neurological status (e.g. GCS <8), which can compromise airway and cause hypoventilation.
- Chest wall trauma caused by flail segment, ruptured diaphragm, or chest burns, which can impair the effective functioning of the respiratory muscles.
- Respiratory/neuromuscular disease resulting in apnoea and respiratory distress, and an ↑ partial pressure of carbon dioxide in arterial blood ($PaCO_2$)/↓ PaO_2 levels.
- *Cardiovascular disease:* cardiac arrest, severe shock/sepsis, or pulmonary hypertension that requires fluid resuscitation (>60mL/kg), inotropic support, or inhaled pulmonary vasodilators.

Equipment

- ETT/tracheostomy *in situ.*
- Non-invasive face mask with straps/cuirass jacket with straps.
- Suction unit and suction tubing.
- Appropriately-sized (for ETT/tracheostomy) suction catheters.
- Ventilator with appropriately sized tubing attached (checked by an appropriately trained professional).
- Humidifier.
- Humidifier giving set.
- 1000mL bag water for irrigation.

Procedure

Safety checks

- Check bedside oxygen and suction unit is working.
- Appropriately sized face mask, oropharyngeal airway, and Yankeur sucker available.
- Appropriately sized anaesthetic bagging circuit attached to the oxygen and self-inflating bagging circuit is present at the bedside.
- If invasively ventilated ensure ETT/tracheostomy is well secured with tape/tapes.
- If invasively ventilated with ETT, ensure position has been confirmed on chest radiograph.
- Ensure ETT/tracheostomy tube length and size is clearly documented.
- If tracheostomy *in situ* ensure bedside emergency tracheostomy box contents has been checked.
- Ensure patient is receiving continuous monitoring of:
  - 3/5 lead ECG.
  - Pulse oximetry.
  - Invasive blood pressure or hourly non-invasive BP.
  - End-tidal CO_2.

Commencing mechanical ventilation

- Explain therapy to patient and family.
- Turn on ventilator.
- Ensure ventilator has been set up in correct mode and settings, and the alarms are suitable for patient size and condition.
- Attach 1000mL bag of water to humidifier, prime giving set and fill humidifier dome to appropriate level.
- If delivering mechanical ventilation via non-invasive face mask.
  - Apply the face mask correctly and secure with straps (according to manufacturer's instructions).
  - It is imperative to ensure a good seal between mask and face to achieve effective ventilation.
- Start mechanical ventilator and attach tubing to patient via ETT, tracheostomy, face mask, or negative pressure jacket.
- Observe patient for effective chest movement, and that continuous observations are within normal parameters.
- Obtain arterial/capillary blood gas within 15–30min of commencing mechanical ventilation to ensure pH, PaO_2, $PaCO_2$, and HCO_3 are within acceptable limits.

Ongoing care

- Document ventilator observations at a minimum of hourly intervals.
- Obtain arterial/capillary blood gas within 15–30min of any changes to mechanical ventilation settings.
- For non-invasive ventilation ensure the patient receives a minimum of 4-hourly pressure area, eye, and mouth care.
- If ETT/tracheostomy has cuff check level of inflation at least once per shift.
- Nurse the patient with head of bed/cot elevated to 30–45° to reduce risk of ventilated acquired pneumonia (VAP).
- Humidify inspired gases to the temperature of 37–38°C to prevent inspissation of secretions.

- Management of ventilator tubing:
  - Change when visibly soiled or mechanically malfunctioning.
  - Routinely replace tubing every 7 days or in line with manufacturer's guidance.
  - Prevent tubing condensation from entering patient airway.
- Deep vein thrombosis prophylaxis (anticoagulants and deep vein thrombosis (DVT) stockings) should be considered in large children and adolescents.
- Provide regular oral hygiene (minimum 4-hourly).
- Regular suctioning of respiratory secretions is required (using universal precautions).
- Regularly assess patient for level of pain/comfort using a validated tool (e.g. COMFORT score) and respond appropriately.

Practice tips

If having problems invasively ventilating the patient use the mnemonic **D-O-P-E:**
- **D**isplacement:
  - Is ETT/tracheostomy in the right place?
  - Is it in the oesophagus, right main bronchus, back of throat?
- **O**bstructed:
  - It the ETT/tracheostomy blocked by secretions, blood, or mucus plug?
  - Is the ETT kinked?
- **P**neumothorax:
  - Has patient got equal chest movement, air entry on auscultation, tracheal deviation, hyper-resonance on percussion?
- **E**quipment: is there ventilator/monitor/ETT/electric/oxygen malfunction?
- Patient tidal volumes can be calculated as 5–10mL/kg.
- Prone positioning can improve oxygenation in patients with ventilation-perfusion (V/Q) mismatch.
- Patients requiring non-invasive ventilation via a face mask may rapidly form pressure marks on their face despite regular pressure area relief. Skin can be protected by applying a hydrocolloid dressing to the site, which acts as a barrier between the mask and the skin.

Associated reading

Department of Health (2007). *Saving Lives: reducing infection, delivering clean and safe care.* HMSO, London.
Resuscitation Council UK (2010). *Resuscitation Guidelines.* Resuscitation Council, London.

Multiple colloid infusions

Background
Colloid infusions are an essential part of the resuscitation process.
Colloids are used:
- When more than 40mL/kg of crystalloid has been given with the requirement for more fluid resuscitation to achieve haemodynamic stability.
- As a first line fluid in certain conditions (e.g. 4.5% human albumin solution (HAS) in meningococcal septicaemia).
- In the management of trauma patients who have received 4 × 10mL/kg aliquots of crystalloid and remain haemodynamically unstable (colloid usually packed red cells).

There is much debate about how much and which fluid is required to resuscitate a patient. It is important to understand the benefits of using colloid versus crystalloids:
- Crystalloids diffuse more readily into the interstitial space.
- Crystalloids may be associated with more peripheral oedema.
- Where capillary leak exits, crystalloids allow more water to enter in interstitial space, because of their low osmotic pressure.
- 2–3 times more volume of crystalloids than colloid is required to expand the same vascular space.[1]

Nursing management of multiple colloid infusions
The key to managing patients that require multiple colloid infusions includes:
- Constantly re-assessing the patient's condition prior, during and post-colloid administration and findings are actioned appropriately.
- Ensuring the patient has continuous haemodynamic monitoring.
- Maintaining strict fluid balance of the patient's input and output (including urinary catheterization).
- Ongoing monitoring and management of electrolytes.

Types of colloids
- Synthetic colloids: gelofusin.
- Blood product colloids:
  - HAS 4.5%.
  - Packed cells.
  - Fresh frozen plasma (FFP).
  - Cryoprecipitate.
  - Platelets.

Patient assessment and continuous observations
- Pulses both centrally and peripherally.
- Colour/pallor/perfusion.
- Central and peripheral capillary refill time.
- *Heart rate (HR)*: ECG 3- or 5-lead.
- BP.
- Temperature.
- Pulse oximetry.
- Urine output.

Setting up for colloid transfusions

- Use the hospital policy when administering blood products.
- Utilize the paediatric intensive care unit (PICU) pharmacopoeia for guidance on indications for use, dosing and infusion compatibility.
- When accessing central lines use the ANTT. You will need two registered nurses for this procedure (see 📖 Aseptic non-touch technique, p. 174).

Equipment

- Name band on patient.
- Prescription.
- IV giving set (appropriate for type of fluid).
- 50mL syringe.
- Electronic infusion device.
- Dispenser pins.
- Air inlet needle (for HAS 4.5%).
- Warming device.

Procedure

- Assess patient.
- Assess the colloid fluid requirement in consultation with medical staff.
- Explain procedure and need for fluids to patient/parents/carers.
- Warn patient and family of possible side effects.
- Check prescription with patient and patient identification.
- Ask if they have any known allergies to blood or blood products.
- Ensure access device (e.g. pressure volume catheter (PVC), CVL) is patent and secure.
- Check the blood product unit as per local hospital policy for administration of blood products.

❶ Please note: it is important that all members of staff involved in the administration of blood products have completed appropriate training as per local hospital requirements.

- Ensure any blood products are compatible with patients own blood type (Table 11.2).

Table 11.2 Blood products and compatibility with patient's own blood

Patient's ABO blood group	Patient's plasma contains	Compatibility
O	Anti A + B	O
A	Anti B	A O
B	Anti A	B O
AB	Neither	A B AB O

- Wash hands.
- Using ANNT spike bag with appropriate giving set.
- Prime the line with the colloid.

- Alternatively depending on the volume, type, and rate of fluid to be administered use a dispenser pin and 50-mL syringe to withdraw the required fluid.
- Attach to patient, ideally via a central venous line.
- Observe patient for sign of any transfusion reactions.
- If administering blood, a set of observation needs to be performed prior to administration, 15min after commencement and on completion of transfusion. Most transfusion reactions occur within the first 15min of transfusion.
- Reassess patient.
- More fluid may be required. Consult and involve medical staff in the process.

Problems and pitfalls

- 40mL/kg of fluid resuscitation can result in significant haemodilution, requiring packed red cell transfusion.
- Multiple colloid transfusion can cause coagulopathy, such as micro vascular bleeding, dilutional coagulopathy, and disseminated intravascular coagulation (DIC), therefore regular testing of FBC and coagulation is required.
- Children are difficult to obtain IV access in emergency situations. If vascular access is not obtained in less than 90s or 2 attempts then an intra-osseous (IO) needle will need to be inserted.
- Once fluid resuscitation occurs then appropriate access (large bore PVC or CVL) needs to be established to allow for further fluid administration.
- The larger vessels where the access device is situated, the less risk of extravasation during administration of large volumes of fluid at fast rates.

Large transfusion volumes of colloids can cause:
- Hypothermia and therefore close temperature monitoring is essential. Hypothermia can be reduced by warming the fluids and/or the patient, however this can be problematic in itself as it can cause vasodilation and shifting of intravascular volume into the peripheries resulting in hypotension.
- *Acidosis:* caused by anion gap.
- *Hypocalcaemia:* may need correcting.
- *Hyperkalaemia:* may need correcting.
- Acute respiratory distress syndrome (ARDS).
- Pulmonary oedema.

Things to consider

- If fluid resuscitation exceeds 60mL/kg inotropic support may be indicated.
- If fluid resuscitation exceeds 60mL/kg mechanical ventilatory support may be indicated (varies depending on medical staff).
- Where to admit the patient and who takes over the responsibility of continuing care should be considered as early as possible.
- Involvement of paediatric high dependency unit (PHDU)/PICU may be indicated for monitoring.
- PICU may be indicted for mechanical ventilation.

- Central access should be obtained as soon as possible. This not only allows the administration of fluids but the monitoring of central venous pressure (CVP) that could give indication of adequate intravascular volume.
- Arterial line insertion is indicated as this allows for invasive blood pressure monitoring enabling accurate haemodynamic status evaluation. It also allows for blood sampling and arterial blood gas sampling to assess patient's electrolytes and acid-base balance.
- Need to assess and address what has caused the requirement of multiple colloid infusions and any other underlying issues (e.g. haemorrhage or sepsis).
- Minimum urine output should be: neonate = 2mL/kg/h; infant = 1.5–2mL/kg/h; child = 1mL/kg/h; adolescent = 0.5–1mL/kg/h.

Associated reading

[1] Advanced Life Support Group (eds) (2005). *Advanced Paediatric Life Support: The Practical Approach*, 4th edn. Blackwell Publishing Ltd, Oxford

Capillary blood gas sampling

Background
Arterialized capillary blood gas sampling may be preferable to arterial puncture for children and infants as the procedure is less painful. The heel is commonly used for infants; the finger or earlobe is used for older children. This procedure should only be performed by a practitioner trained in the skill as inaccurate results can occur due to poor technique.

Equipment
- Non-sterile gloves.
- Warming device.
- Automated lancing device.
- Gauze swabs.
- Heparinized capillary tube.
- Blood gas analyser/procedure tray.
- Small adhesive plaster.
- Sharps disposal bin.
- Suitable distraction aids for age of child.

Procedure for heel sampling (infants)
- Use the plantar heel surface outside the medial and lateral limits of calcaneous bone.
- Position the infant and use distraction aids as appropriate.
- Gather and prepare the equipment.
- Disinfect hands and apply gloves.
- Warm the heel using warm and moist cloth or warming pads.
- Wash the heel with soapy water and dry.
- Use the automated lancing device. Wipe away first drop of blood.
- Collect the blood into the capillary tube by holding tube horizontally.
- Apply pressure and use gauze to dress site.
- Insert blood sample into analyser or in procedure tray if not immediately available.
- Dispose of equipment safely.
- Complete nursing and/or medical documentation.

Procedure for finger sampling (older children)
- Use the medial and lateral aspects of the distal finger.
- Reassure the child, explain the procedure, and use distraction aids as appropriate.
- Gather and prepare the equipment.
- Disinfect hands and apply gloves.
- Warm the finger using warm and moist cloth.
- Wash the finger with soapy water and dry.
- Use the automated lancing device—wipe away first drop of blood.
- Collect the blood into the capillary tube by holding tube horizontally.
- Apply pressure with gauze swab, apply plaster (if not allergic).
- Insert blood sample into analyser or in procedure tray if not immediately available.
- Dispose of equipment safely.
- Complete nursing and/or medical documentation.

Procedure for earlobe sampling (older children)
- Aim to puncture 3mm from the edge of the earlobe.
- Reassure the child, explain the procedure, and use distraction aids as appropriate.
- Remove any earrings and pull hair back from site.
- Gather and prepare the equipment.
- Disinfect hands and apply gloves.
- Warm the earlobe using a warm and moist cloth, or vasodilating cream.
- Wash the ear lobe with soapy water and dry.
- Use the automated lancing device. Wipe away first drop of blood.
- Collect the blood into the capillary tube by holding tube horizontally.
- Apply pressure with gauze swab, apply plaster (if not allergic).
- Insert blood sample into analyser or in procedure tray if not immediately available.
- Dispose of equipment safely.
- Complete nursing and/or medical documentation.

Practice tips
- Positioning the infant or child is important to prevent needle stick injuries. Swaddling infants keeps the correct position and may reduce the pain. Ask an assistant or chaperoning adult to hold the child as appropriate; they can also assist by using distraction aids.
- Warming the site may help to stimulate blood flow. If you use a warm moist cloth, ensure you dry the area thoroughly or the blood will not form a drop. Vasodilating creams are often used for older children, but check local protocols as they are not licensed for this purpose.
- Use an appropriate sized automated lancing device for the child or infant's age and size; see manufacturer's guidance.
- The blood needs to form a 'drop' before introducing the capillary tube; if the blood stops flowing, wipe the site surface to clear any clots.
- Regularly remove the tube from the well of blood, and tilt to mix blood and remove air bubbles that may otherwise alter the results.

Pitfalls
- Capillary blood gas sampling is not reliable for critically ill children or for neonates under 24h old due to poor peripheral perfusion. In these circumstances, arterial blood gases are required.
- Using the finger site for infants may cause nerve damage.
- Using the heel site is contraindicated for infants that have started walking and have callus development.
- Squeezing the site increases pain and can cause haemolysis of sample, thereby causing inaccurate results.

Obtaining and analysing arterial blood gases

Background

Blood gases indicate the efficiency of ventilation, gas exchange, and acid base status. Obtaining an arterial blood gas is usually done either by arterial stab, a one off sample, or by sampling from a continuous arterial line. An arterial stab is most likely to be painful and cause anxiety; therefore, the continuous line is usually the preferred method in children.

The vessels most commonly used are:

- *Neonates:* umbilical artery.
- *Infants and children:* radial, brachial, dorsalis pedis, axilla, or femoral.

Indications for sampling

- Deterioration in patient's clinical condition.
- For frequent blood samples, particularly in the shocked/hypotensive child.
- Following any increase in oxygen therapy/ventilation.
- After ventilation changes, but not within 15min of the changes.
- Prior to extubation.
- Half-hourly following extubation until clinically stable.
- Current practice indicates 4-hourly, if the child is stable, unless otherwise instructed—check local policy/guidelines.

Equipment
- Pair of clean gloves and apron (non-touch technique—check local guidelines and policy).
- Disposable tray.
- Pre-heparinized syringe (1mL).
- 2-mL syringe.
- Sterile wipes (2% chlorhexidine, 70% alcohol).
- Continuous monitoring (heart rate, blood pressure, oxygen saturations).
- Arterial giving set:
  - Infants (<10kg) 50-mL syringe of flush infusing at 1–1.5mL/h.
  - Child (>10kg) 500mL bag of flush.
  - Pressure at 150mmHg or, if child profoundly hypertensive, 300mmHg.

Procedure
- Assess limb perfusion prior to blood sampling.
- Consider patients/parents/carers awareness of procedure and explain as appropriate.
- Open syringe packets ensuring that the syringes are not removed from their packets until immediately prior to use.
- Clean port of 3-way tap with sterile swab for 10s and allow to dry.
- Insert 2mL syringe. Turn tap off to the flush system and withdraw 2mL of blood. ❶ If you feel resistance try repositioning the limb, if resistance remains stop procedure and seek medical advice.
- Turn tap half way between the patient and intraflow (heparinized saline).
- Remove syringe and place back into wrapper.
- Insert *heparinized* syringe in to port.
- Withdraw 0.5mL of blood.
- Turn half-way to patient and intraflow then remove syringe.
- Return the 2mL in syringe with blood to port, ensuring that there are no air bubbles entering the system and give all blood back to the patient.
- Close tap off to patient, withdraw:
  - 2mL flush for children over 10 kg.
  - 1mL for children under 10 kg from intraflow system.
- Open tap to patient and push the flush slowly to avoid blanching.
- Turn tap midline to re-establish flush system.
- Clean bionnector with sterile wipe.
- After arterial blood gas analysis, dispose of all equipment in yellow clinical waste bin.
- Wash hands as per trust policy.

Post-procedure
▶ Assess limb perfusion post accessing of line—look for signs of blanching or congestion to associated periphery.

▶ Ensure that waveform on the monitor has returned to its previous status and alarms are functioning.

▶ The arterial line site should be visible at all times.

Analysis

Carbonic anhydrase

$$H_2O + CO_2 \Leftrightarrow H_2CO_3 \Leftrightarrow H^+ + HCO_3^-$$

Lungs buffering in RBC renal tubules fast (Hb, phosphate) slow
- *Lungs:* major stabilizer of acid base balance.
- *Kidneys:* eliminate acids, but take several days to adjust.
- Look at the pH (7.35–7.45kPa)—is it acidotic, alkalotic or normal?
- Then pCO_2 (4.5–6.0kPa or 35–45mmHg)—is it high, low or normal?
- Then base excess (BE, −2–+2) or bicarbonate (22–26mmol/L)—is it high, low, or normal?
- Finally, look at the pO_2 (10–14kPa or 75–100mmHg)—is it high, low, or normal?
- Oxygen saturations are dependent on Hb, temperature and pH.
- A pH below 6.8 and above 7.8 is classically incompatible with life.

Common Causes

See Table 11.3.
- *Respiratory acidosis:* hypoventilation (CNS depression, obstructive airway disease, artificial ventilation), irritability, decreased conscious level.
- *Respiratory alkalosis:* hyperventilation (raised ICP, meningitis, hypoxia, pulmonary embolus, or oedema), confusion, coma, muscle cramps, paraesthesia.
- *Metabolic acidosis:* chronic diarrhoea or intestinal fistula, renal tubular acidosis, diabetic ketoacidosis, lactic acidosis, renal disease.
- *Metabolic alkalosis:* vomiting, potassium deficiency, diuretic therapy, over treatment with sodium bicarbonate.

Table 11.3 Common causes

Respiratory acidosis	↓ pH	↑ CO_2	−ve base excess or bicarbonate
Metabolic acidosis	↓ pH	↑ CO_2	−ve base excess or bicarbonate
Respiratory alkalosis	↑ pH	↓ CO_2	+ve base excess or bicarbonate
Metabolic alkalosis	↑ pH	↓ CO_2	+ve base excess or bicarbonate

Practice tips

- Try to keep the limb straight when aspirating for the blood gas sample.
- Ensure there is enough blood for the sample and avoid bubbles.
- Minimize delay in analysis of the sample otherwise the O_2 and CO_2 readings will be deranged.
- Look at the clinical state of the patient; what will the gas tell you? Consider the patients' vital signs, clinical history, medications/ treatment, urea and electrolytes (U&Es), red blood cells (RBC), clotting and examine.
- With normal renal function most acidoses will correct themselves.

Common pitfalls

- If a delay is anticipated, then place sample on ice.
- Always use a hepinarized syringe, otherwise the analyser will clot.
- Bubbles in the same will affect the analysis.
- Show the nurse in charge/doctor the blood gas results.
- If the blood gas is normal, but the patient's clinical condition is worsening, start a thorough ABCDE and examination.

Associated reading

Woodrow P. (2009). Arterial catheters: promoting safe clinical practice. *Nurs Stand* **24**(4), 35–40.

Tracheostomy tube change

Background

- The first tracheostomy change should be done by an ear, nose, and throat (ENT) surgeon.
- Humidity is vital in the first week to maintain tube patency, whilst stoma is forming.
- Subsequent changes should be performed weekly by a suitably trained and competent nurse/carer.

Equipment

- Taped tracheostomy tube (same size as that *in situ*).
- Tracheostomy dilators.
- Scissors.
- Lubricating gel.
- Towel/roll for under shoulders (to extend neck).
- Comforter (i.e. dummy).
- Site dressing if indicated.

Procedure

Should be performed by two people in order maintain safety and ensure a smooth procedure is carried out.

- Explain procedure to child and family and gain consent.
- Use comforter, if required.
- Ensure all equipment required is available.
- Wash hands.
- Extend neck (using towel/roll under shoulders).
- Cut tapes on one side.
- If cuffed tube, deflate cuff.
- Remove existing tube.
- Insert new/clean tube.
- Remove introducer/obturator.
- Inflate cuff.
- Clean neck (see Tracheostomy tape change, p. 308). (see Tracheostomy tape change, p. 308)
- Tie tapes.
- Observe skin around site for excoriation. Consider dressing such as Lyofoam®.
- Reassure child.

Practice tips

- Babies and young children may need swaddling.
- Consider sedation in babies and young children for first tube change.
- Heat moisture exchangers (Swedish noses) should not be used for the first week until stoma tract formed as they do not provide sufficient humidity.

Associated reading

Wilson M. (2005). Tracheostomy Management. *Paediatric Nursing* **17**(3), 38–44.

Tracheostomy tape change

Background
This procedure is undertaken to ensure the tracheostomy is secure, the airway maintained, and for hygiene purposes.

Equipment
- Spare tapes.
- Scissors.
- Site dressing if indicated.

Procedure
- Explain procedure to child and family.
- Ensure child has comforter, if required.
- Wash hands.
- Cut tapes.
- Clean neck (see 📖 Tracheostomy suction/toilet, p. 310).
- Apply tapes to one side of tube: thread through flange then pull tapes through loop (see Fig. 11.11).
- Pull tight to make secure (see Fig. 11.12).
- Pull round neck and tie other side with a bow initially (see Fig. 11.13).
- Sit child up and see if you can get 1 finger in between neck and tapes.
- When happy tapes are tight enough tie with a double knot.
- Observe skin around site for excoriation. Consider dressing such as Lyofoam®.
- Reassure child.

Practice tips
- Two people are needed to maintain safety.
- Should be changed daily or more frequently if lots of secretions.
- Tapes can become loose in mobile children so you may need to tighten tapes more than once a day even if they do not need changing completely.
- Leave enough tapes at end to enable tightening later if required.

Pitfalls
- Caution with velcro tapes as little fingers may undo them; therefore, many hospitals prefer not to use them.
- Bandage scissors can be used to prevent cutting child's skin if nervous carer. However, if you put finger under tapes and cut towards finger not skin this also eliminates risk.

Associated reading
Wilson M. (2005). Tracheostomy Management. *Paediatric Nursing* **17**(3), 38–44.

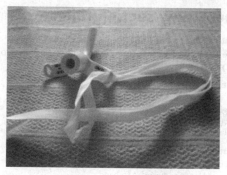

Fig. 11.11 Apply tapes to one side of tube: thread through flange then pull tapes through loop.

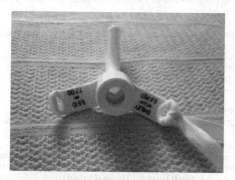

Fig. 11.12 Pull tight to make secure.

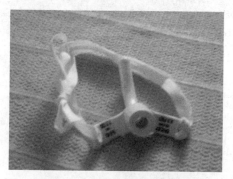

Fig. 11.13 Pull round neck and tie other side with a bow initially.

Tracheostomy suction/toilet

Background
To ensure patency of tracheostomy tube and prevent development of respiratory infection.

Equipment
- Suction catheters (2 × sive of tracheostomy).
- Sterile gloves.
- Syringe (size-dependent on age of child).
- 0.9% saline ampoule.

Procedure
- Explain procedure to child and family.
- Ensure equipment required is to hand.
- Wash hands.
- Put on sterile glove and connect appropriate size suction catheter to suction machine.
- Turn on suction.
- Insert suction catheter into tracheostomy to ½cm before end of tube.
- Pull out of tube and apply suction pressures according to age:
  - 8–10kPa neonate.
  - 10–13 kPa child.
  - 10–16 adolescent.[1]
- Reassure child.

Practice tips
- 0.9% saline instillation should not be used routinely only if secretions thick.
- Change suction tubing daily.
- Wash secretions through tubing with tap water once suction performed.
- Keep measuring tape with length of suction required at bedside to enable pre-measured suction to be performed.

Pitfalls
- Epithelial trauma can occur if deep suction performed.

Associated reading
[1] NHS Quality Improvement Scotland (2008). Best practice statement: caring for the child/young person with a tracheostomy. NHS Scotland, Glasgow.

Management of external ventricular drains and intrathecal catheters

Management of external ventricular drains and intrathecal catheters

Background

External ventricular drains (EVD's) are inserted for a variety of reasons. They are used to regulate excessive production, or inadequate circulation, or absorption of cerebral spinal fluid (CSF). They are infrequently used for the monitoring and control of ICP. They can also be inserted for diagnostic purposes to allow sampling of CSF.

Care of intrathecal catheters differs to that of EVD. They can be in either of two forms:
- An internal port inserted in theatre under GA.
- An external catheter that can be inserted in theatre or a ward environment.

Both have the same main purpose which is to enable the administration of intrathecal medication in accordance with local policy.

Equipment
- Spirit level.
- Drip stand.
- CSF measurement chamber.
- EVD drainage bag.
- Gloves and antiseptic wipes for bag change.
- Small adhesive dressings.

Procedure
- The insertion of the EVD is always performed in theatre by a neurosurgeon.
- It is the responsibility of the neurosurgeon to give instruction on the level at which the drain is to be set.
- Ensure the zero point on the drainage chamber remains level with the bridge of the nose and the upper tip of the ear at all times, which anatomically is level with the Foramen of Munro.
- Read, record, and empty the drainage chamber every hour.
- Record neurological observations at a maximum of 4-hourly intervals depending on the condition of the child.
- Ensure the entry site remains covered by a sterile dressing at all times according to local policy.
- Empty the drainage bag when ¾ full using aseptic non-touch technique (see 📖 Aseptic non-touch technique, p. 174).
- Ensure the drainage catheter is free from obstruction to allow free flow of CSF.

Practice tips

- Ensure the drain is never placed horizontally unless the chamber is empty and the drain clamped, as CSF may block the filter and prevent it from draining.
- Educate patients and parents/carers in how to correctly clamp the drain when moving their child, but to inform trained staff when the drain needs repositioning.
- Patients can get headaches and vomiting post insertion of EVDs or intrathecal catheters due to low ICP so regular analgesia and anti-emetics may be required.
- It is important that drains do not run over cot-sides of the bed.
- EVDs can be used to administer intrathecal antibiotics by a trained member of medical staff without further invasive treatment. The EVD must remain clamped for an hour post-administration to prevent the drug draining out in the CSF.

Pitfalls

- It is essential that children with EVDs *in situ* are closely monitored by staff and parents/carers. Should they alter position without the drain being clamped the EVD may over drain and in some circumstance lead to subdural haematomas.
- Children require constant close supervision to prevent the EVD from becoming dislodged.
- A main risk with EVDs is infection, so it is essential that the patient is observed for any symptoms such as a pyrexia. A CSF sample can be obtained from the drain according to your local policy, for confirmation.

Associated reading

Dunn T. (2002). Raised intracranial pressure. *J Neurol Neurosurg Psychiat* **73**(Suppl 1), i23–7.
Tobias J. (2000). Applications of intrathecal catheters in children. *Paediat Anaesthes* **10**, 367–75.

Inotropic support

Background

Inotropes are indicated in any circumstances where cardiovascular insufficiency (i.e. poor tissue perfusion, hypotension, etc.) is persistent despite fluid resuscitation. Inotropes should be considered where volumes of resuscitation fluids exceed >60mL/kg have been administered (however, this may vary depending on clinician).

Inotropes support the cardiovascular system by:
- Restoring adequate intravascular fluid volume.
- Improving myocardial activity.
- Treating abnormal vascular capacitance and resistance.
- Correcting abnormal heart rate.

Nursing management of inotropes

The key nursing management of patients requiring inotropic support includes:
- Calculating the drug dose and titration.
- Setting up of inotrope infusions.
- Titrating drug to achieve desired effect.
- Stopping of inotrope infusion.
- Practical points.

Calculation

Rate (mL/h)

= dose (micrograms/kg/min) × weight (kg) × 60 (min)/concentration (micrograms/mL)

Or

Dose (micrograms/kg/min)

= rate (mL/h) × concentration (micrograms/mL)/weight (kg) × 60 (min)

NB. All units must be the same

Setting up and changing the inotrope infusion

- Use the hospital drug policy when administering medicines.
- Utilize the PICU pharmacopoeia for guidance on indications for use, dosing and infusion compatibility.
- When accessing central lines use the aseptic non-touch technique (ANTT). You will need two registered nurses for this procedure.

Equipment required

- Drug of choice (prescribed).
- Dilution fluid (e.g. 0.9% NaCl/5% dextrose).
- Prescription.
- 50mL luer lock syringe.
- 10mL luer lock syringe.
- Sterile field.
- Alcohol wipe.
- 3-way taps (you will need one per inotrope).
- Infusion pump line.
- Programmable infusion driver pump.
- Line and syringe labels.

Procedure

- Assess patient.
- Assess inotropic requirements in consultation with medical team.
- Explain the need for the drug, what the drug is, any side effects that could occur as well as the process of the procedure to patient/parent/carer.
- Wash hands.
- Inotropes must be changed one at a time.
- Use aseptic non-touch technique for accessing central lines.
- Check prescription is correct.
- Dilute the inotrope as per prescription to a volume of 50mL.
- With the inotrope drawn up in the syringe, attach it to line and prime.
- Connect the line to the 3-way tap and prime the hub of the 3-way tap ensuring it is full.
- Label both line and syringe.
- Program your pump with weight of child, dose of drug you wish to administer, and volume and dose in the syringe in accordance with prescription.
- Place the syringe in the pump and purge the syringe by 1mL, taking up the slack in the line. This can prevent any surge or dip in blood pressure.
- Continuing to use either the non-touch or aseptic technique attach infusion to the patients' CVL.
- Start the inotrope at a low dose, in consultation with medical staff.
- Titrate the infusion to achieve acceptable haemodynamic status for the patient.
- Reassess patient.

Changing of infusion

- Follow previous procedural steps.
- Start the new infusion and titrate the infusions (both by increasing rate of new infusion and by decreasing rate of expired) to maintain adequate blood pressure.
- Titrate the infusions as the blood pressure allows.
- When BP is stable and the expired infusion weaned to minimal dose place it on hold until child is stable. Placing it on hold allows it to be still attached in case on an emergency or where the BP fluctuates.
- When stable, turn expired infusion off.
- Reassess patient.

Stopping inotropes

- Once an inotrope has been stopped and is no longer required the infusion needs to be safely removed from the patient to prevent accidental administration. This requires removal of the inotropic drug that is left in the dead space of the line and can only be undertaken when all inotropes have been stopped via that lumen of the CVL.
- Use ANTT to access the line.
- To remove the inotropic drug in the line, it is necessary to remove twice the estimated dead-space within the line.
- Using a 10-mL syringe withdraw the required amount.
- Flush with 5mL normal saline.
- If the line does not bleed back and you are unable to withdraw the inotrope, notify medical team and label the line appropriately. *Do not use.* Ensure this is communicated with the rest of the nursing and medical team.

Practice tips
The patient
- Should be assessed for available access including how many, where, and type.
- Requires strict fluid allowance and balance to be calculated appropriately.

The inotrope
- Should not be interrupted due to the short half-life of the drug—doing so can lead to haemodynamic instability.
- Should not be filtered as the drugs mix in the filter and provide an inaccurate rate of the drug.
- Should never be bolused or purged, whilst attached to the patient. It causes surges in BP and heart rate.
- Should be checked for expiry date, concentration, reflect the prescription and how much is left in the syringe. Check compatibility with IV fluids. Be organized and prepared to change the infusion.
- Should be changed using the double pump technique as explained previously to prevent cardiovascular instability.
- Should be weaned slowly to prevent swings in blood pressure.

Access
- When administering inotrope central access (i.e. CVL/longline) is always the preferred route of administration. This is due to the risk of damage to the smaller blood vessels, the reliability of smaller vessels and cannula's for continuous delivery of the drug and the strength of the inotrope administered.
- The bigger the vessel in which the inotrope is administered there is less risk associated with administration.
- It is necessary to consider the amount of dead space within your access and the site and the position it is in.
- Hypovolaemia needs correcting prior to commencement of inotropes.
- Ensure adequate oxygenation for increased myocardial oxygen demand and consumption.

Monitoring
A patient receiving inotropic support requires the following monitoring:
- Invasive BP.
- CVP.
- 3- or 5-lead ECG.
- Oxygen saturations.
- Urine output.
- Fluid balance.
- Capillary refill both central and peripheral.
- Peripheral and central temperatures.
- Neurological observation.

Pitfalls

- Neonates/small children are sometimes difficult for access.
- Inotropes dopamine and dobutamine can be given peripherally, but need to be diluted × 10, which has implications for fluid requirements.
- Arterial lines are not always available, reliability of cuff blood pressure is appropriate for a short period, but arterial line monitoring is standard care for a child requiring inotropes.
- The side effects of inotropes include the development of pressure ulcers and necrosis of tissue.
- Children requiring inotropes have often had multiple fluid boluses and due to illness may become oedematous. This needs clarification and explanation to parents/carers.

Associated reading

Davies JH and Hassell LL. (2007). *Children in intensive care: a survival guide*, 2nd ed. Churchill Livingstone Elsevier: Oxford.

Hazinski MF. (2008). *Nursing care of the critically ill child*, 2nd ed. Elsevier Mosby: Missouri.

Stack CG. (2004). *Essentials of paediatric intensive care*. Cambridge University Press: Cambridge.

Retrieval of the critically ill child

Background

Paediatric intensive care within the United Kingdom has been centralized into lead centres, where expert care can be delivered. The result of this configuration has resulted in critically ill children presenting in smaller district hospitals where paediatric intensive care is not provided. These children need to be stabilized by the local team and then transported to the nearest paediatric bed by an appropriately skilled team. The ultimate aim of this team is to provide intensive care throughout the whole transfer.

It is important to remember that the retrieval team is not a resuscitation team and these skills are required by the personnel at the referring centre.

The team

Commonly the team comprises one medic and one nurse, both of whom are experienced and assessed as competent in retrieval medicine. The patient's condition and stability should also be considered, as those that are perceived to be unstable may require a more experienced team.

The team should aim to mobilize as quickly as possible once the referral is accepted. Once the team is identified, they are responsible for assembling the equipment and drugs required. A checklist of the equipment and checks should form part of the retrieval log.

Equipment required

- Trolley or incubator/baby pod.
- Age appropriate ventilator.
- Suction machine.
- Monitor with age-appropriate leads (should be able to measure heart rate, invasive BP, non-invasive BP, CVP, end-tidal CO_2, respiratory rate, and oxygen saturation).
- Six infusion pumps.
- Age appropriate harness or vacuum mattress.
- Consumables bags, one containing airway and breathing equipment, and one containing circulation equipment.
- Drug boxes.

The equipment should be securely attached to the trolley and should be able to withstand a 10G crash.

Mode of transport

Journeys of less than 2h should be undertaken by road, otherwise air transport should be considered.

If travelling by road, the decision to travel using blue light conditions should be taken by the retrieval team. If the ambulance is able to travel at normal road speed there is little to be gained by using lights and sirens and the team is putting their own safety at risk.

Blue light conditions can be considered when:

- Traffic is at a standstill.
- The patient's condition is deteriorating rapidly and the team's skills are required immediately, as the referring centre is unable to stabilize the patient then the risk to the patient could instigate the use of blue light conditions.
- Life- or limb-threatening conditions during the return journey.

Stabilization

- Follow EU resuscitation guidelines if needed.
- If the patient has been stabilized the team should perform a thorough ABCDE assessment, performing interventions as required.
- Care should be taken to ensure ET tubes and IV access are adequate and secure.
- All assessments and interventions should be clearly documented in the log.
- Once the team is satisfied with the child's condition they should be transferred on to the retrieval trolley and equipment.
- Blood gas should be checked once the child is stable on the transport ventilator before departure.
- Secure child to the trolley using an age appropriate harness that will protect them should the ambulance be involved in a collision.
- The team should also troubleshoot problems that may arise during their return journey and ensure they are prepared to deal with them.
- The retrieval team should work with the referring team to stabilize the patient. Both teams have joint responsibility for the patient during this period.
- The retrieval team does not take full responsibility for the patient until they have left the referring department.
- Ideally the return journey should be undertaken in a safe and calm manner as rapid acceleration and deceleration can worsen the patient's condition.
- Patient assessment, interventions, observations and evaluation should be clearly recorded.

Associated reading

Byrne S. (ed). (2008). *Paediatric and neonatal safe transfer and retrieval: the practical approach. Advanced Life Support Group.* Wiley-Blackwell: Oxford.

Anaphylaxis

Background

Anaphylaxis can be a life-threatening event if it is not managed quickly and appropriately. Anaphylaxis is a rapidly developing problem that can involve airway, breathing, and circulation that can be triggered by food, drugs, or venom. There is a good prognosis if it treated correctly.

Equipment

- High flow oxygen delivery system (non-rebreathe mask or bag/valve/mask).
- Anaphylaxis box (should contain adrenaline 1:1000, chlorphenamine and hydrocortisone).
- IV cannula or IO needle depending on conscious level.
- 0.9% NaCl.
- Monitoring (pulse oximetry, ECG, and blood pressure).

Procedure

- Assess using an ABC structure:
  - **A**irway—assess for swelling, stridor, hoarseness.
  - **B**reathing—assess for increased respiratory rate, wheeze, fatigue, oxygen saturations <95%.
  - **C**irculation—assess for pale, clammy, increased heart rate, drowsy, loss of consciousness.
- If this is a life-threatening problem, administer prescribed dose of 1:1,000 adrenaline IM (see Table 11.4).
- Administer 15L of oxygen via a non-rebreathe mask.
- If circulation is compromised, administer 20mL/kg of 0.9% normal saline after establishing access.
- Administer prescribed chlorphenamine and hydrocortisone (IM or slow IV).
- Keep re-assessing ABC.

Table 11.4 Medication prescribed to treat anaphylaxis.

Age	Adrenaline	Chlorphenamine	Hydrocortisone
Over 12yrs	0.5mL	10mg	200mg
6–12yrs	0.3mL	5mg	100mg
6 mths–6yrs	0.15mL	2.5mg	50mg
Less than 6 mths	0.15mL	250microgram/kg	25mg

Practice tips

- If there is airway compromise they may be better sitting up than lying down. Nebulized adrenaline 5mL of 1:1,000 maybe prescribed every 10min to assist. If the parent or carer is present, involve them if at all possible. The child will feel much safer and comforted by someone familiar.
- If there is breathing compromise they may be prescribed nebulized salbutamol 2.5mg <5yrs, 5mg >5yrs.
- If the circulation is involved, repeated doses of 20mL/kg normal saline may be required, so get them ready—be one step ahead if you can.
- IM adrenaline may need to be repeated every 5min via the intramuscular route. Have it drawn up ready in a labelled syringe.
- Working as a team is imperative to ensure the child or infant is treated appropriately.
- Make sure the time of arrive is noted so you can keep an accurate record of the event. If you have a rhesus clock or stop watch start it.
- Make sure there is a team leader allocated to co-ordinate the event.
- Have a vomit bowl at hand. If the trigger was food, they are often violently sick.
- They may develop a wide spread rash that may look like nettle rash or hives. Warn them and their parents if this is developing as it may upset them further.
- Stay calm. If you panic, they will pick up on your anxieties.
- Be prepared for the unexpected.

Pitfalls

- Anaphylaxis can lead to complete airway obstruction, apnoea, and loss of pulse so you may need to use your basic and advanced life support skills.
- If a child has an underlying health problem for example asthma they have an increased risk of death.

Associated reading

Advanced Life Support Group (2010). *Advanced Paediatric Life Support: The Practical Approach*, 5th edn. BMJ Publishing, London.

Resuscitation Council (UK) (2008). *Emergency Treatment of Anaphylactic Reactions: Guidelines for Healthcare Providers*. Resuscitation Council (UK), London. Available at: ℞ http://www.resus.org.uk.

Respiratory system

Respiratory arrest and basic life support

Background

In children, causes of arrest are more commonly respiratory in origin, resulting from hypoxia. The child at first will compensate for respiratory failure by increasing the use of accessory muscles, respiratory rate (RR), and heart rate (HR), but will eventually become hypoxic. The body will then decompensate causing agitation, drowsiness, confusion, eventual loss of consciousness, and respiratory arrest. Early recognition and response to the sick child is vital for a positive outcome.

Equipment

- Bag valve mask ventilation system (ambu bag).
- Oxygen.
- Suction equipment.

Procedure

Basic life support (BLS) follows a sequence of events to ensure that no matter what the situation, one or more rescuers can respond in an effective manner.

Three S's

Safe to approach

Ensure that you are aware of and avoid any hazards, as well as checking the child is in no further danger.

Stimulate the child

- It is important to establish the responsiveness of the child.
- AVPU can be undertaken.
  - Alert.
  - Responds to Voice.
  - Responds to Pain.
  - Unconscious.
- Clothing that can be easily removed or opened to expose the child's chest should also be carried out at this time.

Shout for help

Ensure that anyone around you is aware of the situation and has summoned further help.

A for airway

- Approach the child/young person and perform an airway opening manoeuvre:
  - Head tilt/chin lift.
  - Jaw thrust.
- See 📖 Airway opening manoeuvres, p. 266.
- Infants will need to be in a neutral position, a child in a 'sniffing' position.
- The rescuer should then look in the child's mouth, noting any obstruction. Do not perform a blind finger sweep.
- If trauma is suspected the child's head and neck should be supported at all times and the jaw thrust method used to open the airway.

B is for breathing

- *Look:* observe any movement of the chest, count RR.
- *Listen:* for respiratory noises such as wheeze, stridor.
- *Feel:* place cheek alongside the child to feel for any breath.
- This should all take 10s.
- If no breath sound or shallow gasping breathes are noted, assisted breathing should take place.
    - 5 rescue breaths, ensuring a good seal and delivered over 1–1.5s for each breath.
    - If no chest rise the rescuer should gently change the head position to try to open the airway.

C is for circulation

- Check for signs of life such as response to stimuli, normal breathing, and spontaneous movement.
- Pulse should be checked to assess if circulatory assistance is needed.
    - Pulse can be felt at the carotid artery for children and in the brachial artery for infants (up to aged 1yr).
    - Femoral pulse may be used in both age groups.
- Assessment should take <10s.
- If there are no signs of life or the pulse rate appears to be <60 beats/min (bpm) then commence chest compressions. Palpation of pulse cannot be the sole determinant for chest compressions; if there are no signs of life and a rescuer is uncertain of pulse, then compressions should be commenced.
- Chest compressions should be aimed at producing an adequate circulation with an emphasis on breathing and should have a ratio of 15 chest compressions to 2 assisted breaths, i.e. 15:2.
- Chest compression should be at least a third compression of the chest at 100 bpm.
- The landmarks for chest compression are one finger breadth above the xipsternum.
    - Use two fingers for an infant under 1yr.
    - Alternatively use your hands to circle the chest and your thumbs laced on the sternum.
    - Use one or two hands for a child over 1yr.
- As part of a circulation assessment capillary refill, feeling of peripheries, and BP may be assessed in a hospital setting.

Recovery

An unconscious child whose airway is clear and who is breathing normally should be turned onto his/her side into the recovery position, ensuring:

- A stable position.
- Free drainage of fluid from their mouth.
- Non-compression of the chest.
- An awareness of cervical spine injuries.
- An easily accessible airway.

Practice tips

- Chest compressions should be delivered over the lower half of the sternum to prevent trauma caused by slipping of the sternum, and causing a fractured rib or penetration injury.
- If there is only one rescuer, undertake cardiopulmonary resuscitation (CPR) for 1min prior to going for help, unless a sudden collapse is witnessed, as defibrillation may be required, and assistance should be sought immediately.
- Have one person leading the resuscitation to ensure all aspects are covered, and roles are clear.

Pitfalls

- When using a bag and mask, correct positioning, and size of mask are vital to maximizing the child's chances of gaining oxygen.
- Giving chest compressions is tiring, so consideration of rotation between rescuers is important.
- Follow the BLS sequence one stage at a time.
- In a hospital setting the sequence continues beyond 'C' with D for disability and E for exposure.

Associated reading

🔖 http://www.resus.org.uk.

❶ Please note that these are brief guidelines. Further reading and training should be undertaken.

Respiratory care at home, school, and in the community

Background
With ever more sophisticated technology within medical care today we have a steady increase in the number of children who are cared for in the community with respiratory conditions. Service provision can range from a supply of oxygen, inhaler, and peak flow teaching, to full 24h life-sustaining ventilation.

Parents and carers are often able to manage their child's respiratory condition at home, with the support of specialized children's community nurse (CCN) teams, GPs, physiotherapists, and the hospital specialist team. The inter-professional team needs to work together to ensure the child and families holistic needs are met.

At home
The many services provided by CCN include:
- Provision, teaching, and maintenance of equipment.
  - Suction.
  - Oxygen.
  - Nebulizers.
  - Monitoring systems.
- Undertake comprehensive risk assessments of the child's respiratory status, and its implications on home and school life.
- Encourage philosophies of health promotion and education of the child and family.
- Complete home oxygen order forms—choosing suitable delivery. A child may use an oxygen concentrator at home, but as these are heavy and bulky they may take a light weight oxygen cylinder or liquid oxygen to school.
- Help develop individual care plans and escalation procedures in case of deterioration.
- Provide family support and respite. There is a critical need for respite amongst families who care for children with long-term respiratory conditions. This provision will have an effect on the whole families' physical and mental health and wellbeing.
- Undertake pulse oximetry or 'sleep study' monitoring where the child's oxygen saturations and HR are monitored over a 12–24h period, usually during sleep.
- Refer for physiotherapy provision.
- Initiate and co-ordinate continuing care packages for children with tracheostomies, long-term life-limiting, or life-threatening conditions, and those children on life-sustaining ventilation.
- Practice nurses, school nurses, and GP's have a vital role to play in the detection and management of acute respiratory conditions, such as croup or the exacerbation of asthma.

At school

It may be necessary to train a designated carer to attend to a child's respiratory needs at school, such as:

• Suctioning.
• Administration of oxygen.
• Administration of nebulizers.
• Management of an emergency tracheostomy change.
• Management of life sustaining ventilation.
• Initiation of basic life support.

Practice tips

• Oxygen suppliers may offer a holiday order service to be requested by the CCN. The child and family only need take enough oxygen for the journey and their permanent supply will be waiting for them on arrival (throughout most of Europe and USA).
• Children who require respiratory support in the community may need to take medications during school hours. The CCN should request the child have two prescriptions, one for home and one for use at school. This will avoid parents needing to repack medicines and ensures they will not be forgotten.

Pitfalls

• Working autonomously in the community means you will need to rely heavily on your skills of assessment. As children's nurses we should not depend solely on machinery to inform us of a child's changing clinical condition. If you are concerned a child's respiratory condition has deteriorated, refer to the appropriate clinician without hesitation.

Associated reading

Department of Health (2004). *National Service Framework for Children, Young People and Maternity Services. Key issues for Primary Care.* DoH, London.
Department of Health. (2010). *National Framework for Children and Young People's Continuing Care.* DoH, London.

History taking and assessment

Background

Respiratory disease and disorders are common in children, due to their respiratory system not fully developing until 8yrs old. Respiratory symptoms can be acute or chronic and appropriate questions need to be asked dependent on presenting symptoms. Knowledge of the paediatric respiratory system is imperative in order to be aware of the normal physiology and subsequent pathophysiology.

Equipment

- Medical and nursing notes.
- Paper for documentation.
- Pen.
- Stethoscope.
- Oxygen saturation monitor (if appropriate).
- Swabs or universal container (if considering infection and a sputum sample or respiratory swab is required).
- Spirometer/peak flow meter (if appropriate).

Procedure

History taking

- Welcome/introduce self to parent/carer and child/young person.
- Ask parent and/or child to explain what has been happening, date of onset of symptoms, pattern of symptoms.
- Clarify points during the consultation.
- Response from questions will direct the consultation and the headings given here may act as a prompt.

Respiratory symptoms

- Cough (pattern, duration, and nature of cough).
- Wheeze (in response to a trigger? heard by healthcare professional, audible?).
- Shortness of breath? (precipitating factor? In response to exercise?).
- Other respiratory sounds, e.g. stridor, grunting.
- Response to treatments tried: either prescribed or over the counter?
- Other non-pharmacological measures taken.

Past medical history

- *Birth history*: gestational age, birth weight, mode of delivery, need for oxygen therapy, or special care as a neonate.
- *Feeding*: breast- or bottle-fed, evolving food allergy, presence of gastro-oesophageal reflux (treated or not).
- Immunization history, including BCG if applicable.
- Exposure to infectious disease, e.g. pertussis.
- Details of any regular infections (especially ear, chest, or skin) or repeated need for antibiotics.
- Stool pattern (in particular pale or oily or constipation).
- Details of any other medical conditions.
- Presence of atopy (include asthma, eczema, food allergy).

- Record height and weight and plot on growth chart (faltering growth, thriving, obese) (see 📖 Measuring weight, height, and body mass index, p. 86).
- Family history, family tree, past/present medical history of biological parents, siblings, or other close relatives.
- Social history.
- Discuss home environment: consider possible triggers, which may include damp or mould, pets, or exposure to passive cigarette smoke.
- Discuss school and/or child care arrangements.

Assessment
- It is crucial to allow a period of time to observe a child when making a respiratory assessment. Ideally, this should be carried out without the knowledge of the child and can often be done whilst taking the history.
- When assessing a child a look, listen, and feel approach is beneficial.

Look
- Observe and record a child's respiratory rate over a full minute.
- Observe respiratory effort and use of respiratory muscles. Subcostal, intercostal, and sternal recession, tracheal tug, nasal flaring, head-bobbing, see-sawing.
- Observe colour, e.g. cyanosis, pallor.
- Observe child's behaviour and interaction with parents/carer.
- Observe chest shape. Consider pectus excavatum, pectus carinatum, Harrison's sulcus, or hyperinflation.
- Observe hands, e.g. signs of clubbing.
- If appropriate obtain oxygen saturation levels (see 📖 Oxygen saturation monitoring, p. 334).

Listen
- Listen for audible respiratory sounds.
  - Wheeze, stridor, grunting.
  - ❶ Silence—immediate help needed.
- If a child can speak, can they speak in a full sentence?

Feel
- Auscultation and/or percussion of the chest. Listen for any respiratory sounds throughout all lung fields such as wheeze, crackles, creps.
- Equal chest rising.

Practice tips
- Ensure the environment is adapted to make it welcoming.
- Provide toys or other forms of distraction to entertain the child.
- Take notes throughout the consultation.
- Do not rush the consultation–it is important to allow adequate but not excessive time to take a proper history that also allows parents and the child/young person to voice concerns and questions.
- Ideally, children should hardly be aware they are being examined/observed.
- Warm the stethoscope prior to placing it on a child's chest.

- Use distraction techniques to keep child relaxed during examination. It is very difficult to make an assessment or auscultate the chest if a child is crying or distressed.
- If a child is co-operative ask them to cough. This can give an indication of the nature of the cough (dry/moist) and may also move secretions, which could alter findings on auscultation.
- Leave any upsetting procedures to the end, e.g. examination of the throat.

Pitfalls

- ❶ Never assume; it may be helpful to listen to the parent/young person and paraphrase in order to ensure you have correctly understood what they have said.
- Try to ask open questions and allow adequate time for answers.
- Living with symptoms on a daily basis can often distort perception—some parents and children may over report or exaggerate symptoms and vice versa.
- In some languages it is difficult to find an adequate translation for the symptom.
- Recording of respiratory rate needs to be over a full minute to ensure there are no inaccuracies.
- Auscultation of the chest is an advanced nursing role and requires practice and patience when carrying it out on children. Findings from an unskilled practitioner may not be reliable.

Associated reading

Barnes, K. (2003). *Paediatrics: A Clinical Guide for Nurse Practitioners*: Butterworth and Heinemann, Edinburgh.

Bradley, R. (2007). Improving Respiratory Examination Skills. *J Nurse Practit* **3**(4), 276–7.

Duderstadt, K. (2006). *Pediatric Physical Examination: An Illustrated Handbook*. Mosby Inc., Maryland Heights.

Listening to breath sounds

Background

Breath sounds are the noises produced by the structures of the lungs during breathing. The skill of listening to breath sounds on infants and children can be both useful and at times life-saving. In BLS it is taught that you look, listen, and feel when carrying out your breathing assessment during the algorithm. The listen part is basic—can you hear any breath sounds? If you don't have any equipment to hand, using the skill of listening is all you need.

Equipment

- A stethoscope.
- A quiet room (hopefully!).
- Some form of distraction if infant/child conscious.

Procedure

- Obtain informed consent from the child/young person or carer.
- Warm the stethoscope to make the procedure more pleasant.
- Remove the upper clothing, protecting dignity, and privacy.
- The trained practitioner will:
  - Use the stethoscope to listen to the lung sounds (auscultation).
  - Listen for abnormal breath sounds such as crackles (sometimes known as rales), rattles (sometimes known as rhonchi), and wheezes.
  - Listen to each side and compare what you hear.
  - Listen front and back.
- An assisting practitioner/parent will:
  - Help to keep the child/infant comfortable.
  - Use distraction techniques to aid the examination.
- Ensure the child's dignity and privacy is protected.
- Document and report all findings.

Practice tips

- A calm, compliant infant/child will make the examination so much easier. Use a teddy or doll to demonstrate the procedure on first.
- Try and keep the infant/child distracted and happy with books/bubbles and mobiles.
- Involve the parents/carer—a young child is likely to feel more confident sitting on a lap, rather than being examined on a bed.

Pitfalls

- Listening for breath sounds in an infant/child can be a difficult procedure to do if they are crying, uncooperative or combative.
- Transmitted sounds are often heard and this can be confusing and misleading.
- One full breath should be listened to in each location.
- Infants/children will sometimes not tolerate sitting still for any length of time.

Oxygen saturation monitoring

Background

Oxygen saturation monitoring or pulse oximetry is a simple and non-invasive method of recording peripheral arterial blood oxygen saturations and is recorded as SpO_2 as a percentage. The oxygen saturation machine works on the principles of measuring the light absorbency of haemoglobin. When haemoglobin is well saturated with oxygen it is red and has the capacity to absorb more light from the infrared sensor probe. Haemoglobin will change to a bluer colour when oxygen levels are lower which will reduce the amount of light absorbed by the sensor. Normal saturation levels are >95%; if a child has saturation levels <92% the medical team should be informed and oxygen therapy considered (see 🕮 Oxygen administration, p. 336).

Equipment

- Saturation monitor.
- Sensor probe.
- Detergent wipe (if using a reusable probe).

Procedure

- Assemble equipment and wash hands/use alcohol rub.
- Explain the procedure to the child and parent/carer, and obtain informed consent.
- Place the sensor probe on a warm and well perfused site.
  - In older children sites include finger, big toe, or earlobe.
  - In smaller children sites can include across the palm of the hand close to the base of the little finger, on the foot on the outer aspect close to the base of the little toe.
- Ensure that the infra-red diodes and detector are directly opposite each other on the site, with the infrared light shining down through the skin onto the photo-detector.
- Ensure adequate trace on the machine (bar indicator or waveform).
- Compare manual HR with the measurement on the machine to confirm reliability.
- Record results as per local policy.
- If monitoring continuous oxygen saturations, set alarm limits to agreed upper and lower limits:
  - Some saturation monitors have factory set parameters for HR and oxygen saturations.
  - Ensure alarm limits are set using agreed parameters for the individual child/young person dependent on their medical condition.
- Ensure the sensor probe position is changed every 4h (check manufacturers guidelines):
  - It is possible to cause damage to the skin if a sensor probe is left in position for prolonged periods of time when monitoring continuously.
  - Probe change should be documented.

Practice tips

- Where oxygen saturation monitoring is indicated, respiratory assessment and measurement should be made and recorded simultaneously in order to give a complete respiratory assessment.
- Saturation monitoring is recommended for children undergoing procedures requiring sedation.
- Some children are frightened of the red light omitted by the sensor probe; it is important to let the child see the probe and discuss the light prior to placing it on the desired site.
- Alarms can cause concern to parents and children/young people and they will often require reassurance.
- Oxygen saturation values will vary between different devices and can lead to errors of up to ±4% in the range 70–100%.[1] When <70% the accuracy of the reading will fall.
- Ensure the sensor probe is appropriate for the weight/size of the child. Disposable probes should be single patient use and discarded when no longer required.
- It can be useful to cover the probe site with a sock/bandage as this reduces the amount of ambient light. It can also help to keep the probe in position, the site of the probe warm and well perfused and out of site of the child if they are distressed by the probe light.
- In the event of smoke inhalation oxygen saturation monitors will prove inaccurate. Carboxyhaemoglobin absorbs a similar amount of light as oxyhaemoglobin, which will lead to an overestimation of results.

Pitfalls

- Alarms on the monitor should only be silenced when the child has been visually assessed. Parents should be cautioned about resetting their own child's machine if it alarms, as this is unsafe practice.
- Using a monitor that can adapt to movement will help to reduce alarms if monitoring continuously; probe position is also important.
- The probe should be clean, in good working order, and fully compatible with the pulse oximeter.
- The probe should be attached to a clean site, which is free from nail varnish and well perfused.

Associated reading

Chandler T. (2000). Oxygen saturation monitoring. *Paediat Nurs* **12**(8), 37–42.

Orr, J. 2010. *The respiratory system*. In: Coyne I, Neill F, Timmins F. (eds) *Clinical Skills in Children's Nursing*. Oxford University Press, Oxford.

Royal College of Nursing. (2007). *Standards for Assessing, Measuring and Monitoring Vital Signs in Infants, Children and Young People. RCN Guidance for Children's Nurses and Nurses Working with Children and Young People*. RCN, London.

[1] Medicines and Healthcare Products Regulatory Agency. (2010). *Top Tips for Pulse Oximetry*. Department of Health, London.

Oxygen administration

Background

Oxygen administration is common for both acute and some chronic illness in children/young people. Young children have lower pulmonary reserves, and high oxygen consumption, leading to rapid falls in blood oxygen levels.[1] In the absence of sufficient oxygen, hypoxia occurs eventually leading to cell death. However, oxygen can be toxic if used inappropriately, and should only be administered following a respiratory assessment, taking into account the child/young person's condition which may affect if, and how much, oxygen can be administered, e.g. in some cardiac conditions.

Oxygen is measured as the fractional inspired oxygen concentration (FiO_2). When being administered, the flow rate and concentration should be documented,[2] the child nursed on an oxygen saturation monitor (see 📖 Oxygen saturation monitoring, p. 334) and regular respiratory assessments taken.

Equipment

- Oxygen.
- Oxygen flow meter. Consider if need to use a low flow meter, although if this is the case, a high flow meter should always be ready in case of an emergency.
- Oxygen delivery system.
  - Nasal canulae and tape.
  - Simple and non-rebreathe mask and oxygen tubing.
  - Venturi specific mask, barrels, and oxygen tubing.
  - Headbox, oxygen tubing, oxygen analyser, consider humidification (see 📖 Humidification, p. 340).
- Observation chart, Paediatric Early Warning Score (PEWS).
- Oxygen saturation monitor and probe.

Types of oxygen therapy

Nasal canulae

- Delivers 0–2L of oxygen flow/min. Do not deliver >2L via this method.
- Consists of 2 soft prongs that arise directly from the oxygen tubing and are inserted into the patient's nares, prongs pointing downwards. Tips of the prongs should never be cut.
- Comes in different sizes.
- Good for delivering low flow.
- Use an appropriate dressing to secure the canulae and protect the skin.
- Humidification is not required.
- Can easily get blocked with secretions.
- Can cause dry mucous membranes.

Simple mask

- A flow rate of >4L/min is needed to prevent re-breathing of exhaled carbon dioxide.
- Adjust flow rate to deliver different concentrations.
- Tight seal is needed for high concentrations.
- Not suitable for long term use.

Venturi mask

- Accurately able to deliver varying concentrations of oxygen of 24, 28, 35, 40, and 60%.
- Concentration depends on colour of barrel chosen and oxygen flow.
  - One side of barrel indicates percentage of oxygen, the other side litres to set the flow meter at, e.g. 35%, 8L.
  - To increase or decrease oxygen, change barrel and flow meter accordingly.
- Due to accuracy, able to assess and communicate if the child/young person's oxygen requirement is increasing or decreasing.
- Requires tight seal.
- Noisy.

Non-rebreathe mask

- The use of valves in the reservoir bag and the mask's oxygen port can increase the inspired oxygen concentration level up to 99% with a flow of 10–15L.
- The patient draws gas from the oxygen rich reservoir and displaces gas through the exhalation ports.
- A flow rate of between 10–15L/min is required to prevent carbon dioxide being inhaled.
- Ensure that the flow is adequate to keep the bag from completely deflating on inspiration. The bag should always be inflated prior to use.
- Used in emergencies.
- Short-term therapy only.
- Not always tolerated.
- Good seal required.

Headbox

- Suitable for small infants (<8 months old) requiring higher levels of oxygen.
- Can deliver >95% FiO_2.
- Calibrate and use an oxygen analyser to measure percentage of oxygen being administered, which should be placed as close to the infants airway as possible.
- Ensure adequate flow and ventilation for the removal of carbon dioxide.
- Do not cover all gas escape routes, e.g. do not pile up blankets around headbox entrance.
- Non-invasive, but limits interaction with carer; seek opportunities for parents/carers to have interaction, e.g. when sheets need changing they could hold their child with a non-rebreathe mask, whilst the nurse changes the sheets.
- Not well tolerated by older babies.
- Misting of the headbox can make observation difficult and can contribute to pyrexia.
- Potential for cold stress in small infants when cold gas is directly delivered, and can lead to bradycardia.
- Removal of headbox leads to rapid fall in oxygen concentration.
- Often requires humidification (see 📖 Humidification, p. 340).

Practice tips
- With the venturi system, the barrels are different colours and this can be utilized to gain the child's interest and co-operation.
- When transferring a child in hospital and using a portable oxygen cylinder, ensure you have sufficient oxygen to last the transfer/procedure and that it is at least half full (refer to local policy as some will require >three-quarters full).
- The 'wafting' method is not accurate and not advised; however, some children will not allow nasal cannulae or a mask near their face. If necessary, it is ideal for the mask to be placed opposite the sternum, although, again, with some children this may be difficult.

Pitfalls
- Oxygen should be prescribed, except in emergencies when it is appropriate to administer oxygen without a prescription.
- Oxygen should be weaned and discontinued as soon as possible.
- Increased oxygen requirement is a sign of a deteriorating child and should generally be reported to medical staff.

Associated reading

Chandler, T. (2001). Oxygen administration. *Paediat Nurs* **13**(8), 37–42.

[1] Resuscitation Council. (2007). *Paediatric Immediate Life Support*. Resuscitation Council (UK), London.

[2] BNFC (2008). *BNF for Children*. BMJ Group/RPS Publishing/RCPCH Publications Ltd, London.

Humidification

Background

The inspired air is normally heated and moistened in the nasal cavity. Inspired air is normally heated at body temperature, warmed and humidified from the nasal mucosa. If the air is delivered, problems may arise, the mucosa may dry and be prone to cracking, then in cells, oxygen dries, and the hygroscopic mucosa can be drying to tissue. This can lead to accumulation of mucus plugs and retention of secretions and blockage of small airways. Airways may be retained and blockage of airways and oxygen, which if left unhumidified, may be used if humidification likely necessary to administer humidification therapy include the following:

- Water
- Oxygen
- Sterile water
- Sterile humidifier or disposable single-use
- Tubing
- Delivery source of oxygen tubing
- Prescription and equipment
- Face mask
- Oxygen flowmeter or flow outlet
- Humidifier bottle or device
- Oxygen

Procedure

Plan the procedure as appropriate to the following:

Cold humidification

- Place mask
- Fluid should be added to the humidifier using sterile water
- Humidification is in reservoir

Hot and humid

- Equipment is attached and the mask fixed and used water in the reservoir. The water should be at 50 to 60°C within the patient discomfort

Heat and moisture exchanger

- Heat and moisture exchanger to replace the function of the upper

Nose and mouth

- Prescribed oxygen should be given
- Ensure the humidifier is fixed and is left the oxygen system

Oxygen delivery

- Attach the prescribed oxygen system to the patient
- The humidification from the mask and lower rate
- Plan to cover patient's nebuliser can comfortably are maintained whilst comfortable oxygen administration and humidification and microbes

Humidification

Background

The function of the nose is to heat and moisten inspired gases. If this is bypassed, e.g. in mouth breathing, or via a tracheostomy, water and heat are lost. Consequently, the air breathed in becomes very dry; the mucus in the airways becomes dry and sticky, there is cilia dysfunction and the respiratory mucosa can become damaged. This can lead to accumulation of secretions, an increase in infection risk, and blockage of small airways. During many respiratory illnesses supplemental oxygen, which is dry, is administered to children. Even with small concentrations, it may be necessary for humidification. However, when to commence humidification can vary, so always consult local policy.

Equipment

- Heater/humidifier.
- Sterile water.
- NaCl 0.9% (with syringe and needle to draw up).
- Prescription chart.
- Nebulization equipment.
- Oxygen mask or nasal cannulae.
- Elephant and oxygen tubing.
- Head box.
- Oxygen concentration monitor (oxygen analyser).
- Saturation monitor and probe.
- Oxygen.
- Air.

Procedure

Brief descriptions of some humidification systems follow:

Cold humidification

Nebulizers
- Should be used to loosen thick, sticky secretions.
- Normally NaCl 0.9% is used.

Closed system
- Oxygen/air is attached and bubbled through a cold water bath/ container of sterile water and delivered to the patient via nasal cannulae or an oxygen mask.

Warm humidification

Heated humidification is most effective as particle size is smaller.

Closed system
- These are similar to the closed cold water system.
- Oxygen is attached to an aerosol heater, which is also linked to a water bath or sterile water.
- Air/oxygen is warmed before it reaches the patient.
- The heater is either electric or battery powered.
- There are many systems available, please consult local policy and manufacturer instructions when setting up and administering via this method.

Headbox
- Usually used for infants, e.g. in bronchiolitis.
- Head is enclosed in a headbox/oxygen tent.
- Oxygen is delivered into the headbox after it has been through a closed system. This again may vary, so please refer to local policy.
- The concentration of the oxygen delivered is monitored within the headbox via an oxygen analyzer.

Heat and moisture exchangers (HME)
- These are used for tracheostomies.
- They consist of hygroscopic paper filters encased in a plastic case.
- Many different types and sizes are available; some contain viral/bacterial filters.
- They function by withdrawing heat and moisture from the respiratory gases expired. This is then resupplied to the gas that the patient breathes in on the next inspiration.
- Oxygen can be delivered through these if required.

Practice tips
- In order to maintain humidification, it is vital to ensure the patient has the correct level of hydration.

Pitfalls
- Cold water systems may cause bronchospasm.
- In warmed systems temperature needs to be monitored as overheating can occur.
- Tubing and masks/cannulae can be heavy and bulky.
- Rain out can occur with water baths/bubble through humidifiers. Tubing needs to be observed and potentially emptied with adjustments made to settings on the water bath.
- Water baths/humidifiers and associated equipment are a source of infection and need to be changed as per hospital policy.
- HME's should be appropriately sized, as there is a small increase in dead space, thus some increase in airway resistance.
- HMEs can become dislodged and also become clogged with secretions.

Associated reading
Goldsmith A., Shannon A. (2009). Humidification devices. *Anaesthes Intens Care Med* **10**(10), 465–7.
Poolacherla R., Nickells J. (2006). Humidification devices. *Anaesthes Intens Care Med* **7**(10), 351–3.

Performing suctioning

Background

Performed to remove excessive or retained secretions from the respiratory tract, or obtain specimens for laboratory examination, following a respiratory assessment. It may be performed as a single procedure by experienced and competent nursing and medical staff (or by suitably trained parents/carers), or may be incorporated into a chest physiotherapy regime. The frequency of suctioning is determined by the child's clinical condition; however, the principles are the same for suction via the pharynx or via an artificial airway, e.g. tracheal tube or tracheostomy.

Equipment

- Suction unit (piped vacuum system or a portable unit) and tubing.
- Suction catheters of appropriate size and type:
  - Rounded tip.
  - 2 or 3 (but no more than 3) lateral holes which should be smaller than the distal hole.
  - Integrated vacuum control. A 'Y' connector should be placed between tubing and catheter where there is no integral control.
  - Catheters should not exceed 50% of the airway's internal diameter (other than when a Yankauer sucker may be used to clear thicker matter from the mouth).
  - If suctioning via a tracheostomy or endotracheal tube (ETT), the suction catheter can be measured by doubling the size of the internal diameter, e.g. 3.0mm diameter, use a 6FG suction catheter.
- Approximate guide to catheter selection for a natural airway are:
  - Infant 5–6 FG.
  - Child <5yr 6–8 FG.
  - Child >5yr 8–10 FG.
  - Each child should be individually assessed.
- Irrigant (if deemed appropriate/necessary).
- Non-sterile gloves.
- Apron.
- Bowl of clean tap water.
- Tissues.
- Disposal bag.
- Labelled specimen container (if required).
- Blanket (for holding child if necessary).
- Oxygen.

Preparation of child and family

- Explanations to both child/young person and family should be given appropriate to their age and condition.
- Explanations should include:
  - Reason for suction and what it will entail.
  - Potential risks.
  - Duration.
  - Expected outcome.

- Child and family should be told that appropriate holding may be necessary.
- Individual requirements of the child should be addressed, e.g. nebulized medication, pre-oxygenation.
  - Pre-oxygenation may be deemed necessary for some children.
  - Adequate hydration of the child should be ensured and/or humidification of inspired gases.
  - Hyperinflation may be required for some ventilated children. This must only be performed in consultation with medical staff, and by a suitably experienced nurse or physiotherapist.

Procedure

- Check all equipment to ensure it is fully operational.
- The negative pressure of the unit must be checked and altered if necessary prior to attaching the catheter.
- Recommended pressures (subject to individually assessed needs) are:
  - Infant 6–9kPa (60–80mmHg).
  - Child 9–11kPa (80–100mmHg).
  - Older child 11–15kPa (max. 120mmHg).
- Ensure resuscitation equipment is readily available.
- Place child on their side (if possible)—2 people may be required, one to perform the procedure and the other to hold the child. If not appropriate to place on side, the child/young person can be placed with their face up, and neck slightly extended.
- Perform clinical handwash (see 📖 Hand hygiene, p. 168).
- Pre-oxgenate child if required.
- Put gloves on. The catheter should only have contact with the child's airway and the practitioner's glove.
- Remove suction catheter from packaging and attach to suction tubing.
- Turn on suction at appropriate pressure.
- Ensuring that no negative pressure is being applied (i.e. keeping integral vacuum control or 'Y 'connector/port open) introduce catheter gently into airway.
  - For natural nasal airway suction, the distance from the level of central incisors to the angle of the lower jaw is determined–the catheter should be inserted just beyond this point.
  - For artificial airway suction, length of the airway should be measured and recorded and the catheter inserted just beyond this point.
  - Medical staff may instruct a different insertion distance, e.g. post-tracheal surgery.
  - If suctioning with a Yankeur, then it should be inserted via a convex angle along the roof of the pharynx, with no 'blind' suctioning.
- Apply negative pressure as individually assessed by occluding the port.
- Withdraw catheter from airway, avoiding any rotation.
- The maximum duration of each suction attempt should be determined by child's response, but should be no more than 10s.
- Removal of viscous secretions may be aided by use of an irritant–but these should not be used routinely–only on medical advice. NaCl may be instilled, or saline nebulizers administered.

- Monitor child continuously throughout procedure:
  - Respiratory rate and quality.
  - Colour.
  - HR.
  - SaO_2.
  - Quantity, colour, and viscosity of secretions.
- Take immediate appropriate action if condition deteriorates.
- Catheters are designed for single use only; catheter and glove should be changed on each pass, unless in an emergency.
- No more than 3 suction passes are recommended. Always allow recovery of the child between each pass. Seek medical advice if suctioning is not effective after 3 attempts.
- If the child is receiving oxygen therapy, recommence oxygen delivery as soon as procedure is completed.
- Clean child's nose/mouth as required and ensure that they are comfortable.
- Give reassurance and information as appropriate to both young person/child and family.
- Suction tubing and flow controls should by flushed with clean water.
- Discard Personal Protective Equipment (PPE) according to local policy.
- Perform clinical handwash.
- Record procedure in health record, including details of aspirate obtained and any clinical reactions. Inform medical and nursing personnel as appropriate.
- Suction tubing and jars should be regularly emptied and washed or changed as per local policy.

Practice tips

- Catheters should not be kinked prior to insertion as a method of vacuum control.
- When removing glove, wrap the used catheter around the gloved hand, pull glove back over soiled catheter and discard safely.
- When a child requires regular suctioning, keep spare gloves and an ample supply of correct sized suction catheters at the bedside.

Pitfalls

- Airway suctioning can lead to tracheobronchial trauma, hypoxia, pneumothorax, cardiovascular changes, intracranial pressure alterations, bacterial infection, and other complications.
- ❶ There may be specific complications when there is a head injury.
- Use of irritants should only be considered on the advice of medical staff—not all the solution is recovered on suctioning, there is a risk of inhalation, and it is frightening and uncomfortable for the child.
- Yankeur's are not to be used for nasal suctioning.
- Physiotherapists may utilize airways, and deep suctioning techniques; these should not be used unless the person is appropriately trained and understands the further risks.

Associated reading

Moore, T. (2003). Suctioning techniques for the removal of respiratory secretions *Nurs Standard*. **18**(9), 47–53.

Obtaining a nasopharyngeal aspirate

Obtaining a nasopharyngeal aspirate

Background

A nasopharyngeal aspirate (NPA) is a procedure where a sample is taken from the nasopharyngeal space by inserting a suction catheter into the nostril. It is most commonly taken to detect the presence of respiratory virus in conditions such as bronchiolitis.

Equipment

- Suction unit and tubing.
- Correct size suction catheter. Catheter should be <50% size of nostril.
- Oxygen.
- NPA collection pot.
- Blanket.
- Vial/ampule NaCl.
- Non-sterile gloves.
- Sample request form.

Procedure

- Explain procedure to parent/carer and gain informed consent. Discuss with the parents/carer whether they would like to stay or leave as some would prefer not to be present for procedure.
- Collect and prepare the equipment.
- The procedure may require two staff; one to perform procedure, whilst the other can assist holding the child still.
- If patient is an infant, wrap in blanket.
- The child should be in either a lateral position so if the child vomits there is less risk of aspiration, or a supine position with head slightly extended.
- Put on gloves.
- Ensure suction is working and set to correct pressure (see 📖 Performing suctioning, p. 342).
- Attach suction catheter and suction tubing to NPA collection pot.
- Switch on suction.
- Insert catheter into the nostril to the pharangeal space without applying suction pressure.
- Occlude suction port to apply negative pressure to obtain sample.
- Withdraw catheter, whilst keeping port occluded.
- Suction up to 5mL of 0.9% NaCl to ensure collection of sample is in the pot, and check there are visible secretions.
- Turn off suction.
- Place separate lid onto the NPA pot to secure sample and place equipment into appropriate clinical waste.
- Remove gloves and wash hands.
- Label NPA and send to laboratory immediately. If this cannot be done, store the NPA in a specimen fridge and send at the earliest opportunity.
- Throughout the procedure monitor the child for any signs of respiratory distress and ensure the child is safe and reassured at the end of the procedure.
- Document in the nursing notes.

Practice tips

- Ensure it is clearly documented when the NPA was taken and sent, and that results are chased. Often the result of the NPA will not alter nursing care given, e.g. in the case of suspected bronchiolitis, but parents/carer are often anxious to receive results, and the sample may indicate a different virus is present, affecting where the patient can be nursed.
- The sample should be taken in the morning; often the laboratory needs to receive the sample early to process it that day.
- Think about when you take the NPA and liaise with parents/carer, e.g. do not take immediately after a feed.
- When a NPA is required, ask medical staff to write the request form pre-procedure so the sample can be sent immediately afterwards.

Pitfalls

- Do not remove your finger from occluding the port on the suction catheter until the suction pressure has been turned off as you may lose the sample into the suction unit bottle and have to repeat the procedure.
- Ensure you obtain an adequate aspirate, as otherwise the laboratory will report insufficient sample, and the procedure will have to be repeated.

Associated reading

Heikkinen T, Marttila J, Salmi A, et al. (2002). Nasal swab versus nasopharyngeal aspirate for isolation of respiratory viruses. *J Clin Microbiol* **40**(11), 4337–9.

Inhaler and spacer use

Background

Children and young people with asthma use reliever inhalers to combat the symptoms of an exacerbation of asthma episode. These inhalers contain bronchodilator medication, which opens up the airways to improve breathing, for example salbutamol. Preventer inhalers can also be used; these are taken regularly to stop exacerbations from occurring. It is important they are used twice a day as the effect is cumulative. They normally contain corticosteroids, which work to reduce airway inflammation, for example beclometasone. There are many different inhaler devices; which inhaler a patient uses is dependent on their age and personal preference. Children <6yr are normally unable to use the turbohaler or accuhaler as they require a strong breath in to be effective.

Equipment

- Inhaler.
- Spacer.
- Prescription chart, if in hospital setting.

Procedure

To ensure that the dose is correctly delivered a child or young person using any type of inhaler should stand or sit up in order to open up their airway.

Pressurized metered-dose inhaler

- Most common type of inhaler.
- To administer one dose shake the inhaler first. This ensures that the inhaler is primed.
- The patient should exhale and place the mouthpiece of the inhaler in their mouth.
- They should then breathe in at the same time as pressing down once on the dispenser.
- They should continue to breathe in slowly and then hold their breath for 10s.
- Before taking another dose wait 30s. This gives the patient the chance to receive the dose, recover and prepare for the next dose.

Turbohaler (dry powder inhaler)

- An inhaler device that is increasingly being used.
- Remove the lid and check the number of doses left on the counter.
- Twist the bottom around and then back again until it clicks.
- The patient should exhale and then placing the mouthpiece between their lips, inhale deeply.
- They should then take it out of their mouth and hold their breath for a further 10s.

Accuhaler (dry powder inhaler)

- Check the counter for the number of doses available.
- Hold it horizontally and open the case by pushing the thumb grip until it clicks. Then push up the lever letting it click.
- The patient should exhale and place the mouthpiece in their mouth and take a deep, slow breath in.
- Then remove from the mouth and hold breath for 10s.

Autohaler

- Looks similar to the pressurized metered-dose inhaler but it is breath activated.
- To administer a dose, remove the cap and shake.
- Click the lever on the top of the autohaler.
- The patient should exhale and place the mouthpiece in their mouth.
- They then breathe in until they hear a click.
- They should continue taking their breath in and then hold their breath for a further 5s.
- Remove from mouth and breathe out.

Spacer devices

- Can be used with pressurized metered dose inhalers.
- In comparison to using the inhaler alone, more medication reaches the lungs.
- Spacers are also useful with poor inhaler technique, as the need for co-ordination is reduced.
- NICE[1] recommend that a spacer device and mask should be used with pressurized metered-dose inhalers when given to children <5yrs.
- There are two types of spacer: large volume and small volume. The child or young person's age and personal preference will determine which size is used.
- A mask can be attached to the spacer when it is being used for a baby or very young child (usually <3yrs old).
- To use the spacer, remove the cap from the inhaler, shake it and then attach it to the back of the spacer.
- The patient should then breathe out and place the mouthpiece in their mouth. If a mask is being used ensure that it covers the patient's nose and mouth and is held firmly in place for a good seal.
- Press down on the inhaler to administer one dose.
- The child should tidal breath for 5–6 breaths, or 10s.
- Remove spacer from mouth and breathe out.
- Wait at least 30s before administering another dose. Only one dose should be administered at a time.
- Spacers should be washed in warm soapy water once a month and left to air dry. More frequent cleaning should be avoided as it causes electrostatic charge.
- Spacers should be replaced every 12 months.

Practice tips

- There are many types of inhaler devices, if you are unsure how to use one, contact a specialist nurse or manufacturer for training.
- It is easier to use an inhaler after you have seen a demonstration, offer to show your patient/their carer how to use their type of inhaler. Ensure that your clinical area has spare inhalers for demonstrations.
- If young children are refusing to use an inhaler or spacer involve a play specialist.
- Steroid containing inhalers can cause problems with a patient's mouth, such as thrush. To prevent this it is important for children and young people to brush their teeth and wash their mouth out after using this type of inhaler.

Pitfalls

- Incorrect inhaler technique is very common and results in the child/young person not receiving the correct dose of their medication. Assess the patients/carers technique. Do not assume they are taking it correctly because they use it at home.
- Patients may be unaware of the variety of inhaler devices available, particularly if they have used one type for a long time.
- Patients using the turbohaler may think they have not had a dose as they may not taste anything.

[1] National Institute of Clinical Excellence. (2000). *Guidance on the Use of Inhaler Systems (Devices) in Children Under the Age of 5 years with Chronic Asthma*. NICE, London.

Nebulizer types and use

Background

Nebulization transforms a solution of a drug into a fine mist for inhalation. This method delivers higher doses of a drug than can usually be achieved by inhaler devices, although handheld inhalers with spacers are often as effective. The fine mist produced is breathed in by the child during inspiration via a close fitting face mask, tracheostomy mask or mouth piece. Nebulization therapy may be part of acute care for the child in respiratory distress or used for the chronically ill child with a long term respiratory condition (see Table 12.1).

The most common delivery system is via a jet nebulizer. This uses an extrinsic gas flow (e.g. piped oxygen, air, or a nebulizer compressor) forced through a narrow orifice to create a pressure that draws a drug from a liquid as a mist. Jet nebulizers are most commonly driven in the hospital setting by piped oxygen set at 6–0L/min.

Table 12.1 Common nebulized drugs for children

Diagnosis	Nebulized drug	Considerations
Exacerbation of asthma	Salbutamol (beta2 agonist bronchodilator)	Must be driven by oxygen in acute exacerbation of asthma 6–8L/min
	Ipratropium bromide (Antimuscarinic bronchodilator)	Must be driven by oxygen in acute exacerbation of asthma 6–8L/min
Severe croup	Adrenaline (alpha and beta adrenoceptor agonist properties)	Close monitoring required. The effects of adrenaline last for up to 3h. Obstruction may reoccur after this period
		Must be driven by oxygen 6–8L/min
	Budesonide (corticosteroid)	Candidiasis may be avoided if you clean the child's teeth or rinse mouth with water after nebulization
		Must be driven by oxygen 6–8L/min
Chronic respiratory purulent infection, e.g. cystic fibrosis	Colistin (antibacterial)	Protection against Gram –ive organisms
		Often administered by nebulizer compressor
	Dornase alpha (mucolytic)	Reduces sputum viscosity or 'stickiness' Normally used pre-physiotherapy
		Often administered by nebulizer compressor
		Mouthpieces should be used so the drug does not deposit on the child's face
Tracheostomy or palliative care	Normal saline 0.9%	Loosens secretions. Normally used pre physiotherapy
		Often administered by nebulizer compressor

Equipment

- Gas flow.
- Oxygen tubing.
- Nebulizer mask, mouthpiece, or system.
- Nebulizer acorn.
- Nebulizer solution.
- Nebulizer dilutant (if required).
- Syringe, needle, and sharps bin if solution requires drawing up.
- Prescription.
- Monitoring equipment.

Procedure

Following correct drug administration protocol:

- Undertake a complete nursing assessment of the child's respiratory condition.
- Obtain informed consent from the child/young person and/or parent/carer.
- Prepare the nebulizer solution you will require (You may need to dilute the drug with NaCl 0.9% to achieve a minimum volume). Nebulized drugs should not be mixed and given simultaneously unless expressly instructed on the prescription sheet and interactions confirmed.
- Ensure the child is sitting comfortably upright to allow for maximum lung expansion.
- Undertake a pre nebulizer peak flow recording if the child is clinically and developmentally able to do this (see 📖 Recording peak flow, p. 354).
- Put the nebulizer solution in the nebulizer 'acorn', attach the oxygen tubing at the bottom of the acorn and to your piped oxygen supply and comfortably fit the facemask over the child's nose and mouth.
- Increase the oxygen flow gradually to achieve 6–8L/min, or turn on the compressor if using compressed air to drive the nebulizer.
- Allow the nebulizer to run until almost all of the fluid has disappeared.
  - This should take approximately 10min.
  - There will be a residual volume; check with the specific manufacturer's instructions to ascertain how much.
- Undertake a complete nursing assessment of the child's respiratory condition post-nebulizer.
- Wash and dry the nebulizer pot after use in accordance with the manufacturer's instructions. Nebulizer consumables are usually single patient use.
- Undertake a post-nebulizer peak flow recording if the child is clinically and developmentally able to do this.
- Document administration and how the child tolerated the procedure.

Practice tips
- Consider what pre- and post-procedural intervention the child may require, e.g.:
  - Use of play specialists.
  - Demonstration of the procedure and listening to the nebulizer before use using a child's chosen toy. Young children are often frightened by the sudden noise of a nebulizer.
  - Age appropriate rewards such as certificates and stickers.
- A good position for nebulization is to hold the child on the parents lap, facing them towards the parent with their head on/over the parents shoulder. The nebulizer face mask can then be held close to the child's face behind the parent. This position allows for optimum lung expansion, reduces anxiety, and causes minimal disruption to the sleeping child.
- If a child is in respiratory distress and have positioned themselves comfortably sitting upright, do not attempt to move them. The child may well be compensating and moving them into an 'optimum position' may cause deterioration.

Pitfalls
- Comprehensively assess the child during nebulization. The child who cries throughout the procedure will tire easily, conversely the child who tolerates the procedure very well may be compensating.
- The proportion of drug that actually reaches the lungs during nebulization is often as low as 10%. The solution that does not reach the lungs is left in the acorn as residual volume or forms droplets on the delivery system.
- Face masks should be an appropriate size, or mouth pieces used to minimize nebulized particles near the eyes.

Associated reading

BMJ. (2009). *BNF for children*. BMJ, London.
The British Thoracic Society. (2009). *British Guideline on the Management of Asthma*. RTS, London.

Recording peak flow

Background

This is a simple test which gives an immediate indication of expiratory muscle strength and airway calibre. The peak expiratory flow rate (PEFR) is defined as the maximum flow achieved on forced expiration from a position of full inspiration and is measured in litres per min (L/min). Peak flow measurements are most frequently used as a tool to diagnose or monitor asthma control. However, they may also be used during respiratory assessment of a child, over the age of 5yrs, to provide additional information when airflow obstruction is suspected.

Equipment

- Peak flow meter.
- Disposable cardboard one–way mouthpiece.
- Detergent wipes (for cleaning between patients).
- Peak flow chart.

Procedure

- Wash and dry hands/use alcohol rub.
- Assemble equipment.
- Explain the procedure to the child/young person and parent/carer and obtain informed consent.
- Ensure pointer on meter is set at zero and hand meter to child.
- Ask the child to:
  - Stand or sit upright in a comfortable position.
  - Gently exhale.
  - Take a deep breath in through mouth.
  - Hold the meter horizontally and place lips around mouthpiece ensuring a tight seal.
  - Breathe out as hard and fast as possible into the meter.
  - Remove mouthpiece from mouth.
- Record the reading and return the pointer to zero.
- Allow child recovery time of a few seconds.
- Repeat procedure twice more.
- Document the highest of the three readings.
  - If peak flows are required regularly at home, they should be completed at the same time of the day.
  - If peak flows are taken as part of an exacerbation of asthma episode, they can be taken 15min pre- and post-bronchodilator inhalation to indicate response to treatment.

Practice tips

- Since September 2004, all peak flow meters have been manufactured to the European Standard EN 13826. There are many different types of peak flow meters available.
- Peak flow meters are labelled 'single patient use' when prescribed by a GP, however, as long as an appropriate peak flow meter is used with the recommended disposable cardboard one-way mouthpieces, meters can safely be used for multiple users. A local decontamination policy should be in place.

- The predicted peak flow value of children is determined by height.
- Peak flow values vary in children. Some children attain values in excess of their predicted value and vice versa when well. It is important to be aware of a child's best peak flow (or baseline) as during exacerbations this will help to determine the severity of the illness with increased accuracy.
- The technique of blowing into a mouthpiece may be difficult for some children. Demonstration of the technique by a healthcare professional may be helpful prior to the child undertaking the procedure.
- Encouragement of the child to blow harder can produce greater results.
- Children may need to have the procedure repeated more than 3 times if the reproducibility of results varies vastly.

Pitfalls

- Children, especially younger children, can find the technique of blowing into a peak flow meter difficult thus obtaining poor results. Technique is best taught when a child is well and regularly recorded in the home to monitor progress.
- The reliability and reproducibility of the result needs to be considered prior to it guiding clinical care.
- Potential errors resulting in unreliable results also include:
  - Lack of effective seal around the mouthpiece (need to consider size of mouthpiece especially in small children).
  - Blocking of the mouthpiece with teeth or tongue.
  - Failure to take a deep enough breath on inspiration.
  - Incorrect technique when blowing out, e.g. coughing or spitting.
  - Child's willingness to co-operate with the procedure.

Associated reading

Booker R. (2007). Peak expiratory flow measurement. *Nurs Standard*. **21**(39), 42–43.
Jevon P. (2007). Respiratory procedures. *Nurs Times*. **103**(33), 26–7.
Orr J. (2010). *The Respiratory System*. In Coyne I, Neill F, Timmins F. (eds) *Clinical Skills in Children's Nursing*. Oxford University Press, Oxford.

Recording spirometry

Background

Spirometry is a test that measures airflow and lung volumes during a forced expiratory manoeuvre from full inhalation. A spirometer measures two basic volumes:

- Forced expiratory volume in 1s (FEV_1); the volume of air expired in the first second of a forced expiration from maximal inspiration.
- Forced vital capacity (FVC), the total volume of air expired forcefully from maximal inspiration to maximal expiration.

Spirometry provides a more robust measurement of airflow obstruction than peak expiratory flow and can be used to diagnose both obstructive and restrictive lung disorders. Almost all children aged five and above can perform spirometry.

Equipment

- Calibration syringe, if required.
- Spirometer.
- Nose clip, if required.
- Filtered mouthpiece.
- Detergent wipe.
- Documentation.

Procedure

- Calibrate the spirometer (this is not always necessary; refer to local policy and guidelines).
- Explain the test to the child in language appropriate to cognitive level and obtain informed consent.
- Obtain child's height and weight (see 🕮 Measuring weight, height, and body mass index, p. 86).
- Ask about any recent illness and medication use (especially bronchodilators).
- Wash hands.
- Demonstrate the technique to child/young person, this should include:
  - Correct posture with head slightly elevated.
  - Inhale rapidly and completely.
  - Position of mouthpiece.
  - Exhale with maximum force.
- Ask child/young person to sit or stand upright. Feet should be placed firmly on the floor.
- Explain the necessity of a nose clip (for consistency) and attach. Nose clips are not always used, again, refer to local policy.
- Ask child/young person to inhale rapidly.
- Place mouthpiece in mouth and ask them to close their lips around it to form a seal.
- Ask the child/young person to 'blast' out the air in their lungs until no more air can be exhaled whilst maintaining upright position.

- Record measurements.
- Repeat procedure a minimum of 3 times.
- Record best measurements from the tests undertaken.
- Dispose of mouthpiece and nose clip.
- Clean spirometer with detergent wipe and wash hands.

Practice tips

- Children require careful instruction in the technique before beginning the test, with reinforcement and encouragement between measurements. 'Keep going' is often repeated throughout the procedure.
- Use of incentive spirometry may improve success rate and quality of manoeuvres.
- Testing children in an adult environment is discouraged.
- A minimum of three and a maximum of eight manoeuvres need to be carried out in order to obtain reproducible results. Reproducible results would be defined as the best of two measurements of FVC and FEV1 being within 5% or 100mL, whichever is greater.
- Each manoeuvre needs to be followed by a short break to allow for normal respiratory pattern to resume.
- Predicted values are referenced for Caucasian children. Adaptation of results needs to be considered for other ethnic groups.
- Quality control and calibration of equipment are vital. A log of calibration results should be maintained. All repairs or other alterations to equipment should be documented along with updates in computer software or hardware (if applicable).
- All practitioners performing spirometry should have received training.

Pitfalls

- Ensure the mouthpiece is an appropriate size for the child.
- Ensure the child does not obstruct the mouthpiece with their teeth or tongue.
- Posture is important to achieve repeatability of results—children need to be encouraged to adopt the correct position and ensure they are not leaning on chairs or tables.
- Children with neuromuscular disease may require manual assistance to guarantee an adequate seal on the mouthpiece. This intervention should be documented.
- Results need to be interpreted in association with a holistic assessment of the child to ensure an appropriate clinical decision is made.

Associated reading

Booker R. (2009). Good use of spirometry in general practice. *Practice Nurse.* **20**(10), 490–5.
Miller MR, Hankinson J, Brusasco V, et al. 2005. Standardization of spirometry. *Eur Resp J* **26**(2), 319–38.
Rosenthal M, Bain SH, Cramer D, et al. (1993). Lung function in white children aged 4 to 19 years: I—Spirometry. *Thorax* **48**(8), 794–802.

Chest physiotherapy

Background

Chest physiotherapy uses various airway clearance techniques to aid the removal of excess mucus from inside the lungs in an attempt to assist coughing, enhance effective breathing and improve ventilation of the lungs. Standard chest physiotherapy is very labour intensive and time consuming and many patients refuse to continue their programmes at home. In recent years devices have emerged which offer more independence to the patient, and are less time consuming. The paediatric physiotherapist will assess every child, suggest and plan methods and techniques to be used and help teach carers and the child as necessary. Children should be reviewed regularly and treatments altered accordingly.

Equipment

- Pillow, wedge or tilting bed (postural drainage, PD).
- Towel (percussion).
- Positive expiratory pressure (PEP) mask/mouthpiece and manometer (PEP) or oscillating positive expiratory pressure devices (OPEP) device.
- OPEP devices, e.g. flutter, acapella, or cornet.
- Stethoscope.

Procedure

Brief descriptions of chest physiotherapy techniques follow:

Postural drainage

- Uses gravity and body positioning to aid the drainage of secretions from the small airways to the large airways to be coughed up or suctioned out. Often used in conjunction with other techniques.
- The positioning of the patient depends on which lobe of the lung is affected, e.g. to clear lower lobes the child is tilted head down.

Percussion

- Form of rhythmic clapping (patting) to the chest wall to vibrate the lungs and help loosen secretions.
- Ensure the hand of the person performing the physiotherapy is cupped.
- Use a towel or layer of clothing between the hand and the chest.
- Repeated patting of the chest wall should not be painful.

Active cycle of breathing techniques

- Consists of three steps which aim to help move secretions from the smaller to larger airways.
- Breathing control (abdominal breathing) is a period of relaxed breathing keeping shoulders and upper chest relaxed.
  - Placing the child's hand on the abdomen and allowing their hand to rise gently with the breath in helps the child to understand abdominal breathing.
  - Sigh out gently, keeping shoulders relaxed.
  - Repeat.

- Deep breathing (thoracic expansion). The Upper chest should remain relaxed with most movement occurring in the lower chest.
  - Sitting in an upright position, take a very slow deep breath in through the nose to the absolute maximum possible.
  - Pause at the end of the full breath for 3–4s.
  - Breathe out through the mouth actively using tummy muscles, but without force.
- Forced expiratory technique (Huff), a forced, breath out.
  - Squeeze abdominal muscles while keeping the mouth and throat open.
  - One or two huffs are followed by a period of breathing control.

Autogenic drainage

- Autogenic drainage (AD) is a series of breathing techniques that uses controlled breathing and minimal coughing to increase the flow of air in the lungs, moving secretions.
- Begins with a period of breathing control followed by three stages:
  - *Mobilizing phase*—breathe out as far as possible, take a small breath in; resist any desire to cough. Repeat at least 3 times. Crackles may be heard.
  - *Collecting phase*—change to medium sized breaths as the sound of the crackles gets louder. Repeat at least 3 times.
  - *Clearing phase*—take long, slow, full breaths to absolute maximum. Repeat for at least 3 breaths. Follow with gentle, but active huffs or cough.
- AD should be continued until mucus is cleared, or the child needs a rest.
- Devices such as the flutter or cornet valve can be used.

Positive expiratory pressure

- Helps to open up airways and get air behind secretions.
- A number of devices are available to give PEP.
- The PEP device has a range of coloured expiratory resisters and a manometer to check the pressure at which the child is breathing out. As the child breathes out the resistance splints open the airways.
- With mask tight against mouth, or via mouthpiece, take a normal breath in and out. Repeat 8–10 times.
- Follow this with 1–2 huffs/cough.
- Period of breathing control.
- Repeat cycle until chest feels clear, usually about 15min.

Oscillating positive expiratory pressure devices

- These devices combine vibration of the airways with PEP.
- Includes the Flutter, the Acapella, and the Cornet.
- *The Flutter*: a small pipe shaped device which contains a metal ball in a cone. During the breath out the ball moves up and down in the cone and interrupts the flow of air, giving an intermittent "back pressure" to the airways as well as causing them to vibrate.
- *The Cornet*: a curved hard plastic tube within which sits a soft flexible rubber tube. The degree of PEP and vibration can be altered by changing the twist in the rubber tube.

- *The Acapella:* consists of a plastic outer shell, inside which is a lever and magnets. The lever action and the attraction between the magnets during the breath out provide vibration and PEP. The degree of PEP and vibration can be altered by a dial at the end of the device.
- All the OPEP devices are used in the same way. The cycle is repeated until the chest feels clear, usually about 15min:
  - Usually from a sitting position instruct the child to slowly inhale to 3/4 maximum breathing capacity.
  - Hold breath for 2–3s then exhale over 3–4s not too forcefully, through the device.
  - It is important to inhale slowly, breath hold and suppress the urge to cough.
  - Perform about 10 breaths. Complete with 2–3 huffs/coughs.

Practice tips

- Techniques require the child/young person's tolerance; try to negotiate a programme or device that they want to use and can be used at home.
- If the child/young person is prescribed bronchodilator inhalers, make sure the patient has these at least 10min before physiotherapy starts.
- Physiotherapy is more effective when secretions need clearing.
  - Early in the morning before getting out of bed can be a good time.
  - Leave about 1h after a meal and 30min after a drink.
- Thorough cleaning and drying is vital for all physiotherapy devices as unwashed devices can harbour bacteria.
- Breathing exercises can be as simple as playing games like blow football, blowing bubbles, playing a wind instrument gently, swimming. A large exercise ball can work well in postural drainage.
- With the Flutter device the steel ball inside can be a choking hazard; do not allow young children to play with this device.

Pitfalls

- Chest physiotherapy is contraindicated where there has been a head injury, frank hemoptysis, fractured ribs or brittle bones, recent surgery where child is in pain or irritable, spinal cord injury or the child is unstable from a cardiac or respiratory perspective.
- Patients should be observed for increased respiratory distress evidenced by changes in vital signs or hypoxemia, and treatment slowed or discontinued if warranted.

Associated reading

Prassad SA, Orska T, Ferguson K, et al. (2007). *Physiotherapy Treatment. Airway Clearance Techniques.* Cystic Fibrosis Trust Factsheet. CFT, Bromley.

Morrison L, Agnew J. (2009). Oscillating devices for airway clearance in people with CF. *Cochrane Database Syst Rev* **21**(1), CD006842.

Tracheostomy care

Background

Equipment

Technique

Tracheostomy care

Background

A tracheostomy is an artificial opening made into the trachea through the anterior neck, where the tube then sits, providing an airway on either a temporary or permanent basis. Reasons for a tracheostomy include obstruction, trauma or a congenital abnormality. There are different types of tubes, some cuffed/uncuffed (cuffed tubes are less common as there is a risk of stenosis),[1] plastic/metal (often plastic), some with an inner tube. This will alter care, so ensure you are familiar with the tracheostomy the child/young person has.

Equipment

- Suction catheter of correct size.
- Suction equipment (see 📖 Performing suctioning, p. 342).
- Oxygen equipment, including a tracheostomy mask.
- HME.
- Gauze.
- Normasol sachet.
- Gallipot.
- Dressing if necessary.
- Neck roll.
- Gloves.
- *Emergency equipment:* ensure emergency tracheostomy equipment is kept at the patient's bedside at all times, and is taken with them on excursions:
  - A spare tracheostomy tube of same size and make.
  - A tracheostomy tube that is one size smaller, same make.
  - Spare inner tube (if required).
  - A water-based lubricant.
  - Round ended scissors.
  - Tracheal dilators (this will vary due to potential damage caused, refer to local policy).
  - Spare tracheostomy tapes.
  - 2mL syringe and 0.9% NaCl.

Tracheostomy care

The following is required as part of tracheostomy care:
- Tube change (see 📖 Tracheostomy tube change, p. 306).
- Tape change (see 📖 Tracheostomy tape change, p. 308).
- Suction (see 📖 Performing suctioning, p. 342).
- Humidification (see 📖 Humidification, p. 340).
  - Normal humidification does not occur as upper airway is bypassed, therefore humidification is necessary.
  - HME's are used, although not in the first week of tracheostomy formation.

- *Care of the stoma site:*
  - This is to ensure the tracheostomy site is kept clean and dry in order to prevent development of respiratory infection and to avoid secretions from irritating and causing breakdown of surrounding skin as well as preventing fungal skin infection.
  - Should be undertaken daily.
  - Examine the site and neck for any redness, rash, or signs of infection, including the back of the neck.
  - Swab if infection suspected.
  - Clean with normasol and non-shearing gauze, moving from the stoma site outwards.
  - Do not use cotton wool as fibres may enter stoma site.
  - Generally a clean technique can be used, but refer to local policy.
- Teaching parents/carers in all aspects of tracheostomy care for preparation for home is vital.
- Always consider the comfort of the child, and use of play specialist as appropriate.
- Commencement of feeding, and use of speaking valves will be decided with a consultant, and speech and language therapy.
- Document all care.

Practice tips

- Dressings should only be used when needed and not routinely due to risk of tube displacement and infection. Gauze as a dressing should not be used as fibres may enter the stoma site.

Pitfalls

- Care of the tracheostomy in the first week of formation is specific and differs to normal care that proceeds after this period, thus the child/ young person should be cared for in an appropriate environment by nurses that are competent to do this.
- Ensure those caring for a child with a tracheostomy have sufficient knowledge and training or are supervised by a nurse who is; if you identify that you require further skills in this area seek out education and supervised practice.

Associated reading

NHS Quality Improvement Scotland, 2008. *Best practice statement: caring for the child/young person with a tracheostomy.* NHS Quality Improvement, Scotland.

[1] Wilson M. (2005). Paediatric tracheostomy. *Paediat Nurs* **17**(3), 38–44.

Using non-invasive ventilation

Key concepts

Non-invasive ventilation (NIV) is commonly used in high dependency care or intensive care settings to treat both acute and chronic respiratory failure in children. The aim of NIV is to prevent worsening respiratory failure/distress whilst minimizing the patients' discomfort. The need for intubation or a tracheostomy is thus reduced and the risks associated with mechanical ventilation are avoided. The use of NIV for children on long-term ventilation at home or in hospital means that it can be used in settings other than paediatric intensive care.

NIV can be used for children with a variety of clinical conditions such as acute respiratory failure, obstructive sleep apnoea, neuromuscular disease, chronic lung disease, cardiac disease, and weaning from invasive ventilation.

The 3 most frequently utilized methods of NIV in children are: negative pressure, continuous positive airway pressure (CPAP) and bi-level positive airway pressure (BiPAP).

Negative pressure

- The Hayek RTX respirator (biphasic cuirass ventilation) is the optimum method of delivering negative pressure ventilation.
- Biphasic cuirass ventilation (BCV) works using a non-invasive cuirass or shell, attached to a power unit which actively controls both phases of the respiratory cycle (the inspiratory and expiratory phases).
- Inspiration is initiated by an extra thoracic negative pressure which leads to the lungs expanding and drawing in air.
- The result is an increase in the patient's functional residual capacity (FRC) if there is constant negative pressure throughout the respiratory cycle.
- Advantages of BCV are that it avoids any interference with the airway, it is most like the normal physiology of respiration and it has minimal haemodynamic disturbance.
- The main disadvantages are the noise of the machine; the cuirass jacket can be frightening difficult for the small child.

Continuous positive airway pressure

- The indications for using CPAP are primarily to promote respiratory function, decrease the work of breathing, and improve oxygenation.
- CPAP is delivered by a set flow of continuous positive pressure in order to prevent alveoli collapse.
- The aim of CPAP is to increase the FRC, which is the volume of air in the lungs at the end of expiration, thereby increasing the surface area available for gas exchange.
- CPAP is most likely used for infants with bronchiolitis, apnoea, or for children with obstructive sleep apnoea.
- There are several different machines that are available which can deliver CPAP both non-invasively and invasively. Commonly, the infant flow system is used for infants (<10kg) and the nippy junior for children (>10kg).

- CPAP can be delivered with a face mask or nasal prongs or in some cases, invasively through an endotracheal tube or tracheostomy.
- Advantages to using CPAP are that it decreases the work of breathing, improves oxygenation and gas exchange and if tolerated, can avoid the need for intubation.
- Disadvantages are that it may not be well tolerated, causing agitation, and compound the respiratory distress.
- NIV CPAP is contraindicated in the patient who is not spontaneously breathing or who has a reduced level of consciousness because there is no back up breath rate.

Bi-level positive airway pressure

- The indications for using BiPAP are predominantly the same as for CPAP (see 🕮 Continuous positive airway pressure, p. 364).
- BiPAP works by combining the benefits of pressure support ventilation (PSV) and CPAP, and keeps the lungs open during the entire respiratory cycle.
- Inspiratory pressure causes lung inflation and expiratory pressure prevents alveolar collapse and both can be manipulated and set on the BiPAP machine. Rate and spontaneous timed mode can also be controlled (back-up breaths are delivered if the patient's rate of breathing falls below a preset level).
- Using BiPAP has a number of advantages: improve minute ventilation, improve oxygenation, decreased work of breathing, avoidance of intubation, sedation, and anaesthesia.
- Different machines will use different interfaces for delivery. Most commonly used in paediatrics are the nasal mask and the full face mask covering nose and mouth.
- The full face mask can be frightening for the small child, causing discomfort so attention should be paid to explanation and not adding to their distress.
- As with using CPAP, signs of agitation, haemodynamic instability, increase CO_2, confusion, pooling of secretions are signs that BiPAP is not being tolerated and medical advice and intervention is required immediately.

Procedure

Whichever method of non-invasive ventilation is used you should ensure that:

❶ Only those who are trained and assessed as competent should be involved in these procedures.

- There is an appropriate size ambubag and face mask, Guerdal airway, and suction at the bed space and that in the O_2 outlet, there is a dual bar with an oxygen meter and Schrader valve.
- That the machine is correctly set up according to the manufacturers' guidelines.
- The ventilation mode, pressures, and alarm parameters are set according to the Registrar/Consultants' prescription and Humidification is set.
- The settings, pressures, humidification temperature, and water level should be checked hourly and recorded.
- There is continuous ECG and SaO_2 monitoring.

- RR, effort, HR, SaO_2 should be recorded hourly and BP at least 4-hourly.
- There should be at least 1 peripheral intravenous (IV) cannulae and the nasogastric tube (NGT) on free drainage.
- On commencement of non-invasive ventilation a blood gas should be taken after approximately 30min. Thereafter, dependant on the child's clinical condition (minimum 4–6-hourly) or if changes are made to the settings.
- Document the bonnet size and prongs/and cuirass jacket size.
- A vest or T-shirt should be worn under the Cuirass jacket to aid with the seal and avoid pressure marking.
- Consider the need for pain relief and/or sedation and administer, if required, as per prescription monitoring the effect.

Practice tips

- If you know how to set up NIV, you will know how to troubleshoot if it alarms or if your patient's condition worsens.
- The treatment of underlying pathology should be attended to.
- Continuous monitoring of SaO_2 and CO_2 (either transcutaneously or end-tidal) are vital.
- The clinical condition of the child will dictate if the child requires intubation and intensive care, so close monitoring and assessment are crucial.
- In small children when using NIV, try to cluster cares and avoid constant handling as this can increase their oxygen demand and worsen their distress.
- When using the nasal prongs, observe for oral breathing as this can sometimes affect the delivery of the CPAP or BiPAP.
- In the older child, spend time explaining to them and their parents how the machine and interface work.
- Consider position changes 4–6-hourly and relieving the pressure of the prongs or mask.
- Use duoderm/granuflex for skin protection on the cheeks if using nasal prongs or on the bridge of the nose if using the mask.
- If NIV is not being applied as a life support or in acute situation, monitoring can be discontinued once the correct settings have been achieved.

Pitfalls

- Consider early use of NIV to avoid further respiratory deterioration and exhaustion.
- In accurate sizing of nasal prongs/mask/cuirass jacket.
- Ensure the water level in the humidifier is checked regularly so as to avoid thickening secretions.
- Agitation, abdominal distension, and decreasing SaO_2 can lead to poor delivery of NIV and worsen respiratory distress.

Further considerations

- It must be considered that if the child is requiring NIV their condition may worsen and therefore Invasive Ventilation would be required. This decision would be made by the consultant in charge and in collaboration with the Retrieval Service (see local guidelines).
- Indications for intubation are spontaneous breathing rate <8bpm, respiratory arrest, potential, or upper airway obstruction, decrease in airway protection due to poor neurological function, anticipation of worsening respiratory state due to shock, acute respiratory failure, chest trauma, hypoxaemia in spite of supplemental oxygen, inadequate respiratory muscle function, or ventilation, and unstable chest wall.
- Management of a child requiring invasive ventilation should be in an acute care setting, such as High Dependency or A&E where appropriate monitoring and staffing can be ensured until the child can be stabilized prior to transfer by the retrieval team to paediatric intensive care unit (PICU).
- As with NIV, gaining information about the underlying pathology and any previous admissions is vital to ensure that prompt, effective treatment occurs in a timely manner.

Associated reading

Corrado A, Gorini M, Villella G, et al. (1996). Negative pressure ventilation in the treatment of acute respiratory failure: an old non-invasive technique reconsidered. *Eur Resp J* **9**, 1531–44.

Samuels M, Bolt P. (2007). Non-invasive ventilation in children. *Paediatr Child Health* **17**(5), 167–73.

Thomson A. (1997). The role of negative pressure ventilation. *Arch Dis Childh* **77**(5), 454–8.

O'Neill N. (1998). Improving ventilation in children using bi-level positive airway pressure. *Pediat Nurs* **24**, 377–82.

Hazinksi MF. (1992). *Nursing Care of the Critically Ill Child,* 2nd edn. Mosby, St Louis.

Teague WG. (2005). Non-invasive positive pressure ventilation: current status in paediatric patients *Paediat Resp Rev* **6**(1), 52–60.

Assisting tube thoracostomy

Background

A tube thoracostomy or chest drain is a flexible plastic tube that is inserted through the side of the chest wall into the pleural space by a suitably trained professional. Tube thoracostomy is a traumatic procedure for child, family, and professionals. The nurse plays a vital role in preparing the child and family for the procedure, and ensuring that someone stays with the child to keep them completely still, talk to them, and divert them from what is happening.

Indications

To remove air, i.e. a pneumothorax from the pleural space, or remove fluid, i.e. a pleural effusion from the pleural space.
- Chylothorax is a collection of lymphatic fluid.
- Haemothorax is a collection of blood.
- Empyema is a collected of infected pus.

Equipment

- Sterile gloves and gown.
- Skin cleansing solution.
- Chest drain insertion kit.
- Chest drain of appropriate size—small bore drains are more comfortable 8–14 FG.
- Connecting tubing and closed drainage system-sterile drainage bottle, filled to prime level with sterile water, two chest drain clamps.
- Selection of sterile syringes and needles.
- Scalpel and blade.
- Suture material.
- Dressing.
- Specimen pots to obtain any samples for microscopy, culture, and sensitivity.
- Prescription chart and local anaesthetic, premedication, and pain relief.

Procedure

- Observations of temperature, pulse, respirations, blood pressure, oxygen saturation should be performed pre procedure.
- Administer analgesia as prescribed prior to procedure and allow time to take effect.
- This is an aseptic technique.
- The child is positioned with their arm behind their head to expose the axillary area. If this is not possible then the child can sit upright leaning over a bed table with pillow.
- The skin over the insertion area is cleaned and draped with sterile gauze.
- Local anaesthetic will be administered to the area of insertion and the underlying muscle by the person carrying out the procedure. They may also attempt to aspirate fluid from the pleural space. Any aspirate should be documented on the child's fluid balance chart.

- Once the anaesthetic has taken effect insertion of the chest drain will continue. The nurse assisting will hand over scalpel, artery forceps, drain of correct size, and connecting tubing as asked.
- Once the drain is *in situ* it will be sutured and the nurse can attach the closed drainage system to the drain.

Practice tips

- Chest drain insertion has been reported to be a painful procedure; therefore, it is vital that premedication is given and adequate pain control. Unless it is in an emergency if available use the skills of the play specialist.
- Ensure that emergency resuscitation equipment is available and accessible throughout the procedure.
- Observation of the child is vital throughout the procedure particularly respiratory assessment.
- If there is a leak from the insertion site use occlusive dressing.

Pitfalls

- The child must remain completely still during the procedure. Any movement may cause an error on the operator's part when defining the track for the drain to follow.
- It is vital that the closed drainage system is checked regularly to ensure patency of the tube as clogging can cause serious complications such as tension pneumothorax, empyema (see 📖 Care of an underwater seal chest drain, p. 374).

Associated reading

Kinjal N, Sethuraman KN, Duong D, et al. (2011). Complications of tube thoracostomy placement in the Emergency Department. *J Emerg Med* **40**(1), 14–20.

Laws D, Neville E, Duffy J. (2003). BTS Guidelines for the insertion of a chest drain. *Thorax* **58**(11), 53–9.

Roberts JR, Hedges RJ. (2004). *Clinical Procedures in Emergency Medicine*. WB Saunders Co Philadelphia.

Performing tube thoracostomy

Background

A tube thoracostomy or chest drain is a flexible plastic tube that is inserted through the side of the chest wall into the pleural space. The British Thoracic Society recommends the tube is inserted in an area described as the 'safe triangle', in the 5th intercostal space slightly anterior to the mid-axillary line (Fig 12.1). The free end of the tube is usually attached to an underwater seal, below the level of the chest. This allows the air or fluid to escape from the pleural space, and prevents anything returning to the chest.

Indications

To remove air, i.e. a pneumothorax from the pleural space, or to remove fluid, i.e. a pleural effusion from the pleural space
- Chylothorax is a collection of lymphatic fluid.
- Haemothorax is a collection of blood.
- Empyema is a collection of infected pus.

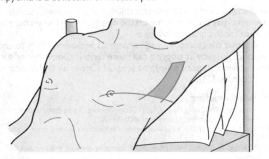

Fig. 12.1 The 'safe triangle' for insertion of a chest drain. Reproduced from *Thorax* 2003 Laws, Neville and Duffy 58 suppl II (copyright notice 2011) with permission from BMJ Publishing Group Ltd.[1]

Equipment

- Sterile gloves and gown.
- Skin cleansing solution.
- Local anaesthetic.
- Chest drain insertion kit.
- Chest drain of appropriate size—small bore drains are more comfortable 8–14 FG.
- Connecting tubing and closed drainage system—sterile drainage bottle, filled to prime level with sterile water, two chest drain clamps.
- Selection of sterile syringes and needles.
- Scalpel and blade.
- Suture.
- Dressing.
- Specimen pots to obtain any samples for microscopy, culture, and sensitivity.
- Prescription chart with appropriate premedication and pain relief.

Procedure

All staff should be trained, have had a period of supervision and be assessed as competent in the insertion of chest drain. Prior to procedure the following should be performed:

* Observations of temperature, pulse, respirations, blood pressure, oxygen saturation.
* Coagulation status: if a child is prescribed anticoagulants or is known to have coagulopathy or platelet defect.
* Administer analgesia as required prior to procedure and allow time to take effect.
* Radiological confirmation of site of insertion.
* This is an aseptic technique.
* Thorough explanation and consent should be obtained from the parents/child.
* Premedication.
* Positioning- the child is positioned with their arm behind their head to expose the axillary area. If this is not possible then the child can sit upright leaning over a bed table with pillow.
* The skin over the insertion area is cleaned and draped with sterile gauze.
* Local anaesthetic is given to the area of insertion and the underlying muscle.
* The amount and type of any fluid aspirated should be documented in the child's records and the volume recorded on the child's fluid balance chart.
* Once the anaesthetic has taken effect an incision is made just above and parallel to the rib. The incision should be slightly bigger than the professional's finger and drain.
* A track is now made through fat and muscle using curved artery forceps until the parietal pleura is reached.
* Connecting tubing and drain should be ready.
* The pleura is then breached further by pushing the forceps up over the ribs, a pop will be heard.
* The drain is inserted through the track which has been made.
* The tube is sutured in place, dressing applied, and attached to closed drainage system.
* The tube will remain in position until air; fluid has completely drained from the pleural space.
* Repeat chest X-ray to ensure correct position of drain.

Practice tips

* Chest drain insertion has been reported to be a painful procedure therefore it is vital that premedication is given and adequate pain control. Unless it is in an emergency if available use the skills of the play specialist.
* Ensure that emergency resuscitation equipment is available and accessible throughout the procedure.
* Observation of the child is vital throughout the procedure particularly respiratory assessment.
* If there is a leak from the insertion site use occlusive dressing.

Pitfalls

- The child must remain completely still during the procedure. Any movement may cause an error on the operator's part when defining the track for the drain to follow.
- It is vital that the closed drainage system is checked regularly to ensure patency of the tube as clogging can cause serious complications such as tension pneumothorax, empyema (see ☐ Care of an underwater seal chest drain, p. 374).

Associated reading

Kinjal N, Sethuraman KN, Duong D, et al. (2011). Complications of tube thoracostomy placement in the Emergency Department. *J Emerg Med* **40**(1), 14–20

Laws D, Neville E, Duffy J. (2003). BTS Guidelines for the insertion of a chest drain. *Thorax* **58**(11), 53–9.

Roberts JR, Hedges RJ. (2004). *Clinical Procedures in Emergency Medicine*. WB Saunders Co Philadelphia.

---

[1] Laws D, Neville E, Duffy J, Pleural Diseases Group, Standards of Care Committee, British Thoracic Society (2003). BTS guidelines for the insertion of a chest drain. *Thorax* **58**(Suppl. 11), ii53–9.

Care of an underwater seal chest drain

Care of an underwater seal chest drain

Background

Chest drains are inserted into the pleural space, under sedation. The indication for inserting chest drains in children is either a significant pleural fluid collection or, less commonly, a pneumothorax. The British Thoracic Society[1] recommend that children who require a chest drain insertion should be transferred to a tertiary paediatric respiratory unit for the procedure, provided the child is well enough to transport.

Equipment

- 2 non-toothed clamps.
- A bowl or similar, for chest drain bottle to safely sit it.
- Documentation.

Procedure

The following summarizes care needed whilst the chest drain is *in situ*:

- Check regularly that the tube is draining well (for frequency, refer to local policy).
- Ensure it is clearly documented the amount of fluid drained, if it is swinging, and the colour:
  - The drainage bottle should be observed for swinging to indicate that air is being evacuated from the pleural space.
  - This will decrease as the lungs re-inflate, usually over 24–72h.
- Fibrinolytics may be prescribed and administered; consult local policy.
- The chest drain bottle should not be >three-quarters full, and when changed should be done so aseptically. Clamping of the tubing is required for changing bottles.
- Ensure there is the minimum level of sterile water in the water seal chamber.
- Monitor vital signs (at least 4-hourly).
- Observe patient regularly for changes to colour, pain, or unequal chest movement. If any gasping or shortness of breath, instantly call the emergency medical team.
- Insertion of a chest drain is both painful and traumatic for children. Pain assessment and control must be given regularly throughout.
- The catheter will be stitched in place; however, a suitable dressing should be applied to prevent air entry:
  - Use of key hole dressings are recommended, and no or very light strapping to prevent undue pulling on the surrounding skin.
  - The wound site should be kept dry.
- For maximum benefit the child should be sat upright, lent towards the drain, supported by pillows.
- Educate the child and family around ensuring that the drainage bottle remains below chest height and that tubing is not kinked.
- Clamping of the tubes during movement is no longer necessary; however, ensure 2 non-toothed clamps that can be quickly applied are by the bed side in case of accidental disconnection of the tube. Never clamp a bubbling chest drain.

- Encourage patient to mobilize, with support, and have physiotherapy input where this is appropriate. If suction assistance is in operation it is likely that movement will be restricted.
- Offer mental and physical stimulation to the child, e.g. games, DVDs.
- Ensure that a chest X-ray is carried out prior to removal of catheter.

Suction
- The indications for suction remain unclear; however, the belief is that suction can aid lung re-expansion.
- Prescription of suction is a medical responsibility.
- Purpose made low grade suction units should be used when applied to a chest drain. Standard high volume, high-pressure suction units should not be used.

Practice tips
- The child/young person and family will need to be reassured constantly around the care of the drain and wound site.

Pitfalls
- The underwater seal drainage system should never be lifted above chest or wound height, as water and debris will by gravity drain back into the lungs.
- Milking and stripping the tube are now not recommended practice.

Associated reading

Balfour-Lynn IM, Abrahamson E, Cohen G, et al. (2005). *BTS Guidelines for the Management of Pleural Infection in Children*. British Thoracic Society, London.

[1] British Thoracic Society. (2008). *Guidance for the implementation of local trust policies for the safe insertion of chest drains in children, following the NPSA rapid response report*. NPSA/2008/RRR003.

Cardiovascular system

History taking and assessment

Background

As with any history taking, it is essential to gain subjective information from the child and/or parent about what they believe any problem to be. An infant or child presenting with a cardiac problem, may not be clearly identifiable to the parent, but is likely to have key information within their history that is suggestive such as:

- Difficulty breathing, particularly at rest or following feeding.
- Inability to complete a feed, or even feed at all.
- Sweating.
- Unusual weight gain or 'puffiness'.
- Parents may have observed colour change, such as pallor or cyanosis.

Cardiovascular assessment

Initial inspection would include observation for:

- Dysmorphic features.
- Skin colour, e.g. signs of cyanosis, mottling, anaemia.
- Oedema.
- Clubbing of the extremities.
- Respiratory distress.

Following observation of the infant or child, the nurse should palpate the child's pulse and record all vital signs. Palpate the pulse for 1min. In infants and children under 2yrs the brachial pulse is generally the easiest to palpate, in older alert children the radial pulse is usually chosen, or the carotid. When palpating the pulse you are examining the rate, rhythm, volume, and character, from absent, weak, normal, to bounding.

Obtaining an accurate blood pressure (BP) recording can be a challenge with young children and infants, as available equipment has limitations and mobile wriggling children do not necessitate an accurate recording. To aid this consider:

- Cuff selection (see manufacturers instruction for size guidance).
- Cuff position, generally argued as 2/3 of the distance between elbow and shoulder.
- The use of distraction to enable accurate recording.

Associated reading

Gill D, O'Brien N. (2007). *Paediatric Clinical Examination Made Easy*, 5th edn. Elsevier Churchill Livingstone, Edinburgh.

Trigg E, Mohammed T. (2006). *Practices in Children's Nursing: Guidelines for Hospital and Community*. Elsevier Churchill Livingstone, Edinburgh.

Cardiac monitoring

Background

Cardiac or electrocardiogram (ECG) monitoring measures the electrical activity within the heart, enabling an ECG complex to be transmitted onto the cardiac monitor, recorded or printed.

Once recorded, the electrical impulses will provide information including the rate and rhythm of cardiac activity, allowing the sequence to be analysed for any sign of abnormality.

❶ There are a large variety of monitors/machines available, both on the market and within practice areas, so it is important that anyone using a cardiac monitor is aware of the individual machine's functions and capabilities, and has been trained and assessed as competent in its use.

Reasons for possible cardiac monitoring

- History of cardiac disease, such as:
  - Abnormalities of conduction.
  - Ischaemic damage.
  - Hypertrophy.
- Pre- or post-cardiac surgery.
- History of syncope (fainting, loss of consciousness).
- Shocked patients or those with electrolyte disturbance.
- To monitor the potential effects of medication, either prescribed or following ingestion.

Arrhythmias

Within infants and children cardiac arrhythmias are relatively uncommon. A normal cardiac rhythm, *sinus rhythm,* is generally regular and would display a rate that is within the child's expected range for their age.

Abnormalities which may be seen with cardiac monitoring include:

- Sinus tachycardia (fast, but normal rhythm).
- Sinus bradycardia (slow, but normal rhythm).
- Supraventricular tachycardia (rate generally exceeding 220 beats per min (bpm), possibly as high as 300 bpm).
- Asystole.
- Junctional rhythm.
- Forms of heart block.

Associated reading

Advanced Life Support Group (2005). *Advanced Paediatric Life Support: A Practical Approach*, 5th edn. BMJ Books, London.

Coyne I, Neill F, Timmins F. (2010). *Clinical Skill's in Children's Nursing*. Oxford University Press, Oxford.

Davies JH, Hassell LL. (2007). *Children in Intensive Care: A Survival Guide*, 2nd edn. Churchill Livingstone, London.

12-lead electrocardiogram recording

As with 3-lead continuous cardiac monitoring, a 12-lead ECG records the electrical activity within the heart, however a 12-lead ECG provides a graphic recording of this activity and enables the heart to be examined more specifically recording information from different angles and planes.

In some cases, a 10-lead ECG will be performed.

Limb leads view the heart from the frontal plane and chest leads transversely, i.e. from the front and left side. By examining the heart from different angles, areas of concern can be isolated. Specifically leads II, III, and aVF show inferior surface activity, V1–V4 anterior surface, and leads I, aVL, V5, and V6 the lateral surface.

❶ Incorrect information may be recorded if a 12-lead ECG recording is not performed correctly therefore in order to prevent error this skill must only be performed by appropriately trained and proficient personnel.

Electrocardiogram interpretation

Before performing an ECG it is essential that you are familiar with both the normal anatomy and physiology of the heart, and the cardiac cycle. Within children's nursing, it is less common for general children's nurses to have a wealth of experience of either ECG recording or interpretation; however, it is essential that any nurse performing an ECG can interprete the basic information. This can be aided by asking the following questions:

• What is the patient's heart rate?
• Is the rate regular?
• What is the rhythm?
• Do the QRS complexes appear normal?
• Do the ST segments and T waves appear normal?

Procedure of recording a 12-lead electrocardiogram

• Gather all equipment required and ensure that you are familiar with how to operate the 12-lead ECG machine.
• Ensure you have gained the consent of the child and family, and that you have explained what you are about to do.
• You will need to position the infant or child lying down, in a warm environment, although you must protect dignity, especially with adolescent patients. You will need to access the child's chest, therefore also request that clothing is minimal or removed above the waist.
• Prepare the skin, which needs to be clean and dry, to ensure that the electrodes/probes adhere to the skin.
• Attach the limb and chest leads, as directed:

This is often very challenging in very small infants. If you find that the adhesive tabs used to attach the leads are too large to fit across the chest, and smaller paediatric alternatives are not available within your organization/practice area you may find you can cut the tabs lengthwise, as long as the lead can still be successfully attached.

- To ensure correct identification and documentation, enter the patient's details into the machine.
- Check the machine details, such as date and time are correct.
- In co-operative able children, ask them to relax and lie as still as possible. In infants and very small children attempt to encourage them to lie as still as possible. This may be achieved by sucking or feeding.
- Record the ECG. See Fig. 13.1 for a normal ECG trace.

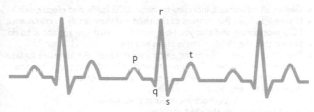

Fig. 13.1 A normal ECG trace (sinus rhythm).

Positioning of limb leads
- *Red/RA lead:* right forearm, proximal to the wrist.
- *Yellow/LA:* left forearm, proximal to the wrist.
- *Green/LL:* left lower leg, ideally proximal to the ankle.
- *Black/RL:* right lower leg, ideally proximal to the ankle.

Positioning of the chest leads
- *C1/Red (V1):* immediately right of the sternum, 4th intercostal space.
- *C2/Yellow (V2):* immediately left of the sternum, 4th intercostal space.
- *C3/Green (V3):* position in between V2 and V4.
- *C4/Brown (V4):* mid-clavicular line, 5th intercostal space.
- *C5/Black (V5):* horizontal to V4, anterior axillary line.
- *C6/Purple (V6):* remain on same horizontal line as V4 and V5, but mid-axillary line.

Associated reading

Advanced Life Support Group (2005). *Advanced Paediatric Life Support: A Practical Approach*, 5th edn. BMJ Books, London.

Coyne I, Neill F, Timmins F. (2010). *Clinical Skill's in Children's Nursing*. Oxford University Press, Oxford.

Davies JH, Hassell LL. (2007). *Children in Intensive Care: A Survival Guide*. 2nd edn. Churchill Livingstone, London.

Positioning of electrocardiogram electrodes

Background

Three-lead ECG monitoring is generally chosen for continuous ECG monitoring.

Procedure

- Gather all equipment, including monitor, ECG leads, and electrodes.
- Ensure you have the consent of the child and their family to commence ECG monitoring, and that you have explained what you are about to do.
- Ensure that the child's chest is clean and dry.
- Remove the backing from the electrodes to reveal the adhesive surface and stick the first two electrodes to both left and right shoulders and position the third on the left side of the lower chest/abdomen or if necessary left leg.
- The leads are usually colour-coded and positioned:
  - With the red to the right shoulder.
  - Yellow to the left shoulder.
  - Green to the abdomen.
- Occasionally, the monitor may have a fourth black lead, which is then positioned opposite the green lead on the right side of the abdomen.

There are a number of rhymes to help you remember lead placement such as:

Ride Your Green Bike, (Red, Yellow, Green, Black) or following the sequence of traffic lights. However, when doing this it is important to remember the rhyme or sequence follows a clockwise (as you are looking at the patient) circular motion starting from the patients right shoulder.

- Once the electrodes are positioned the leads can then be attached to the patient via the electrodes and connected to the machine to commence ECG recording.
- In order to record the ECG, switch on the machine and ensure that all aspects are working, and that a power supply is available. Check which lead is presently monitoring the patient; commonly, continuous monitoring will be recorded through lead II.

Central venous pressure monitoring

Background

Provides an indicator of child's haemodynamic state. Used commonly in paediatric intensive care units (PICUs) and high dependency (HD) areas. Pressure is monitored via a central venous catheter (see 📖 Managing central venous catheters, p. 238). As these are central access devices, those managing these lines must follow a strict aseptic technique. The trace will be shown as a softly undulating wave on the monitor. Central venous pressure (CVP) reflects the pressure of the blood returning to the right side of the heart.

Equipment

- Central venous catheter (CVC, double or triple lumen) *in situ*.
- Physiological monitor with CVP capacity.
- Non-disposable compatible pressure lead.
- Disposable pressure transducer monitoring kit.
- Pressure infuser bag or syringe driver/pump.
- Normal saline/heparinized saline (local policy).
- Sterile three-way tap.
- Sterile wipe.

Procedure

- Undertake comprehensive nursing and medical assessment.
- Discuss need for monitoring with child and family, and gain consent for procedure.
- Gather and prepare all equipment.
- Apply strict aseptic technique at all times.
- Follow local infection control policy.
- Check the prescribed fluids and prepare. Either prepare syringe or set up a pre-made bag in a pressure infuser bag.
- Label and document as per local policy.
- Prime fluid through disposable pressure transducer line ensuring the line is free from bubbles. Collect in gallipot to prevent spillage.
- ❶ NB. Most sets have an internal flush system which needs to be used to allow priming to occur.
- Inflate pressure bag (if using) to 150–200mmHg or syringe to 1–3 mL/h dependent on prescription/local policy.
- Connect non-disposable pressure lead to monitor, a CVP display should be evident.
- Connect other end of non-disposable pressure lead to the disposable pressure transducer.
- Clean end of CVC with sterile wipe and flush (according to local policy) to ensure patency. Connect with primed line.
- Commence the infusion at the prescribed rate.
- Open 3-way tap to allow infusate to flow.
- Position line so transducer is level with heart/mid axilla.
- Ensure patency of line (not trapped or kinked).
- The transducer must be calibrated at zero pressure.
- A wave form will be evident on monitor.
- Scale to be set so whole wave form can be seen and limits set.
- Normal values 0–5mmHg.

Practice tips

- Following insertion CVC position should be confirmed by X-ray/ ultrasound scan (USS).
- Document following insertion of line and commencement of monitoring.
- Zero CVP and monitor each shift and document.
- Low CVP readings indicate hypovolaemia.
- Measuring the trend is important to gain an understanding of the child's fluid status.
- High CVP reading indicates fluid overload.
- Falling CVP:
  - Fluid loss (haemorrhage, vomiting, burns, ketoacidosis).
  - Inappropriate use of diuretics.
  - Systemic vasodilation (medication, sepsis, neurogenic shock).
- Elevating BP:
  - CVC occlusion.
  - Fluid overload.
  - Systemic vasoconstriction.
  - Heart failure.
  - Increased intrathoracic pressure.

Pitfalls

- Observe for ectopic beats following insertion of CVC as tip of catheter may be resting against cardiac tissue. If this occurs CVC should be repositioned.
- CVC can also be used for administering drugs and obtaining blood samples. If regular blood gases are needed then an arterial line should be placed.
- Ensure 3-way tap is correctly used to prevent potential exsanguination and contamination of line.

Associated reading

Woodrow P. (2002). Central venous catheters and central venous pressure. *Nurs Stand* **16**(26), 45–51.

Blood pressure measurement

Background

- Blood pressure measurement can be used to diagnose chronic conditions, such as chronic kidney disease or cardiac disease.
- It can also be used to assess a child's condition following or during treatment.
- Blood pressure should be measured at least once per hospital attendance to obtain a baseline measurement for each child.

How is blood pressure measured?

Invasive

BP measurements, such as arterial BP monitoring enable continuous direct readings to be obtained, via an arterial line connected to a monitoring system. This is commonly used in critical care areas, but it is not practical or 'child friendly' for most environments.

Non-invasive methods

These are more appropriate for clinics and general environments. Two types are commonly used:

Automated (oscillometric) methods

- Provide readings with little intervention from the nurse.
- Pressure changes in the cuff are compared with BP data stored in the machine and readings provided accordingly.
- The machines pump up to pre-determined levels, and if the child is mobile and/or upset several attempts may be made to obtain a reading.
- Some machines pump up higher with repeated attempts.

Manual sphygmomanometers

More labour intensive for the nurse, requiring the interpretation of sounds heard either via stethoscope or Doppler ultrasound device. However, the nurse has more control over the reading, and can increase accuracy and comfort of the patient accordingly.

What are the readings required?

The systolic pressure is the higher number and related to the contraction of the heart muscle. During manual measurement this is identified when the first pulse sounds are heard returning. This is known as Korotkoff Phase 1.

The diastolic pressure is associated with the heart muscle relaxing. This is not heard when using a Doppler device. Using a stethoscope it is identified by the disappearance of all noise (Phase 5 Korotkoff sound) in most patients. Phase four, when sounds appear to become muffled should be used in patients in whom the sounds do not disappear.

Procedure

- Explain procedure appropriately and gain consent.
- The child or young person should sit down for 3min before a reading is taken, as exercise can cause a false high reading.
- The child should be comfortable and the limb used for measurement supported and relaxed.
- Where possible an arm should be used for the reading.
- The same limb and cuff should be used each time to ensure each reading is comparable.
- The cuff should be selected to ensure that the inflation area/bladder covers at least 80% of the limb circumference. Most modern cuffs have a range indicator to assist in selection. If several cuffs fit, select the cuff with the longest width. Cuffs that are too small will give an inaccurately high reading and vice versa.

Good practice specific to manual measurement

- Estimate systolic pressure by palpating the pulse whilst pumping the cuff. The systolic pressure is determined when the pulse disappears. Release the pressure.
- Pump to 30mmHg over the estimated pressure once stethoscope or Doppler applied. This ensures the most accurate reading possible.
- Deflate the cuff at 2mmHg/s listening for the sounds appearing and then disappearing. Release all of the pressure within the cuff once the second sound is heard.
- Ensure the child is comfortable.
- Record the reading to the nearest 2mmHg, do not round up or down, to ensure the most accurate possible record is made.

When a Doppler device is used with small children it may be necessary to use two nurses as this ensures accuracy, particularly if the child is moving during the procedure. The systolic reading only can be heard.

Interpretation of readings

- Treatment should not be commenced based upon a single BP reading in isolation.
- The environment, stress and anxiety, discomfort, and equipment functioning amongst other factors can affect the accuracy of readings.
- Trends in BP and consideration of other influencing factors and patient observations should always be considered.
- BP increases with age and size of child.
- Centile charts for BP are available for reference to ensure the correct norm is used for comparison, see 📖 Associated reading, p. 387.

Associated reading

National High Blood Pressure Education Program Working Group on High Blood Pressure in Children and Adolescents (2004). The Fourth report on the diagnosis, evaluation, and treatment of high blood pressure in children and adolescents. *Pediatrics*, **114**, 555–76.

Cardiopulmonary arrest and basic life support

- Cardio-respiratory arrest is much less common in children than in adults.
- There are distinct differences between the arrest of cardiac origin, seen predominantly in adults, and the asphyxial arrest, which occurs commonly in children.
- Where children do suffer cardiac arrest it is more likely to be secondary to respiratory aetiology.

❶ All health professionals working with children should receive regular training and update on basic life support (BLS) procedures.

National guidelines on resuscitation are published by the Resuscitation Council (UK) (℘ http://www.resus.org.uk/pages/guide.htm) and include guidance and algorithms for:

- Basic life support.
- In-hospital resuscitation.
- Advanced life support.

Procedure

- Ensure the safety of rescuer and child.
- Check the child's responsiveness:
  - Gently stimulate the child and ask loudly, 'Are you all right?'
  - Do not shake infants or children with suspected cervical spine injuries.
- If the child does not respond:
  - Shout for help.
  - Turn the child onto his back and open the airway. Use the neutral position for infants up to 1yr; sniffing position for child above 1yr and up to 8yrs; full head tilt for those over 8yrs (see Box 13.1).

❶ Take great care if you suspect neck injury, but remember that establishing an open airway is imperative.

- Keeping the airway open, look, listen, and feel for normal breathing for no more than 10s:
  - Look for chest movements.
  - Listen at the child's nose and mouth for breath sounds.
  - Feel for air movement on your cheek.

In the first few minutes after cardiac arrest a child may be taking infrequent, noisy gasps. Do not confuse this with normal breathing.

- If the breathing is not normal or absent:
  - Carefully remove any obvious airway obstruction. Do not put fingers into mouth as the delicate palate of the infant could be damaged or a foreign body pushed further in.
  - Give five initial rescue breaths.
- Assess the child's circulation (signs of life). Take no more than 10s to:
  - Look for signs of life. These include any movement, coughing, or normal breathing (not abnormal gasps or infrequent, irregular breaths).
  - If you check the pulse take no more than 10s. In a child aged over 1yr feel for the carotid pulse; in an infant, feel for the brachial pulse; for both infants and children the femoral pulse can also be used.

Box 13.1 Respiration methods in infants and young children

Rescue breaths for an infant
- Ensure a neutral position of the head
- Take a breath and cover the mouth and nasal apertures of the infant with your mouth, making sure you have a good seal. If the nose and mouth cannot both be covered in the older infant, the rescuer may attempt to seal only the infant's nose or mouth with his mouth (if the nose is used, close the lips to prevent air escape)
- Blow steadily into the infant's mouth and nose over 1–1.5s sufficient to make the chest rise visibly
- Maintain head position and chin lift, take your mouth away, and watch for his chest to fall as air comes out
- Take another breath and repeat this sequence four more times

Rescue breaths for a child over 1yr
- Ensure 'sniffing' position of head
- Pinch the soft part of his nose closed
- Open his mouth a little, but maintain the chin lift
- Take a breath and place your lips around his mouth, making sure that you have a good seal
- Blow steadily into his mouth over about 1–1.5s sufficient to make the chest rise visibly
- Maintaining head tilt and chin lift, take your mouth away and watch for his chest to fall as air comes out
- Take another breath and repeat this sequence four more times.

- If there are no signs of life, unless you are *certain* that you can feel a definite pulse of greater than 60 beats per minute within 10s:
  - Start chest compression.
  - Combine rescue breathing and chest compression.
- For all children, compress the lower half of the sternum:
  - To avoid compressing the upper abdomen, locate the xiphisternum and compress the sternum one finger's breadth above this.
  - Compression should depress the sternum by at least one-third of the depth of the chest.
  - Don't be afraid to push too hard. Push 'hard and fast'.
  - Release the pressure completely, then repeat at a rate of 100–120 beats per minute.
  - After 15 compressions, tilt the head, lift the chin, and give two effective breaths.
  - Continue compressions and breaths in a ratio of 15:2.

The best method for compression varies slightly between infants and children (Box 13.2).
- Continue resuscitation until:
  - The child shows signs of life (normal breathing, cough, movement or definite pulse of greater than 60 beats per minute).
  - Further qualified help arrives.
  - You become exhausted.

Box 13.2 Chest compression methods in infants and young children

Chest compression in infants
- The lone rescuer should compress the sternum with the tips of two fingers
- If there are two or more rescuers, use the encircling technique:
- Place both thumbs flat, side by side, on the lower half of the sternum, with the tips pointing towards the infant's head
- Spread the rest of both hands, with the fingers together, to encircle the lower part of the infant's rib cage with the tips of the fingers supporting the infant's back
- Press down on the lower sternum with your two thumbs to depress it at least one-third of the depth of the infant's chest

Chest compression in children aged over 1yr
- Place the heel of one hand over the lower half of the sternum (as described for infants)
- Lift the fingers to ensure that pressure is not applied over the child's ribs
- Position yourself vertically above the victim's chest and, with your arm straight, compress the sternum to depress it by at least one-third of the depth of the chest
- In larger children, or for small rescuers, this may be achieved most easily by using both hands with the fingers interlocked.

❶ It is vital for rescuers to get help as quickly as possible when a child collapses:
- When more than one rescuer is available, one (or more) starts resuscitation, while another goes for assistance.
- If only one rescuer is present, undertake resuscitation for about 1min before going for assistance.

The only exception to performing 1min of cardiopulmonary resuscitation (CPR) before going for help is in the case of a child with a *witnessed, sudden collapse*, when the rescuer is alone. In this situation, a shockable rhythm is likely and the child may need defibrillation. Seek help immediately if there is no one to go for you. See Box 13.3 for the paediatric basic life support algorithm.

❶ Box 13.3 Paediatric basic life support algorithm

- Unresponsive?
  - Shout for help
  - Open airway
- Not breathing normally?
  - Five rescue breaths
- No signs of life?
  - 15 chest compressions
  - 2 rescue breaths
  - 15 compressions
- ❶ Call resuscitation team.

Practice tips

- Palpation of the pulse should not be the sole determinant of the need for chest compressions. You should also determine the presence or absence of 'signs of life', such as response to stimuli, cyanosis, normal breathing (rather than abnormal gasps), or spontaneous movement.
- The decision to start CPR should take less than 10s from beginning the initial assessment of the child's circulatory status and if there is still doubt after that time, CPR should be initiated.
- Shockable rhythms are unusual in children under 1yr of age and the main focus of resuscitation should be on good-quality CPR.
- Interruptions are minimized by not stopping compressions during defibrillator charging, immediate resumption after shock delivery and continuing without a pause for breaths, once the trachea is intubated.
- To minimize interruptions in CPR, it may be possible to carry an infant or small child, whilst summoning help.

Useful website

Access ℘ http://www.resus.org.uk for full details on:
- Basic life support.
- In-hospital resuscitation.
- Advanced life support.

Feeding the cardiac infant

Background

Meeting the nutritional needs of a needs child/baby with a congenital heart defect (CHD) can present as a challenge for the nurse/carer. This is because:

- Metabolic rate is raised.
- Increased heart and respiratory rates.
- Calorific requirements are greater.
- Fatigue causes inability to take sufficient amounts.

The carer should monitor the infant carefully during feeding, and not allow them to continue to the point of excessive fatigue and exhaustion. Referral to a paediatric dietician within either the hospital setting or community is important to ensure formula is supplemented as per local policy.

Procedure

- Allow the infant to be well rested and fed soon after wakening.
- Feeding 3-hourly works for the majority of infants.
- The feeding regime should be individualized to each infant.
- A teat with a larger hole, making sucking easier and thus decreasing energy expenditure (but not to cause flooding), may be beneficial.
- Position in semi-upright position.
- Rest frequently.
- Stimulate jaw and cheeks by stroking to encourage sucking.
- Limit feeding time to 30min to reduce exhaustion.

Practice tips

- Mothers who wish to breast feed should be encouraged to either alternate each feed with a breast feed and then high calorific bottle feed, or express their milk and supplement.
- Some infants will require feeding via a nasogastric tube (NGT) for a period of time to provide total nutritional support or to supplement oral feeding. Local policy should be adhered to.
- Some infants with severe CHD and a neurological dysfunction may need feeding via a gastrostomy tube.
- Fluid restriction is often required for these infants (post-operatively or during time of times of cardiac failure).
- Feeds should be calculated over a 24-h period and the nurse should aim to feed during waking hours.
- With toddlers and infants it is recommended that fluids are given in small cups to give the appearance of a full container.

Associated reading

Hockenberry M, Wilson D. (2007). *Wong's Nursing Care of Infants and Children*, 8th edn. Mosby, St Louis.

Neurological system

Neurological assessment and observations

Background

Paediatric neurological observations are used to establish the neurological status of a child. This involves carrying out an assessment using an adapted Glasgow or Adelaide coma scale. All patients who require neurological observations will be assessed with regard to limb movement, responsiveness, pupil reaction and vital signs.

Neurological observations should be carried out by a competent healthcare professional who will act appropriately to the findings. Paediatric coma charts are available for use with children of 2yrs of age and under, and for those over 2yrs old.

Equipment

- Neurological observation chart (age appropriate).
- Sphygmomanometer or multi parameter monitor.
- Stethoscope.
- Pen torch.
- Millimeter scale for pupil measurement.
- Temperature monitoring equipment.
- Relevant local procedure documents for recording of neurological observations, blood pressure (BP), pulse, respiratory rates (RR), and temperature recording.

Procedure

- Wash hands and apply alcohol gel.
- Explain procedure to the child and family.

Modified paediatric coma scale

Eye opening

Assess for eye opening, score, and document appropriately.

- *4 Eyes open spontaneously*: recorded when the child has their eyes open without the need for stimulus and indicates arousal mechanisms of the brainstem are active.
- *3 Eyes open to voice*: when eyes open to a clear, loud command, indicating the auditory sensory pathway is functioning. This is an abnormal response indicating a depressed level of consciousness and not to be confused with waking a sleeping child who should receive a score of 4.
- *2 Eyes open to pain:* if no response to voice a painful stimulus is used, see local policy for guidance and ensure an explanation is provided to child and family prior to inflicting this. The requirement for painful stimuli indicates a depressed level of consciousness.
- *1 No eyes opening*: in spite of voice and pain stimulus the child does not open their eyes, indicating the arousal mechanisms of the brain stem are inactive.

Verbal/grimace

Assess verbal/grimace response in line with the child's development and ability, score and document appropriately.

- *Grimace response:* non-verbal/intubated patients.
- *Child/Infant response:* prelingual patients.
- *Adult/Child response:* lingual patients.
- *5:* recorded if the patient has normal facial activity, normal verbal ability appropriate for age, or is able to provide an appropriate verbal response to a question, for example 'What is your name?' This relies on the nurse being aware of what is a normal response for that child and indicates that the cognitive centres of the brain are functioning properly.
- *4:* recorded if the child has, less than usual facial/oromotor activity or is only evident following touch stimuli, or if the patient is unable to answer trigger questions appropriately indicating neurological deterioration.
- *3:* recorded if the child displays a vigorous grimace to painful stimulus; if the child, has an irritable or inappropriate cry; or there is limited or absent understandable conversation.
- *2:* recorded if the child displays a mild grimace to painful stimuli, occasionally whimpers or moans or makes incomprehensible sounds without recognizable words.
- *1:* recorded if the child displays no response to painful stimuli, indicating malfunction of the cognitive centres of the brain.

Motor response

Assess best motor response, score, and document appropriately.

- *6:* the child should be able to obey a simple command and should be able to do this twice, or normal spontaneous movements should be observed.
- *5:* when a patient locates and attempts to remove a painful stimulus.
- *4:* withdraws to painful stimulus without localizing or does not withdraw to touch.
- *3:* abnormal flexion to painful stimulus, decorticate posturing is displayed.
- *2:* abnormal extension to painful stimulus, deccerebrate posturing is displayed.
- *1:* no response to painful stimulus.

Assessment of limb movement

- Assess each limb, score, and document appropriately.
- Assessed in upper and lower limbs by asking the child to perform tasks independently and then again with the assessor applying force in the opposing direction that the limb is moving. In young children assessment of spontaneous limb movement is used.
- Limb strength is graded as normal power, mild weakness, severe weakness.
- If the patient is unconscious central painful stimulus may be applied to elicit movement—ensure local policy is followed.

Pupil assessment
Assess pupil response, score, and document appropriately.
- Reduce external bright light.
- Observe pupils simultaneously using a millimeter scale to assess size and shape. Pupils are normally equal and round any deviation from this may suggest raised intracranial pressure (ICP).
- Shine a torch into each eye moving from the outer aspect of each eye. The pupils should constrict immediately and withdrawal of the light should cause equal dilatation.
- Unequally constricting/dilating pupils indicates constriction of the oculomotor nerve.

Vital signs
Assess and document the child's pulse, respiratory rate, pattern, blood pressure, and temperature in accordance with local policy. The brain has limited compensatory methods when intra cranial pressure is raised; alterations in a child's vital signs indicate utilization of these compensatory methods. Cushing's triad refers to a group of signs and symptoms suggesting the brains compensatory methods are failing and is a pre- terminal sign.
- *Tachycardia* may indicate haemorrhage in a trauma patient or reduction in parasympathetic tone or increase in sympathetic tone in neurological impairment.
- *Bradycardia* is seen in the later stages of increased intra cranial pressure and is indicative of Cushing's triad. NB. This is a pre-terminal sign.
- *BP:* the brain uses an auto-regulatory system to respond to alterations in blood pressure utilizing vasoconstriction and dilatation. When ICP is high cerebral perfusion is reduced, in an attempt to rectify this the systolic blood pressure is elevated however, the diastolic remains relatively stable this resulting widening pulse pressure is indicative of Cushing's triad.
- *Respiratory rate:* changes in the pattern and rate of breathing can indicate alterations in the function of the brain stem.
- *Increased Respiratory rate:* In an attempt to reduce ICP the respiratory rate is elevated the resultant reduction in carbon dioxide causes vasoconstriction which reduced blood flow to the brain.
- *Cheyne stoke and cluster breathing:* respirations are erratic in rate and pattern and indicate a sudden rise in intra cranial pressure, indicative of Cushing's triad.
- *Temperature* alterations may be caused by damage to the hypothalamus which acts as the bodies temperature control centre.
- *Hyperthermia* increases the child's metabolic rate and therefore oxygen and glucose requirement. Carbon dioxide produced as a by-product will cause vasodilatation and an increase in intracranial pressure.
- *Hypothermia* as a result of damage to the brain stem or hypothalamus causes peripheral vasoconstriction increasing blood flow to the brain and may cause worsening bradycardia.

Practice tips

- Awareness of the child's normal abilities is useful when conducting neurological observations. Clear documentation of what is normal for them and collaboration with parents/carers is key to successful and reliable assessment whenever possible.
- An irritable or inappropriate cry is characterized by a high pitched wailing sound and an inconsolable child despite addressing needs of daily living.

Pitfalls

- Patients who have been transferred from other hospitals may have some degree of disorientation which is understandable.
- Some children may always have unequal or abnormally shaped pupils; parents may be able to help with assessment.

Associated reading

Advanced life support group. (2004). *Advanced paediatric life support: the practical approach*. BMJ Books, London.

Kirkham FJ, Newton CR, Whitehouse W. (2008). Paediatric coma scales. *Develop Med Child Neurol* **50**, 267–74.

Waterhouse C. (2005). The Glasgow Coma scale and other neurological observations. *Nurs Stand* **19**, 56–64.

Assisting with lumbar puncture

Background
Performed to obtain a specimen of cerebrospinal fluid (CSF) from the subarachnoid space, to aid diagnosis of meningitis, encephalitis, and other neurological conditions, remove excess fluid, or inject medication. CSF is normally a clear, colourless and sterile liquid.
❶ Performed by an experienced doctor.

Equipment
- Lumbar puncture (LP) set.
- LP needles (appropriate sizes; see Table 14.1).
- Local anaesthetic (LA) agent.
- Sterile containers (according to local protocols) and specimen forms.
- Sterile towels.
- Sterile gloves.
- Small adhesive plaster.
- Antiseptic agent.
- Suitable distraction aids, e.g. story book, tape, etc.

Table 14.1 Appropriate sizes of LP needles

Size of needle (length)	Height of child	Approx age of child
2cm	<50cm	Preterm neonate
3cm	50–80cm	<2yrs
4cm	80–120cm	2–5yrs
5cm	120–150cm	5–12yrs
6cm	150–180cm	>12yrs

Procedure
- Undertake comprehensive nursing and medical assessment.
- Performing a LP is a high risk procedure. The decision to undertake it should be made by senior medical personnel who should explain the procedure and gain informed written consent.
- Consider LA, sedation, or General Anaesthetic (GA) as appropriate.
- Gather and prepare all equipment.
- Monitor all sedated or seriously ill children with continuous pulse oximetry.
- Position child on their side or, at edge of bed and away from operator. Draw knees up to chest, flex neck. Craniospinal axis parallel to bed.
- Apply local anaesthetic cream to area where LA will be injected if used. Allow time to take effect.

Doctor will:
- Prepare skin, after removing local anaesthetic cream.
- Towel up sterile field.
- Locally anaesthetize skin and between spinous process.
- Undertake procedure, aiming to insert needle between L3 and 4 or L4 and 5.
- Discard first few drops of CSF.

Nurse will:
- Allow 1–2mL CSF to flow into each sterile container.
- Usually 3 separate samples collected for:
  - Glucose and protein.
  - Gram stain and culture, and sensitivity.
  - Cell count and differential.
- Apply plaster to site and leave *in situ* for 24h. (Check for allergies prior to plaster application).
- Dispose of equipment.
- Observe child post-procedure for headache, CSF leakage from site, or other complications. Observe vital signs and neurological status. Report any deviations from normal parameters to medical staff and document.
- Complete nursing documentation.

Practice tips
- Correct positioning is vital, with maximizing of intravertebral spaces making it easier to access the subarachnoid space. Take time to get it right, and consider the health and safety issues for the person holding the child—they may need to hold the position for some time.
- An additional member of staff to undertake distraction will be invaluable.
- Headache after procedure will usually settle within 24–48h. Laying the child flat may help. Give paracetamol as prescribed and encourage oral fluids.
- Pencil-point (blunt) needles reduce the risk of headache in adults, but the evidence is not convincing in children. Their use may be appropriate with adolescents.

Pitfalls
- LP is contraindicated when ICP raised as 'coning' (cerebral herniation) may result.
- Insertion trauma may contaminate the sample with blood.
- Overflexing of the neck when positioning may cause respiratory compromise, especially in infants.

Associated reading
Farley A, McLvafferty E. (2008). Lumbar puncture *Nurs Stand* **22**(22), 46–8.

Seizure management

Background

Seizures are episodes of uncontrolled electrical activity in the brain.
Manifestations will depend upon the site of origin and may include:
- Unconsciousness or altered consciousness.
- Involuntary movements.
- Changes in perception, behaviours, sensations, and postures.

Prolonged seizure activity

Will have the following effects:
- Heart rate (HR) increase.
- BP increase.
- Blood glucose levels increase.
- Respirations may be compromised leading to oxygenation decrease.

After about 30min these physiological mechanisms fail and may contribute
to neurological damage.
Ultimately the child may suffer with:
- Hypoxaemia or apnoea.
- Hypoglycaemia from raised metabolic activity in skeletal muscles.
- Cellular destruction.

❶ Prompt and accurate observation and appropriate intervention is
essential to minimize the risk of permanent damage when a seizure is
prolonged.

Procedure

- Ensure that child's health record(s) contains full details of seizure
  history, i.e. on all hospital admissions, outpatient/GP/school nurse
  appointments, etc., update record to provide the fullest picture of
  seizure patterns, manifestations, and treatments, including:
  - Altered, or loss of, consciousness, behaviour.
  - Motor movements, muscular contractions.
  - Eye movements.
  - Duration of seizures and whether they appear to occur in clusters
    or as isolated incidents.
  - Any pre-disposing factors/typical times.
  - Cyanosis.
- Ensure that child's health record(s) contain the child's current weight

During a seizure

- Nurse next to:
  - Working oxygen.
  - Working suction.
  - Appropriate size bag-valve-mask, e.g. Ambu-bag™.
  - Appropriate size airway.
- Administer oxygen if required.
- Nurse child on their side.

❶ Ensure that the environment is safe:
- Move objects that may obstruct child's movement or cause injury.
- Call for assistance, but aim to never leave any child having a seizure.
- Ensure the seizure is timed.
- Administer prescribed rectal/buccal/intravenous (IV) medication according to local guidelines if required, ensuring the correct dosages are administered. Always ensure that drugs are prescribed by the medical staff and that correct policy and procedures are followed.
- Monitor and support child's vital functions.
- Administer further doses of rectal/buccal/intravenous medication according to hospital policies.
- Seek immediate medical assistance if you are concerned that child is not responding to medication and/or vital signs indicate the need for medical intervention.
- Take appropriate emergency action to support life.
- If child is given IV anti-convulsant therapy, they should be closely monitored during administration for:
  - Level of consciousness.
  - Respirations.
  - HR.
  - BP.
  - Temperature.
- Chart, document, and report seizures as appropriate, ensuring that you include the following:
  - Date and time.
  - Full description of activity and effect on child's vital signs, behaviour, and movement.
  - Duration.
  - Nursing intervention.
  - Medication.
- Ensure child is safe and comfortable as they enter the post-ictal phase. Ensure bed rails are in place.
- Continue to monitor and observe closely to determine recovery.

❶ A seizure that lasts for at least 30min or repeated seizures lasting for 30min or longer from which the patient does not regain consciousness is classified as *status epilepticus* and is a medical emergency that requires immediate medical attention.

Associated reading

Appleton R, Chadwick D, Baker G. (2001). *Epilepsy*, 4th edn. Martin Dunitz Ltd, London.

Gastrointestinal system

History taking

Background

The gastrointestinal (GI) system or tract involves the full system from mouth through to anus. Its main physiological function is to enable each of us to acquire the nutrition and fluids we need in order to survive, grow and develop.

When taking a history of GI-related symptoms, there are many facets to consider. GI system symptoms can be related to many other systems within the body. The history will give the clues needed to find the cause of the problem. Subsequent examination will confirm diagnosis.

Procedure: presenting complaint

- What is the main presenting problem? Clarity regarding this is vital.
- It is also beneficial to ascertain the child/young person's view. What is their concern? What do they want to happen? What are they expecting from you?

History of presenting complaint

- Enquire in more depth into the symptoms that have been presented.
- For each symptom ensure all attributes are established.
- There are several mnemonics that can assist with this. Here we will use OLD CART to explore the symptom of vomiting (Box 15.1).

Box 15.1 Mnemonics for taking a history of presenting complaint

- *Onset:* when did the vomiting start? Was there anything of note at the time of onset—new foods, unwell before, any pain noted at time of onset?
- *Location:* more related to pain—where does this occur?
  - Most children over 3yrs should be able to point to where is sore.
- *Duration:* how long has this been going on?
- *Character:* is the vomit the same as the food stuffs, i.e. unaltered? Is it green, yellow? Is the volume more or less than the intake? Is there much retching? Is there any blood present? Is there any mucous present?
- *Aggravating/alleviating factors:* has the family tried to give the child any remedies or medicines? Have these worked? Enquire specifically about any homeopathic treatments that may not have been reported immediately by family members. Has the family tried to give the child fluids of any form? If so, in what form and how has this been tolerated by the child/young person?
  - Does vomiting occur after all food stuffs or only specific foods/fluids?
- *Radiation/related:* are there any other problems related to the vomiting—stomach pains, headaches, rashes, general upset?
  - Has there been any weight loss noted?
- *Timing:* does the vomiting occur immediately after taking oral food stuffs? Does it occur at specific times of the day? Does it occur before, after or during certain activities?

Past medical history

- The past medical history allows you to explore pertinent clues from what has gone before (see 📖 Assessment, p. 406).
- Has the child recently travelled to foreign countries and consumed 'different food'.
- Is there an underlying illness that could explain the current symptoms or alert you to a more urgent diagnosis, i.e. a child with known diabetes presenting with abdominal pains should be assessed for ketoacidosis; likewise a child with known sickle cell disease presenting with abdominal pain should be assessed for sickle cell crisis.
- *In the younger child:* the birth history should be taken. Has the infant recently changed from breast milk to bottles, has new food stuff been added to a weaning diet? When was meconium passed?
- *For older children:* has the young person changed their dietary habits, e.g. become vegan/vegetarian? Has their appetite altered recently?

Practice tips

- Parent/family history is important. Remember to ask about autoimmune diseases, such as Crohns or coeliac disease. Some families will be prone to constipation. There may also be a family history of abdominal migraine.
- It is also important to ask about other siblings: are they well? Do they have similar symptoms?
- Remember to ascertain the child's immunization status and allergy status.
- Is the child on any medication that could be causing symptoms?
- Has there been any contact with known infections/contact with other sources of infection, e.g. farm animals or domesticated tropical pets?
- *If a young person presents with abdominal pain:* assessment and careful questioning regarding sexual activity/substance misuse should be undertaken. These questions may need to be asked in a private setting away from parents/family members.
- When assessing pain, e.g. in the OLD CART example, remember to use an age-appropriate pain assessment tool (see 📖 Assessment of pain, p. 118).

Pitfalls

- Abdominal pain can have many causes, be careful to rule out the common ones before moving onto the less common.

Associated reading

NICE (2009). *Diarrhoea and vomiting in children; Diarrhoea and vomiting caused by gastroenteritis: diagnosis, assessment and management in children younger than 5 years.* NICE Clinical Guideline 84. NICE, London.

Assessment

Background
Assessment is the process of examining the child to confirm or check details and physical signs described within the history taking in order to formulate a diagnosis.

Equipment
- Tongue depressor and light source for examination of mouth.
- Otoscope for examination of ears.
- Stethoscope for auscultation.
- Warm hands for palpation and percussion.
- Distraction toys.
- Blood glucose meter to rule out high or low blood sugars.

Procedure
- Explain the procedure in age-appropriate terms to the child and family, and gain consent.
- The ears, nose, throat, urinary tract, and chest are all related to parts of the GI tract and may produce symptoms within the abdomen; thus, examination is required (see 📖 Assessment of the ear, p. 548, 📖 Examination of the nose, p. 550, 📖 Examination of the throat, p. 552, 📖 History taking and assessment, p. 330, and 📖 History taking and assessment, p. 454).
- Assessment of hydration status (see 📖 Assessing dehydration, p. 94).
- Examination of the abdomen involves inspection, percussion, auscultation, and palpation. (NB. This is a specialist skill and the role of the student/newly qualified nurse is to observe and assist if necessary).
- Begin with inspection, then auscultation before moving on to percussion and palpation which may elicit pain and prevent further examination.
- Approach the abdominal examination from the child's right-hand side.
- The younger child may be more co-operative if left on the parents/carer's lap for the examination, rather than being placed on the couch.

Inspection
- Wash and decontaminate your hands as per hospital policy.
- Observe the child when getting onto the couch; are they guarding the area? Is there pain on movement? Does it stop once the child/young person has stopped moving?
- Look at the shape of the abdomen; is there any asymmetry or notable masses? Are there any peristaltic motions noted? Does the skin over the abdomen look tense/shiny?
- Are there any rashes or lesions over the abdomen?
- Are there any signs of trauma, such as bruising?
- Ask the child/young person to cough and observe for any pain produced within the abdomen.

Auscultation
- Perform this prior to percussion and palpation as they may induce pain and can alter bowel activity.
- Using a stethoscope, listen in the four quadrants for bowel sounds, which should normally be heard 5–30 times/min.
- ❶ A tinkling sound sometimes described like water being poured from one cup to another[1] is indicative of bowel obstruction.

Percussion
- Percussion is used to assess for distribution of bowel gas and to detect any possible areas of dullness that can be palpated.
- Percuss each of the four quadrants in turn, noting sounds obtained for tympany or dullness. Tympany is the hyper resonant sound from bowel gas and dullness is related to masses or solid structures.

Palpation
- Ensure your hands are warm for this part of the examination.
- Palpation can be performed in two stages:
  • First, use light palpation to discover areas of specific tenderness (this can also help gain the co-operation and trust of the child/young person). Work from the right lower quadrant to the right upper, left upper, and finally, the left lower quadrant.
  • Deep palpation follows: work in an order that enables the area now suspected as being most painful, to be examined last. Press deeply with the palmar surface of your fingers identifying any masses and noting their location, size, and shape.
- During this part of the examination rebound tenderness should be elicited by withdrawing your fingers quickly.
- Document all findings within the child's notes and refer any concerns to the appropriate personnel.

Practice tips
- Within the right upper quadrant the liver edge will be palpable on an infant, this should be soft. As the child gets older this should be less easy to palpate and should be investigated further if felt.
- ❶ Rebound tenderness is a sign of peritonitis. If felt over the right lower quadrant this could indicate appendicitis.
- It should be noted that rebound tenderness is not evident in some children who present with appendicitis.

Pitfalls
- Children/young people with appendicitis can present with referred pain. Be alert to pain elsewhere that may be atypical presentation.
- Examine ENT, respiratory, and urinary systems alongside the GI tract to rule out other factors that may be causing abdominal symptoms.

Associated reading
Barnes K. (2003). *Paediatrics: A Clinical Guide for Nurse Practitioners*. Butterworth Heinemann, London.
Bickley S. (2007). *Bates' Guide to Physical Examination and History Taking*, 9th edn. Lippincott Williamson and Wilkins. Philadelphia.

[1] Patient.co.uk (2011) *Abdominal Examination*. Available at: ℘ http://www.patient.co.uk/doctor/Abdominal-Examination.htm.

Managing nausea and vomiting

Background

- *Nausea:* feeling sick with an inclination to vomit. Nausea usually precedes vomiting.
- *Vomiting:* the ejection of matter from the stomach often with considerable force. Vomiting is one of the body's responses to toxins or gastric/intestinal inflammation.
- Vomiting can also occur when a child wishes to resist taking food, liquids, or medicines.

Equipment

If unsure of cause, use of a side room/cubicle should be considered.

- Gloves.
- Vomit bowl.
- Receptacle for disposal of tissues, etc.
- Apron.
- Tissues.
- Mouthwash.
- Toothpaste and tooth brush.

Procedure

It is important to ascertain the cause of nausea and vomiting in order to provide appropriate treatment.

Possible causes include:

- Urinary tract infection (UTI)/acute gastro-enteritis (AGE) cause may be viral (rotavirus or norwalk) or bacterial (*Salmonella* or *Escherichia coli*)/chemotherapy treatment/food allergy/post-operative nausea and vomiting (PONV)/irritable bowel syndrome (IBS)/mesenteric adenitis, and abdominal migraine.
- Potential surgical cases in which vomiting may be a symptom include: pyloric stenosis/appendicitis/strangulated hernia/intersussception/mal-rotation of the bowel.

Treatment

Treatment will depend on the cause.

Management

- Nurse in isolation if appropriate and ensure that all appropriate infection control measures are in place as per hospital policy.
- Ensure the safety of the child's airway:
  - Nurse near working oxygen and suction.
  - If the child is alert tip their head down and observe closely for choking/possible aspiration.
  - If the child is not alert place on their side and observe closely for vomiting/choking/possible aspiration (use of a permanent saturation monitor may be indicated).
- Put on a pair of gloves and a disposable apron.
- Provide tissues and receptacles for both vomit and soiled tissues.
- Obtain specimens for laboratory analysis if required.

- Post-vomiting encourage the child to rinse out their mouth/clean their teeth.
- Reassure/comfort the child and parents.
- Document fluid loss accurately on an appropriate fluid balance chart.
- Observe for episodes of diarrhoea.
- Provide rehydration fluids via appropriate route and ensure a strict fluid balance record is maintained.
- ❶ Observe the child for any signs of dehydration—dry mucous membranes/sunken eyes/sunken fontanelle in babies/increased capillary refill time/decreased urinary output/increased agitation or confusion/cold peripheries/decreased tissue elasticity/increased heart rate/decreased blood pressure (see 📖 Assessing dehydration, p. 94).
- Inform appropriate medical personnel promptly of any concerns and follow local policy/medical guidance as to most appropriate treatment.

Practice tips

Where dehydration is a concern due to AGE (acute gastroenteritis)
- *If a child is receiving oral rehydration fluids:* flavouring the solution with fruit squash can make it more palatable for the child.
- Use of an oral syringe may be necessary in young children or older babies.
- Encourage good hand hygiene and observe for breaches of isolation/infection control policy (see Chapter 7).
- Where appropriate encourage parents/carers to carry out the rehydration regime and record intake, as this is something they can instigate at home.

PONV
This may be related to anaesthetic agents, analgesia particularly opioids or surgical procedure.
- Offer anti-emetic medication if appropriate and as per hospital policy.
- ❶ If the child's jaw has been wired, e.g. following osteotomy, ensure wire cutters are available and easily accessible in case of emergency.

Pitfalls

- ❶ Failing to make an accurate assessment of hydration status.
- ❶ Failing to ensure appropriate rehydration regime is carried out.
- Not clarifying the role of the parents in undertaking the regime.
- Not re-assessing for other possible causes of nausea/vomiting, e.g. testing urine sample for UTI, glucose, ketones, pregnancy, etc.

Associated reading

Barnes K (ed.) (2004). *Paediatrics: A Clinical Guide for Nurse Practitioners*. Butterworth-Heinemann, London.

Clancy J, McVicar A. (2009). *Physiology & Anatomy for Nurses and Health Care Practitioners. A Homeostatic Approach*, 3rd edn. Hodder & Arnold, London.

Lissauer T, Clayden G. (2001). *Illustrated Textbook of Paediatrics*, 2nd edn. Mosby, London.

Stool assessment

Background

There are various factors relating to the pattern of defaecation and characteristics of the stool, such as development, medical conditions, structural abnormalities, diet, exercise, and medication. Collection of samples for analysis in specific circumstances may be requested, e.g. for occult blood, ova and parasites, bacteria, viruses, and for digestive secretions.

Procedure

- Assessment of stool involves general observation of characteristics including colour, consistency (form), volume, odour, and composition. The Bristol Stool Chart[1] is a grading chart that may be used in the assessment of consistency.
- Record history of onset, frequency and duration, medications, associated symptoms, such as nausea/vomiting, recent travel, fluid and dietary history.[2]
- Obtain samples for stool cultures for analysis of bacterial, fungal, or viral cause, and for change in normal stool.

Practice tips

Newborns and infants

Meconium

- Passed in the first 24–36hrs after birth. Failure to pass meconium may indicate atresia, Hirschsprungs disease, or cystic fibrosis.
- Black/dark green.
- Sticky, tarry.
- Odourless.

Transitional[3]

- Passed in first week of life.
- Greenish/yellow.
- Loose.
- Odourless.

Breast-fed milk stool

- Mustard yellow.
- Watery to soft, seedy.
- Odourless.

Formula-fed milk stool

- Yellowish/green.
- Soft, more formed than breast-fed baby stool.
- Slight sharp smell.

Toddlers and pre-school children

- Key developmental milestone is completion of toilet training. The majority of children achieve control of defaecation by 3yrs of age.
- Toddler stools are influenced by their diet. The stools are described as frequent, loose, and explosive containing undigested food.

School age children/adolescents[3]
• By the age of 10yrs, stools are similar to adult stools.
• Light to brown colour resulting from pigments stercobilin and urobilin derived from the breakdown of bilirubin in the intestines.[3]
• Children and young people (CYP) can control and delay defaecation.

Deviations from normal (see Table 15.1)

Table 15.1 Deviations from normal

Observations	Possible cause	Associated conditions
Mucus, blood Loose 'redcurrant jelly'	Inflammation	Inflammatory bowel disease Intussusception (late sign)
Mucus, blood Watery Green/brown Offensive odour	Infection	Gastroenteritis
Greasy, shiny Bulky Pale Foul odour (steatorrhoea)	Malabsorption of fat Wheat/gluten intolerance	Cystic fibrosis Coeliac disease
Nodular Hard	Dietary imbalance Dehydration Stool witholding	Constipation
Visible streaks of blood	Trauma	Anal fissure
Black Tarry (Melaena)	Digested blood Medication, e.g. iron	Oesophagitis Peptic inflammation

Table modified from[3,4]

[1] Lewis SJ, Heaton KW. (1997). Stool form scale as a useful guide to intestinal transit time. *Scand J Gastroenterol* **32**(9), 920–4.

[2] Dougherty L., Lister S. (eds) (2008). *The Royal Marsden Hospital Manual of Clinical Nursing Procedures*, 7th edn. Wiley-Blackwell, Oxford.

[3] Berman A, Snyder S, Jackson C. (2009). *Skills in Clinical Nursing*, 6th edn. Pearson Prentice Hall, New Jersey.

[4] Moules T, Ramsay J. (2008). *The Textbook of Children's and Young People's Nursing*, 2nd edn. Blackwell Publishing, Oxford.

Rectal irrigation

Background

Rectal irrigation is performed to evacuate stool from the rectum and lower colon in the management of faecal incontinence and chronic constipation. It involves introducing water into the rectum and colon via the anus. The water and contents of the rectum and descending sigmoid colon are subsequently evacuated into the toilet. Although initially performed by a parent/carer it is a procedure that the child can be taught to carry out independently. This section is based on using the Peristeen Anal Irrigation system™, as this is the only device currently available and licensed for use in children. Please check local policy regarding what systems are available for use in your own area.

Equipment

- Anal irrigation kit (Peristeen)™ including:
  - Irrigation bag and tubing.
  - Control unit.
  - Rectal catheter (2 sizes small/large).
  - Lukewarm (body temperature) water.
  - Apron and Gloves (non-latex)—if procedure carried out by carer.

Procedure

- Undertake a comprehensive nursing and medical assessment.
- Performing rectal irrigation is not without risk (e.g. perforation of the bowel). The decision to undertake it should be made in consultation with senior medical personnel or the child's GP if to be carried out in the community.
- Explain the procedure to the child and family, and gain valid consent.
- Gather and prepare all equipment. Fill the irrigation bag with lukewarm water and run it through the system until there is sufficient water in the catheter packaging to enable the catheter to become lubricated (the catheter has a coating that lubricates it when wet).
- *If the child is able to stand unsupported:*
  - Insertion of the catheter is best carried out with the child standing next to the toilet.
  - This involves either standing directly in front of the toilet, facing away and leaning slightly forwards or standing to the side of the toilet.
- *If the child is unable to stand:*
  - The child should be positioned on a bed or changing mat for insertion of the catheter and inflation of the balloon.
  - The child can then be lifted onto the toilet or commode using a hoist and toileting sling if necessary.
- If the child is confident sitting on the toilet and has good sitting balance then the catheter can be inserted whilst the child is sitting on the toilet. With time this is a procedure that some children can be taught to do independently.

- Once the catheter has been inserted into the rectum (up to the finger grip to ensure the balloon is fully inflated inside the rectum), the catheter balloon is inflated by turning the dial to the appropriate symbol and using sufficient pumps of the balloon (usually 2–3 for the large catheter, 1–2 for the small catheter).
- The dial is then turned to the water symbol and water is pumped slowly into the rectum—the exact quantity instilled will vary from child to child. In practice the irrigation usually starts with volumes of 100–200mL and increases over a period of time as the child's tolerance increases to an average volume of ~500mL. Confirmation of the volume required must be clarified prior to commencement.
- When the appropriate volume of water has been instilled the dial is turned to the air symbol and the balloon is deflated allowing the rectal catheter to slide out. The water and contents of the rectum and descending colon are subsequently evacuated into the toilet.
- Once the evacuation is complete the child should be assisted to wipe their bottom if able, otherwise this should be carried out by the carer, and the child should be made comfortable.
- The rectal catheter should be disposed of as per local policy, and the remaining equipment cleaned and stored away.
- The results of the rectal irrigation should be documented if necessary.

Practice tips

- The child's privacy and dignity should be maintained at all times.
- As this procedure is designed to take place over the toilet or commode, appropriate toileting aids (such as a seat reducer/step) should be in place if necessary to enable the child to sit comfortably.
- Distraction techniques may be useful for some children to help them relax during the insertion of the rectal catheter.
- If the child is able, encourage them to operate the control unit—this will not only act as a distraction technique, but also help facilitate the child's later independence.
- Some children may experience abdominal cramps during the procedure—try to pump the water more slowly and check the temperature.
- Adjust the volume of air in the balloon if there is leakage of fluid or the catheter is expelled prematurely.

Pitfalls

- ❶ The Peristeen Anal Irrigation system™ is designed to be used in children over the age of 3yrs. Special caution must be used in children under 3yrs.
- ❶ Special caution must also be taken in children with recent abdominal or anal surgery, anal fissure, or inflammatory bowel disease.
- ❶ Rectal irrigation should not be used when there is a known obstruction of the large bowel, or in the acute stage of inflammatory bowel disease or diverticulitis.

Associated reading

Ausili E, Focarelli B, Tabacco F, et al. (2010). Transanal irrigation in myelomeningocele children: an alternative, safe and valid approach for neurogenic constipation. *Spinal Cord* **48**(7), 560–5.
Bohr C. (2009). Using rectal irrigation for faecal incontinence in children. *Nurs Times* **105**(7), 42–4.

Stoma care: how to change a bag

Background
A stoma is a surgical opening made into the bowel; a part of which is then brought out onto the child's abdomen in order to form the stoma. A stoma is always sited above an area of diseased bowel. Stomas may be temporary, until corrective surgery has taken place, or permanent.

Types of stomas
- *Jejunostomy*: a stoma made into the jejunum.
- *Ileostomy*: stoma made into the ileum.
- *Colostomy*: a stoma made into the colon. The surgeon may make a single stoma; a double loop stoma or a proximal stoma with a mucous fistula.
- *Vesicostomy*: a stoma made directly into the bladder and opening onto the child's abdomen.
- *Ileal conduit/urostomy*: a stoma that diverts the flow of urine away from the bladder. The stoma is made using a small piece of ileum into which the ureters are implanted.
- *Ureterostomy*: a stoma to divert the flow of urine away from the bladder. One or both ureters are moved to make a stoma, and the resulting stoma will be small.

Why is a stoma made?
- Neonates require a stoma if they are born with a congenital abnormality, e.g. Hirshsprung's disease, ano-rectal malformation, duplication cysts, ileal or colonic atresia, gastroschisis, cloaca or meconium ileus. Pre-term babies may require an Ileostomy for necrotizing enterocolitis.
- Children and young adults may have a stoma for Hirshsprung's disease, ulcerative colitis, Crohn's disease, abdominal tumours or trauma. Urinary stomas are made for obstructions of the urinary tract system or bladder function problems.
- Waste matter from the stoma may be formed or fluid, depending on where the stoma is placed. Losses from the ileum may be watery, whilst losses from the colon will be more formed.

Equipment
- New stoma bag cut to fit and ready to use. (A template may be available from a previous stoma bag change and this helps to cut the flange to a size suitable for the child).
- Protective pad for the child or baby to lie on.
- Non-sterile gloves.
- White apron.
- Gauze swabs.
- Scissors.
- Warmed tap water.
- Disposal bag.

Procedure

- Ensure all necessary equipment is available.
- Explain the procedure to the child and family, and gain consent.
- Wash and dry hands thoroughly, and apply gloves and apron.
- If the stoma bag contains faeces, it should be emptied prior to removal as this reduces the risk of leakage onto the wound or child.
- Measure and document how much stool has been emptied.
- Once the bag has been removed, wet a gauze swab with warm water and using a push/pull technique remove the old appliance (helps to prevent damage to the peristomal skin and reduces pressure near to the suture line).
- Clean around the stoma to remove any faeces using wet swabs; then dry the area thoroughly.
- Check the flange is cut to the correct size.
- Remove the backing paper from the flange and apply the new bag positioning the stoma in the centre of the flange.
- Once in position press the flange gently onto the skin to ensure the bag sticks securely to the site. The stoma bag flange should fit close to the stoma, but should not touch it. (See 📖 Pitfalls, p. 415.)
- Reassure the child and carer, and answer any questions they may have in order to help them understand the process and prepare them for the next time the bag is changed.
- Dispose of all equipment as per hospital policy.
- Remove gloves; wash and dry hands.
- Record stoma bag change in the child's nursing care plan.

Practice tips

- Consider the use of analgesia when changing a stoma bag for the first time following surgery as the child may have a tender abdomen, especially along the suture line.
- Observe the colour of the stoma on return from theatre and record in the nursing notes. The colour of a healthy stoma is pink/red. Alterations to blood supply of the stoma may cause it to become lighter or darker in colour. Any alterations need reporting to the surgical team.
- If the stoma length changes (retracted or prolapsed) seek advice. ❶ If a prolapse is evident alongside a change of stoma colour, urgent medical advice is required.

Pitfalls

- If the stoma bag flange touches the stoma it may cause trauma to the stoma.
- If the flange of the stoma bag is cut to an incorrect size, e.g. too large the skin may be exposed to faecal fluid and may become excoriated and sore. Pressing the flange into position should ensure it adheres to the skin.

Associated reading

Lyon C, Smith A. (2010). *Abdominal Stoma and their Skin Disorders*. Informa Healthcare, London.
Breckman B. (2005). *Stoma Care and Rehabilitation*. Elsevier/Churchill Livingstone, London.
Paediatric Stoma Nurse Group (UK) (2010). *Standards of Care: Paediatric Stoma Care*, endorsed by World Council of Enterostomal Therapists. Produced by Hollister and Pelican Healthcare, London.

Passing a nasogastric tube/nasogastric feeding

Background

Oral feeding is the preferred method for feeding children. However, if a child is unable to obtain adequate oral intake, enteral feeding may be necessary.

- Enteral feeding = method of supplying the child with fluid and nutrients via a tube into the GI tract.
- NG feeding is the most common method of enteral feeding in clinical practice and the community unless long term use is expected.
- Thousands of tubes are inserted daily without incident, but there is a risk that the tube can become misplaced into the lungs during insertion or move out of the stomach at a later stage.

In February 2005 following reports of patient death/harm caused by misplaced NGT, the NPSA issued a patient safety alert. Between Sept 2005 and March 2010 there were a further 21 deaths and 79 cases of harm reported. Thus, the NPSA has published new updated guidance and recommend that all healthcare professionals involved with nasogastric tube position checks are assessed as competent.[1]

Equipment

- Working oxygen and suction.
- Disposable plastic apron and gloves.
- Clean trolley.
- Sterile water/water-based lubricant.
- Appropriately sized NGT.
- Hydrocolloid dressing.
- pH indicator paper (CE approved).
- Tape to secure tube.
- 2 × 20 or 50-mL syringes.
- Soother (for infants/young children).
- Clean sterile scissors.
- Vomit bowl.

Please note the following guidance is applicable for children and infants. For guidance specific to neonates please refer to local policy.

Procedure

Prior to insertion the following questions need consideration

- Is NGT feeding the right choice for the patient? An assessment should be undertaken to identify the appropriateness of NGT feeding and the rationale for the decision should be recorded in the patient's notes.[1]
- Is this the right time to place the NGT? Is appropriate equipment available? If there is not sufficient, experienced support available to accurately confirm NGT placement (e.g. at night) unless clinically urgent, placement should be delayed until that support is available.[1]

Insertion

- Explain the procedure to the child and family, and gain consent.
- Ensure an assistant is available.
- Ensure working oxygen and suction is easily accessible.

- Wash and dry hands as per infection control policy, and put on apron.
- Clean the work surface, tray, and trolley as infection control policy.
- Place equipment on the trolley maintaining integrity of sterile items.
- Ensure the child has no known allergies, e.g. to tape.
- Ensure there are no contraindications to insertion of the NGT.
- Cut the hydrocolloid dressing and tape to size using sterile scissors.
- Ensure the NGT is intact and not damaged.
- *Position the child appropriately:*
  - Wrap babies in a blanket and hold in the arms of an assistant or lay on their side.
  - Ask older children to help by slightly hyper-extending the neck, keeping still, breathing through the mouth, and swallowing when asked.[2]
- Wash and dry hands, and apply non-sterile gloves.
- Measure the length of the tube to be inserted—place exit port of tube at the tip of the nose and measure from the tip of the nose to the ear and then from the ear to a point midway between the xiphoid process and the umbilicus.[2] Note or hold the marking on the tube.
- Lubricate the end of the tube with sterile water or lubricant.
- Ensure the cap of the NGT is closed.
- Gently introduce the tube into the child's nostril.
- Angle the tube slightly upwards and gently advance over the back of the nose into the nasopharynx, and continue to advance downwards.
- Children may gag as the tube reaches the back of their throat:
  - Encourage older children to swallow or sip water unless contraindicated.
  - Offer young children a soother to encourage them to suck.
- Observe for signs of respiratory distress that may indicate the tube has been passed into the trachea/bronchus—excessive coughing, choking, or cyanosis. If observed withdraw the tube and assess child's condition.
- Advance the tube until the predetermined mark is at the opening of the child's nostril.
- Ask your assistant to place two fingers on the tube to secure position.
- Connect a 20-mL syringe and gently aspirate 0.5–1mL fluid.
- Place a few drops of fluid onto the pH strip and match the colour change to the colour code on the box.
- The National Patient Safety Agency recommends feeding may take place if pH is below 5.5 (❶ practice does vary; refer to local policy).
- ❶ If a satisfactory aspirate is not obtained, refer to the tips given here.
- Once a satisfactory aspirate has been obtained place the hydrocolloid dressing on to the skin on the child's cheek, place the tube over the dressing and secure with tape.
- Flush the NGT with an appropriate amount of sterile water (5–10mL is usual practice, but check local policy).
- Dispose of all equipment as per local policy and wash hands.
- *Document:*
  - pH result obtained.
  - Size and length of tube.
  - External length of tube once secured.
  - Nostril used.
  - Date inserted.

Practice tips

- Smaller syringes cause greater pressure on aspiration; thus, only 20- or 50-mL syringes should be used to aspirate.
- The risk of aspiration is reduced in infants placed on their side.
- NGT used for feeding should be radio-opaque throughout their length and have externally visible length markings.[1]
- pH indicator paper used should be CE marked and intended to test human gastric aspirate.[1]

If no aspirate is obtained

- If possible turn the child onto their left side and retry.[1]
- Advance/withdraw the tube by 1–2cm and retry.[1]
- Give mouth care to patients who are nil by mouth (NBM) as this stimulates gastric secretion of acid and retry.[1]
- Do not use water to flush the NGT prior to positive confirmation that the tube is in the stomach.[1]
- If an aspirate is still not obtained proceed to X-ray. (X-ray is used only as a 'second line test' when no aspirate has been obtained or pH paper has failed to confirm a satisfactory aspirate).[1]
- Following X-ray a competent clinician with evidence of training should document confirmation of NGT position in the patient's stomach.[1]

If aspirate obtained is above 5.5

- Refer to local policy.
- National Patient Safety Agency (NPSA) recommends a second competent person should check the NGT. If satisfactory aspirate is still not obtained proceed to X-ray.
- In some situations, e.g. where patients are fed continuously or receiving acid reducing medication it may not be possible to obtain an aspirate between 1 and 5.5. In such cases refer to local policy and take appropriate medical advice.
- Documentation following pH testing should include:
  - Whether an aspirate was obtained.
  - pH value.
  - Who checked the aspirate pH.
  - When it was confirmed to be safe to administer the feed.
  - Medication.[1]
- Documentation following X-ray should include:
  - Who authorized the X-ray.
  - Who confirmed the position of the NGT.
  - Confirmation that any X-ray reviewed was the most current X-ray for the correct patient.
  - The rationale for the confirmation of position of the NGT.[1]

Pitfalls

- ❶ Do not use the tube until its position has been positively confirmed.
- ❶ NGT should not be flushed and no liquid or feed should be introduced into the tube following initial placement until the position has been confirmed either by pH testing or X-ray.
- Hyper-extension of the neck in infants can occlude the airway.
- KY jelly should not be used as a lubricant as it may affect pH.[1]

- ❶ Auscultation 'whoosh tests' and/or interpretation of the appearance of aspirate should never be used to determine tube position as it is unreliable.[1]
- Litmus paper determines acidity, but not pH level. Do not use.
- ❶ Observe for signs of vagal stimulation while passing the gag reflex:
  - ↓ Pulse.
  - Gasping.
  - Apnoea.
  - Coughing.
  - Cyanosis.
  - Gagging.
  - Vomiting.
  - If symptoms are observed withdraw the tube immediately and assess the child's condition.

Nasogastric feeding: administering bolus and continuous feeds

Background
Enteral feeds can be given via gravity (bolus feeding) or via a pump on either an intermittent or continuous basis.[2] Where possible intermittent feeding is preferred as it mimics normal feeding patterns more closely, and may fit better with a child and families normal routine. In addition, continuous feeds can result in the suppression of gastric acid production, which can lead to the potential for increased bacterial growth.[2]

Equipment
- Disposable plastic apron/gloves.
- Prescribed feed.
- Feed pump if continuous feeding is planned.
- Kangaroo/gravity set for bolus feed.
- 20–50mL syringes.
- Sterile water
- pH indicator paper (CE approved).
- Clean trolley, work surface, or tray.

Procedure
Following initial insertion of the NGT repeat checks of position should be made before administering each feed/before administering any medication/at least once daily if the tube is not in use or the child is receiving a continuous feed (if possible an hour delay without further feeding should be allowed before testing the gastric aspirate).[1]
- Explain the procedure to the child and family and gain consent.
- Ensure the head of the bed is elevated to approximately 45° as this ↓ the risk of pulmonary aspiration and improves gravitational flow.[2]
- Ensure the child is in a comfortable position: small children may be happier to sit on a parents/carer's knee.
- Wash hands and apply plastic apron.
- Clean the trolley, work surface, and tray.
- If using a feed pump, clean the pump as per policy.
- Switch the pump on and test it is in full working order.

- Check the feed prescription chart and ensure that the appropriate feed is administered.
- Check the expiry date of the feed.
- Wipe the top of the feed with an alcohol wipe and allow to dry.[2]
- Check the seal on the lid is intact and shake the feed thoroughly.
- Wash hands and apply non sterile gloves.
- Attach a 20–50-mL syringe to the NGT, gently aspirate 0.5–1mL of fluid from the stomach, and replace the cap.
- Apply a few drops of the fluid onto a pH indicator strip and match the colour change to the colour code on the box.
- NPSA state a feed can be safely commenced if the pH reading is below 5.5. ❶ Some Trusts stipulate lower pH readings—please refer to local policy.
- Once an appropriate aspirate has been obtained flush the NGT with 5–10mL of water depending on the child and then replace the cap.

Bolus feeding
- *If using a Kangaroo set:*
  - Remove the set using non-touch technique, attach a 50-mL syringe, prime the line with the prescribed feed and clamp the set.
  - Kink the NGT, open the cap and attach the kangaroo set.
  - Ensure the syringe and set is filled with feed prior to unclamping.
- *If no Kangaroo set is to be used:* pinch the NGT, attach a 50-mL syringe, fill the syringe with feed, or un-pinch the tubing.
- Allow the feed to flow into the child's stomach via gravity.
- The feed should be administered over the same amount of time as the child usually takes to feed orally. The required height of the syringe to achieve this will vary depending on:
  - The size of NGT.
  - Viscosity of feed.
  - Presence of thickening agents in the feed.
  - Professional judgment with regards correct syringe height must be exercised.
- ❶ Observe the child's condition and respiratory status during the feed.
- ❶ Discontinue the feed immediately if there are concerns and review the child's condition.

Continuous feeding
- Remove the feed-giving set using non-touch technique, prime the line with the prescribed feed and clamp the line.
- Kink the NGT, open the cap, and attach the administration set.
- Fit the administration set correctly into the pump, switch the pump on, set the rate and volume to be infused as per instructions or prescription.
- Set the pump to run and unclamp the administration set.
- ❶ Observe the child's condition and respiratory status closely during the feed.
- Refer to local guidelines in relation to hanging times of milk feeds.
- Label the feeding line (date and time treatment started and the feed running through).

Once the feed is complete
- Flush the enteral tubing as per policy.
- Document the episode of care (volume given, type of feed, and duration).
- Dispose of all equipment as per policy and wash hands.

Practice tips
- NGT used for feeding should be radio- opaque throughout their length and have externally visible length markings.[1]
- pH indicator paper used should be CE marked and intended to test human gastric aspirate.[1]
- Feed administration sets should be changed as per policy (at least 4-hourly in high risk babies).
- Feeds should not be administered too quickly as this can cause discomfort and ↑ the chance of the child vomiting during/after the feed
- Oral mouth care should be performed regularly on all children who are being fed enterally to promote comfort and hygiene.
- In the community setting access to radiology in cases where no aspirate/unsatisfactory aspirate are obtained is difficult. Thus, a full multidisciplinary risk assessment should be made and documented prior to a child being discharged from the acute setting with an NGT. Guidance on the ongoing confirmation of NGT position should be provided by appropriate community staff, communicated to the child/parents and documented within the risk assessment.[1]

Pitfalls
- ❶ In the following circumstances a child should not be fed via the NGT unless a satisfactory aspirate has been obtained or the position has been confirmed by X-ray and documented:
  - Following initial insertion.
  - Following episodes of vomiting/retching/coughing spasms.[1]
  - When there is suspicion of tube displacement (e.g. loose tape/visible section of the tube appears longer).[1]
  - In the presence of new or unexplained respiratory symptoms including a reduction on oxygen saturations.[1]
- ❶ If in any doubt the feed must not be commenced until tube position has been positively confirmed.

Associated reading
Glasper, A. Aylott, M. Battrick, C (2010). *Developing Practical Skills for Nursing Children and Young People.* Hodder Arnold, London.

[1] National Patient Safety Agency (2011). *Reducing the Harm Caused by Misplaced Nasogastric Feeding Tubes in Adults, Children and Infants: Patient Safety Alert* (1253). Available at: ℘ http://www.nrls.npsa.nhs.uk/resources/?entryid45=129640&q=0%c2%acnasogastric+feeding%c2%ac.

[2] Coyne, I. Neill, F. Timmins, F. (2010). *Clinical Skills in Children's Nursing.* Oxford University Press, Oxford.

Gastrostomy feeding

Background

Gastrostomy feeding is often used for children who require the long term administration of enteral feeds, e.g. children with an absent gag reflex, some children with cystic fibrosis.[1]

A gastrostomy is an opening made into the stomach wall through which a tube is inserted. In children, this is usually a surgical procedure performed under general anaesthetic (GA). The decision as to which device is most appropriate depends on the individual child and the surgeon's preference.

Types of device

- Percutaneous endoscopic gastrostomy (PEG). Inserted under endoscopic conditions and can stay *in situ* for up to 2yrs.[2]
- Balloon-inflated gastrostomy tube/button, which needs changing every 3–12 months.
- Non-balloon gastrostomy devices can remain *in situ* for up to 1yr. These devices are inserted using an obdurator.

Equipment

- Disposable apron/gloves.
- Correct extension set that locks into the gastrostomy button.
- Prescribed feed.
- Pump and appropriate giving set if continuous feeding is planned.
- Sterile water.
- 50mL syringe.

Procedure

- The principles for administering a gastrostomy feed are the same as for NG feeding (see 📖 Background, p. 419) with the exception that it is not necessary to check the position of the tube via gastric aspirate prior to administration of the feed each time.[2] ❶ Please refer to local policy as practice may vary.
- It is important, however, to check that the tube does not appear to have moved, fits well, and appears to be intact and in full working order.
- If there is any doubt regarding tube position:
  - An aspirate should be obtained and pH checked using pH paper.
  - Feeding can commence if the aspirate obtained is below 5.5.[3] Again, practice varies refer to local policy.
  - If the aspirate obtained is above 5.5 or no aspirate is obtained, refer to local policy and seek appropriate advice. ❶ Do not use the tube if in any doubt.
- Once happy with tube position feeding can commence. Feeds may be given as a bolus via a syringe or as a continuous feed using an enteral feeding pump. Refer to dietetic feeding plan.
- Prime, clamp, and attach the extension set to the feed port if a button is being used. Ensure that it is securely locked in place:
  - Remove the safety cap from the feeding port.
  - Line up the black line on the extension set with the black line on the button port.

- Gently push the extension set into the button port. Hold the button port with your other hand to prevent undue pressure being exerted on the child's abdomen.
- Turn the extension set clockwise until it stops. The set should now be locked into position.
- Administer 5mL of water prior to feed to ensure the device is patent. Refer to local practice.
- Administer the feed (📖 Background, p. 419)
- *During the feed:*
  - Observe the child's condition and respiratory status in case of vomiting, reflux, and aspiration.
  - Observe for signs of discomfort that may indicate problems, e.g. abdominal distension.
  - Observe for signs of infection.
  - Observe for signs of tube blockage, which is best avoided by flushing the tube well after feeds.
  - Observe for dislodgement of the tube or device (see 📖 Pitfalls, p. 423).
- Once the feed is complete flush the gastrostomy button as per policy, clamp, and disconnect the extension set and replace the stopper.
- Wash and store the extension set as per policy.
- Dispose of all equipment, wash hands, and document episode of care.

Practice tips

- Feeds should be administered at room temperature to promote comfort.
- If a tube becomes blocked the administration of either warm or fizzy fluid can help to unblock the tubing. If this is unsuccessful medical review should be sought.[1]

Pitfalls

- ❶ If there is any doubt in relation to tube position this must be positively ascertained before the tube is used.
- ❶ Feeds should not be administered too quickly as this can lead to 'dumping syndrome'—a condition where ingested food bypasses the stomach too rapidly and thus enters the small intestine mainly undigested.[1]
- ❶ *Dislodgement:* if a tube is accidentally dislodged/pulled out a replacement tube should be reinserted into the stoma as quickly as possible to prevent closure of the stoma.

---

[1] Glasper A, Aylott M, Battrick C. (2010). *Developing Practical Skills for Nursing Children and Young People.* Hodder Arnold, London.

[2] Coyne I, Neill F, Timmins F. (2010). *Clinical Skills in Children's Nursing.* Oxford University Press, Oxford.

[3] National Patient Safety Agency (2011). *Reducing the Harm Caused by Misplaced Nasogastric Feeding Tubes in Adults, Children and Infants: Patient Safety Alert* (1253). Available at: ℘ http://www.nrls.npsa.nhs.uk/resources/?entryid45=129640&q=0%c2%acnasogastric+feeding%c2%ac.

Gastrostomy care: cleaning, caring for, and changing

Background
The following information provides a guide to the general management and care of a balloon-inflated gastrostomy button. Please note it is also important to refer to local policy relevant to your area and manufacturer's guidelines.

Equipment
- Plastic apron.
- Sterile gloves.
- Dressing trolley.
- Sterile dressing pack.
- Alcohol gel.
- Detergent wipes for cleaning trolley.

For cleaning
- Cool boiled/sterile water.
- Sterile galipot.
- Sterile gauze swabs.

For changing
- Replacement gastrostomy device.
- Sterile water for injection.
- Gastrostomy extension set.
- Water based lubricant.
- 5-mL syringe.
- Sterile gauze swabs.

Procedure
This guidance is based on care of an established gastrostomy. Devices that have been recently inserted surgically require specific care. Please refer to local policy pertinent to your area.

Before the procedure
- Explain the procedure fully to the child and family, and gain consent.
- Ensure the child is in a comfortable position.
- Wash hands and apply plastic apron.
- Clean the trolley as per policy and decontaminate hands.
- Open the sterile dressing pack and prepare all required equipment using aseptic non-touch technique (ANTT, see 📖 Aseptic non-treatment technique, p. 174).
- Decontaminate hands as per policy and apply sterile gloves.

Cleaning a gastrostomy button
- Clean the stoma site at least once daily.
- Dip sterile gauze into warmed sterile water and wipe round the site once before discarding the gauze.
- Repeat until the stoma site is clean and document the episode of care.
- The area around the gastrostomy may be cleaned while the child is in the bath.

General care of a gastrostomy button

- Observe the stoma site for:
  - *Proper fit*—should fit flush to child's skin, but not be too tight. (The stoma tract may be measured; seek specialist advice for this).
  - *Signs of sore excoriated skin*—caused by leakage from stoma site.
  - *Signs of infection*—redness/swelling/purulent exudate/pain.
  - *Granulation tissue*—ensuring a proper fit may help prevent this.
  - *Damaged tube/device*—will need immediate replacement.
- The gastrostomy button should be rotated through 360° at least daily to prevent the tube from adhering to the child's skin.
- The water in the retention balloon should be changed weekly or as per manufacturer's instructions.
- Gastrostomy devices should be changed routinely as per manufacturer's instructions or as clinically indicated.
- Document the episode of care.

Changing a gastrostomy button

- Ensure the child is in a comfortable position, lying down is preferable.
- If replacement is routine in nature, assess whether any significant growth has occurred since the last change. If so the stoma tract may need to be measured to ensure insertion of the correct size device.
- Remove the new gastrostomy device from the sterile packaging using ANTT and place on the sterile field.
- Ensure the device is functional. Attach a 5-mL syringe to the balloon port. Insert the required amount of sterile water. Observe for leaks.
- Remove all water from the balloon and cover the tip with a water-based lubricant.
- Gently aspirate all water from the balloon on the device to be removed and document the volume obtained.
- Explain clearly to the child that you are about to remove their button.
- Hold the new device in your dominant hand.
- Using your non-dominant hand gently withdraw the old device and immediately insert the new button.
- Insert the device fully until it is flat against the skin, attach a 5-mL syringe to the balloon port and insert the stipulated amount of water (as per manufacturer's instructions/child's notes).
- Wipe away any remaining gel with sterile gauze and disconnect the syringe.
- *Check the position of the button:*
  - The button should fit snugly, but should not be too tight.
  - Turn the gastrostomy button one full circle to help confirm its position in the gastrostomy tract. If you cannot turn the button seek appropriate help or advice.
  - Attach the gastrostomy extension set and allow a small amount of gastric fluid to flow back into the set. Remove the fluid and test with pH indicator paper (the reading should be < than 5.5).
  - If pH is above 5.5 or no aspirate is obtained remove the button, reinsert and try again. If a satisfactory aspirate is still not obtained refer to local policy and seek appropriate advice, e.g. from medical team or nurse specialist.

- NB. Medications given to reduce acid production may affect pH value and show a reading higher than 5.5. Check with parents or drug card and seek appropriate medical advice.
- If a satisfactory aspirate has been obtained re attach the extension set and flush well with sterile water. (Check local policy for amount required). ❶ For renal patients seek advice from the renal nursing team on the amount of water needed to flush the device.
- While flushing inspect the stoma site for signs of leakage.
- ❶ If, on flushing, water will not go into the stomach or the child complains of pain, discontinue the flush immediately and seek advice as the device may be misplaced.
- Discard all equipment as per policy and wash hands.
- Document the episode of care, including the date inserted and the date the next change is due.

Practice tips

- Ensure the new device is inserted immediately following removal of the old device to preserve the stoma tract.

Pitfalls

- Do not overfill the balloon as this can cause the patient discomfort and damage the balloon.
- Plan to change the gastrostomy button before an enteral feed, otherwise feed will leak out of the stomach.
- ❶ Misplacement of the tube on insertion can be a potentially serious complication. This is when the device visually appears to be in the correct position, but the tip is actually positioned in the abdominal cavity as opposed to the stomach. (Hence, testing of any aspirate obtained following insertion of a new device is recommended).
- ❶ If in any doubt regarding the position of the device do not use the button until tube position has been confirmed.

Associated reading

Coyne I, Neill F, Timmins F. (2010). *Clinical Skills in Children's Nursing*. Oxford University Press, Oxford.

Glasper A, Aylott M, Battrick C. (2010). *Developing Practical Skills for Nursing Children and Young People*. Hodder Arnold, London.

National Patient Safety Agency (2011). *Reducing the Harm Caused by Misplaced Nasogastric Feeding Tubes in Adults, Children and Infants: Patient Safety Alert* (1253). Available at: ℅ http://www.nrls. npsa.nhs.uk/resources/?EntryId45=129640.

Bowel surgery care

Background

Bowel surgery can be necessary to treat varying conditions. Surgery can range from relatively minor procedures such as a herniotomy to much more complex surgery, involving full or partial resection of the bowel and the formation of stomas.

Pre-operative care for children undergoing some elective, bowel surgery may involve clearing the bowel of its contents (see 📖 Pitfalls, p. 429). This is necessary to aid the surgeon's view during surgery e.g. during colonoscopy and may reduce the risk of infection.[1] Washouts, enemas, or laxative preparations are used depending on the surgeon's preference. Laxatives are given orally or via a NGT and enemas are administered rectally to stimulate bowel movements and clear the bowel. Washouts flush the bowel clear of stool. ❶ Increased or excessive stool loss, which may occur following bowel preparation, can deplete the child's body of vital fluids. Regardless of the method of washout used, adequate hydration must be maintained to prevent dehydration, either by giving oral clear fluids or by administering fluids intravenously.[2] Some oral preparations can cause nausea and vomiting so intravenous (IV) fluids would be more appropriate in this circumstance.

As with any surgery/procedure, pre-operative care involves preparing the child and parent/carer for the proposed surgery, and any changes they may be faced with post-operatively.

Procedure

Pre-operatively

- Follow local protocol regarding general preoperative care (see 📖 Pre-operative care, p. 246).
- If bowel preparation is required, explain all stages of the procedure to the child and their carer, and gain consent.
- Allow the child and their parent/carer time to ask questions and express anxieties.
- If the child is toilet trained, ensure that they have access to a toilet for the duration of their bowel preparation.
- Ideally, a private cubicle with toilet facilities should be provided to maintain privacy and dignity.
- Carry out whichever method of bowel preparation is requested by the surgeon as per manufacturer's instructions and hospital policy.
- Measure and record all losses on a fluid balance chart and document all intake to ensure the child remains hydrated.
- Take baseline observations of temperature, pulse, and respirations (TPR) and blood pressure (BP) pre-operatively. Regular observations should continue during bowel preparation to observe for signs for dehydration. (1–4-hourly or as condition/local policy dictates).

Post-operatively

- Undertake regular observations (30min to 4-hourly as condition/local policy dictates).
- Monitor closely for signs of dehydration, bleeding, infection, or pain.

- Ensure adequate analgesia is administered. A morphine infusion or patient/nurse-controlled analgesia (PCA/NCA) may be administered with IV paracetamol to provide effective pain relief. Analgesia may vary between trusts, often dictated by the surgeon, anaesthetist, or pain team.
- Effective pain assessment appropriate for the child's age and cognition should be carried out to ensure pain relief is sufficient ([book] Assessment of pain, p. 118, [book] Pain management, p. 122, [book] Patient-controlled analgesia, p. 124, and [book] Nurse-controlled analgesia, p. 126).
- Post-operatively the child may be kept nil by mouth to allow the bowel to recover. Thus, IV maintenance fluids will be required.
- The child may have a NGT. This aims to reduce nausea and vomiting by removing gastric losses. If losses exceed 20mL/kg/day intravenous replacement will be required.
- Observe the child's wound site for bleeding or signs of infection. Contact the surgeon if there are concerns.
- If the child has had a stoma formed a referral to the stoma care nurse specialist should be made.

Practice Tips
- Infants have a larger surface area than older children or adults and as such can lose heat more quickly. Solution for washouts should be lukewarm prior to use to prevent rapid cooling of the infant/minimize abdominal cramps. ❶ NB special caution is required in very young children. ❶ Over-warming can damage the bowel.
- Positioning children on their left side with their knees drawn up makes insertion of the tube easier and may make distraction more effective as a parent/carer or play specialist can be positioned in front of the child away from the where the procedure is taking place.

Pitfalls
- ❶ The practice of routinely clearing the bowel prior to elective surgery is declining in popularity within the paediatric population and is not without risk. Routine bowel clearing prior to surgery must only be commenced at the specific request of the relevant surgeon.
- ❶ Patients with inflammatory bowel conditions such as Crohns Disease or colitis should not receive bowel washouts prior to surgery due to the risk of perforation or bleeding.[1]
- If saline or enema solution is retained, do not repeat the process. Seek medical assistance.

Associated reading
Trigg E. Mohammed T. (eds) (2010). *Practices in Children's Nursing: Guidelines for Hospital and Community.* Churchill Livingstone, Edinburgh.

[1] Dougherty L, Lister S. (2008). *The Royal Marsden Hospital Manual of Clinical Nursing Procedures,* 7th edn. Wiley-Blackwell, Oxford.

[2] Dykes C, Cash B. (2008). Key safety issues of bowel preparations for colonoscopy and importance of adequate hydration. *Gastroenterol Nurs* **31**(1), 30–5.

Recognizing infection/blockage

Background

Infection or blockage can disrupt the normal functioning of the bowel and prevent stool from passing through the bowel. Blockage can be partial or complete, and may be due to mechanical obstruction (a physical blockage), or an ileus (reduced motility with no structural cause). Infections can occur as a result of a virus or bacteria, and can indicate complications such as ulcerative colitis.

Causes of mechanical obstruction in children can include:

- Hernia (containing bowel).
- Adhesions (scar tissue from surgery or caused by Crohns disease).
- Intussusception (invagination of the bowel, often presenting with intermittent pain and redcurrant jelly-like stool that constitutes a more advanced sign in addition to symptoms of bowel obstruction).
- Tumour.
- Volvulus (an abnormal twist in a loop of bowel).
- Malrotation (non-rotation or incomplete rotation of the mid-gut).
- Severe constipation (can block the lower bowel so causing obstruction).

Ileus can be caused by:

- A chemical or electrolyte imbalance (i.e. hypokalaemia).
- A temporary result of abdominal surgery.
- Decreased blood supply to the bowel (can be caused by constriction of blood vessels or a blood clot).
- Bacterial or viral pathogens.
- Meconium ileus (failure to pass meconium in first 48h of life) may present with bileus vomiting and abdominal distension).
- Paralytic ileus in the newborn may be associated with necrotizing enterocolitis (a condition seen more often in premature babies where part of the bowel becomes necrotic). ❶ This can cause infection in the blood and lungs, and is life threatening.

Symptoms of mechanical obstruction include:

- Abdominal distension.
- Abdominal pain and cramping.
- Constipation.
- Diarrhoea.
- Vomiting (faecal vomiting can occur with severe obstruction).

Symptoms of ileus include:

- Abdominal distension.
- Abdominal pain and cramping.
- Constipation.
- Diarrhoea.
- Vomiting.
- Absent bowel sounds.
- Lack of flatulence.

Symptoms of infection include:
- Vomiting.
- Diarrhoea.
- Abdominal distension.
- Abdominal cramps.
- Pyrexia.

Various procedures can determine diagnosis of an infection or bowel obstruction.

Procedure
- Assessment of symptom history is vital to establish the cause and to determine any relevant past medical history.
- Medical examination to listen for bowel sounds (high pitched sounds suggest obstruction, and absence of sounds is a sign of prolonged obstruction or ileus).
- Assess pain considering the type of pain, duration, and severity.
- Assess for pyrexia, vomiting, and any bowel movements.
- Passing a NGT may relieve distension and vomiting.
- Bloods are taken to identify infection that may then be treated with antibiotics. Ideally, IV access should be secured at the time of taking bloods.
- Abdominal X-ray can detect a blockage in the small or large intestine.
- Abdominal CT scan can distinguish between a partial or complete obstruction and identify restricted blood flow.
- Surgery may be necessary to relieve obstruction or remove necrotic bowel that can be caused by restricted blood supply.
- Treatment will depend on the cause.

Practice Tips
- A patient should be kept nil by mouth until obstruction is ruled out and adequate hydration must be maintained with intravenous fluids.
- ❶ Late presentation may include symptoms of shock due to dehydration and fluid resuscitation may be necessary.

Pitfalls
- ❶ Bileus vomiting in neonates should be treated as an emergency and necessitates an urgent surgical review.
- ❶ Vomiting in the infant can be a sign of pyloric stenosis (obstruction of the pyloric sphincter), particularly if the vomiting is projectile. This also requires an urgent surgical review.

Associated reading
Shalkow J, Florens A, Asz J. (2010). Paediatric small bowel obstruction. Available at: ℘ http://emedicine.medscape.com/article/930411-overview.

Infant feeding: breast feeding

Background

Breast milk contains everything a baby needs for around the first 6 months of their lives. It has the added benefit of helping to protect babies against various infections and diseases, whilst also conferring health benefits to the mother. The longer a child is breast-fed, the longer the protection lasts. Current guidance advises that babies should be exclusively breast-fed for the first 6 months. WHO recommends breast feeding for 2yrs or longer.

Equipment

- Clean cold running water.
- Comfortable chair.
- Nursing bra (for ease).
- Breast pads.
- Drink.
- Cream, e.g. white soft paraffin, purified lanolin.

Procedure

- Immediately after a baby is born skin-to-skin contact should be encouraged as this helps to promote breast feeding.
- Ensure all steps are clearly explained to the mother.
- Mothers may need a lot of support in the early stages.
- Ensure the mother is in a comfortable position.
- The mother should hold the baby's whole body close to her with the baby's nose positioned level with her nipple.[1]
- The mother should allow the baby's head to tip back slightly to allow the babies top lip to brush against the nipple.
- This should encourage the baby to make a wide open mouth.[1]
- At this point the mother should gently bring the baby towards her breast (the baby's bottom lip and chin should touch the breast first).
- When the chin is firmly touching the breast; the mouth is open wide and the nose is clear there will be more of the dark skin of the areola visible above the baby's top lip than below it.
- A baby's cheeks should be full and rounded as they feed.[1]
- If the mother does not feel that her baby has latched on correctly she can gently slide a clean finger into the baby's mouth, gently break the suction and try again.
- Breast feeding should feel comfortable for the mother, the baby should be relaxed, and a soft swallowing sound should be audible.
- Babies will usually come off the breast when they have had enough.
- After the baby has finished feeding they should be winded as appropriate. Breast-fed babies often have less wind than formula-fed babies.

Practice tips

- Women often worry about whether their baby is receiving enough breast milk. Generally, a baby is getting enough milk if:
  - The baby is healthy and gaining weight.
  - The baby is satisfied after the majority of feeds and comes off the breast on their own.
  - The mother's breasts and nipples are not sore.
- Breast feeding is thought to protect:
  - *The baby against*—ear infections, asthma, eczema, chest infections, obesity, GI infections, and childhood diabetes.[1]
  - *The mother against*—breast and ovarian cancer.[1]
- All pregnant women have milk that is ready for her baby at birth. This is known as colostrum and contains antibodies that help to boost a baby's immunity.
- If a woman develops cracked or sore nipples the following tips may help:
  - Squeezing a few drops of milk from the breast at the end of a feed and gently rubbing them into the skin.[1]
  - Breast pads should be changed at each feed. If possible, it is better to use breast pads without a plastic backing.[1]
  - It is advisable to avoid soap as it dries out the skin.
  - It is recommended that breast-feeding women wear cotton bras to ensure air can circulate.
  - Cracks or bleeding may be treated with a thin smear of white soft paraffin or purified lanolin.[1] If lanolin is used it should be applied to the cracks, rather than the entire nipple.
  - Women often feel thirsty when breast feeding; thus, it is advisable that they have a drink close to hand while feeding.

Pitfalls

- The baby not latching onto the breast properly. This could lead to:
  - An unsettled baby who is not receiving enough milk.
  - Weight loss.
  - Cracked sore nipples.
  - Tender breasts, blocked ducts, or mastitis.
- Babies born with a tongue tie can have difficulty in latching on. If there are concerns, the mother and child should be referred to their midwife.
- It is not advisable to give babies dummies until breast feeding is successfully established as this can reduce a mother's milk supply.
- Breast feeding while natural is not always easy to get right. Some women need a lot of support and may feel extremely anxious, tired, and distressed. It is important to be alert to these signs and to remember that breast feeding is not always successful for all women and their babies.

Associated reading

[1] Department of Health (2010). *The Pregnancy Book*. COI. DoH, London. Also available at: http://www.dh.gov.uk/publications.

Expressing and storage of breast milk

Background
All pregnant women should be informed of the benefits of breastfeeding. The UK Government and World Health Organization (WHO) recommend that babies be exclusively breast fed for the first 6 months of life, as breast milk contains all the nourishment a baby will need. If a baby is unable to breast feed, it is important that the mother starts expressing breast milk as soon as possible after birth, preferably within 6h.

Equipment
- Nil if hand-expressing.
- A hand or electric breast pump.

Procedure
Hand expression: first 48h
- Wash your hands before expressing or handling expressed breast milk.
- Gentle breast massage can be used at any time to start the milk flow.
- Find where you need to press to start milk flow. Milk reservoirs in the breast do not actually exist. Instead, ultrasound imaging appears to show that milk ducts expand and contract along their entire length.
- Press a few centimetres away from the nipple, where the breast feels slightly firmer.
- Position the thumb and first finger opposite each other, so that the breast lies between them.
- Compress and release your finger and thumb rhythmically to encourage milk flow.
- It may take a few minutes until the let-down reflex starts.
- If milk stops flowing, move your finger and thumb to a new position, and repeat until milk starts flowing again.
- Repeat until milk stops flowing then repeat on the second breast.

Expression using breast pump
- After 48h use simultaneous pumping with an electric breast pump according to individual manufacturers guidelines.[1]

Storage of Breast Milk
- Store fresh expressed breast milk (EBM) in the fridge at 0–4°C and use within 5 days.[2]
- EBM can be stored in the freezer compartment of a fridge for up to 2 weeks or a freezer at –20°C for up to 6 months.[3]
- Defrost milk by placing in a fridge and use within 24h.[2]
- Once warmed use immediately.
- Although, the clinical significance of organisms in maternal EBM is uncertain, its role as a potential vector for infecting pathogens should be recognized.[2]
- EBM should be used in order of date expressed.
- Once warmed, fresh EBM should be used within 1h.

Practice tips

- Ideally, it is preferable to use fresh breast milk where possible, as freezing may impact on the properties of the milk.
- Prolactin, the hormone that produces milk is at its highest during the night. Expressing at this time will ensure a good ongoing supply.
- Mothers should be encouraged to engage in skin to skin contact with their baby as soon as possible after birth, ideally <45min.[2]
- Whilst in hospital mothers should be shown how to hand express their milk. Written information should also be provided.[2]
- If a baby requires admission to the neonatal unit it is important for mothers to express 6–8 times in 24h to help stimulate good flow.[3]
- Simultaneous pumping has been found to encourage higher prolactin levels, and a greater volume of milk.
- Women, who breast feed, lower their risk of developing breast and ovarian cancer.[4]
- Health benefits conferred by human milk include reduced incidence of diarrhoea and otitis media.[4]
- Children who are exclusively breast fed during the first 3 months are less likely to develop juvenile, insulin-dependent diabetes.[4]
- Breast milk is important for premature babies. Premature breast milk is extra rich in antibodies and growth factors and so can: protect against bacteria and viruses/boost the baby's immune system/protect against stomach and chest infections/is easier to digest.[5]

Pitfalls

- EBM should not be warmed in a microwave as this can result in hot spots.[2,3]
- Avoid teats, dummies, or nipple shields whilst establishing breast feeding as they can cause nipple confusion/interfere with normal sucking.[6]
- For women who do not produce sufficient milk, technical and emotional support is fundamental to reduce stress levels.
- Donor breast milk is available, but due to potential infection risks banked milk undergoes pasteurization and donor mothers are screened for HIV antibodies.[7]

---

[1] Renfrew MJ, Craig D, Dyson L, McCormic F. (2009). Breastfeeding promotion for infants in neonatal units: a systematic review and economic analysis. *Hlth Technol Assess* **13**(40), 1–146.

[2] The National Collaborating Centre for Primary Care (NCCPC). (2006). *Postnatal Care of women and their babies*. Available at: ℘ http://www.nice.org.uk/nicemedia/live/10988/30146/30146.pdf.

[3] Department of Health (2009). *Birth to five*. Produced by COI for the Department of Health, London. Available at: ℘ http://www.dh.gov.uk/publications.

[4] NHS Choices. (2011). *Breastfeeding*. Available at: ℘ http://www.nhs.uk/Planners/breastfeeding/Pages/breastfeeding-benefits.aspx.

[5] ℘ http://www.bliss.org.uk.

[6] UNICEF. *The Baby Friendly Initiative*. [Online]. Available from: ℘ http://www.unicef.org.uk/babyfriendly.

[7] NICE (2010). *Donor Breast Milk Banks*. Available at: ℘ http://guidance.nice.org.uk/CG93.

Infant feeding: formula feeding

Background

Infant formulas are derived from cow's milk that has been modified in order to meet the nutritional requirements of growing infants.[1] Infant formula can be used as an alternative to breast milk, but formula milk does not confer the extra health benefits of human milk (see 📖 Infant feeding: breast feeding, p. 432).

Equipment

- Sterile bottle and teat.
- Sterile plastic teat forceps.
- Sterile bottle of infant formula/powdered milk formula.
- Jug of hot water/appropriate bottle warmer.
- Plastic apron.

Procedure

- Explain the procedure to the parents/carers and gain consent.
- Ensure that the correct infant formula is available.
- Wash hands, put on a plastic apron, and ensure a clean workspace.
- If using sterile ready-made formula:
  - Check the expiry date.
  - Ensure that the button in the middle of the lid remains depressed.
  - Inspect the appearance of the formula for any potential concerns.
- If using powdered formula milk refer to 📖 Making up infant formula, p. 438.
- Remove the sterile bottle and teat from the sterilizing unit, and assemble. Use sterile plastic teat forceps to remove the teat and attach to bottle.
- It is important to use the child's own bottle if possible and the correct sized teat:
  - If the holes in the teat are too small the child will have to work harder to obtain the feed and may tire quickly.
  - If the holes in the teat are too large milk flow will be quicker and the child may be at greater risk of choking.
- Pour the sterile milk formula into the sterile bottle, and fix the teat and lid. Ready-made formula can be given to term infants at room temperature; however, many infants prefer it to be warmed.[1]
- Warm the formula to the required temperature by placing the bottle into a jug of warm water or an appropriate bottle warmer.
- Test the temperature of the milk by applying a few drops onto the underside of your wrist. The milk should feel warm, but not hot.
- If appropriate, ensure that the child's nose is clear of mucous and secretions as infants will often not feed well if their nose is blocked.
- Take the infant in your arms, and ensure that both you and the baby are sat in a comfortable position.
- Ensure that the child is positioned with their head above their stomach to reduce the risk of accidental aspiration/regurgitation of milk.
- Gently put the teat of the bottle to the infant's lips.

- If they appear reluctant to accept the teat, try stroking the side of the child's mouth with the teat.
- Once feeding, observe the child for any signs of distress that might indicate a problem, such as gulping, excessive movement of extraneous limbs, a worried expression, a change in colour.
- Maintain eye contact and observe the child continually during the feed. Stop the feed immediately if any of the signs listed here are noted.
- The bottle should be held in a position that ensures the teat remains full of milk to minimize the amount of air swallowed by the child.
- Stop the feed to wind the infant at an appropriate point. Most infants can take approximately half the volume of their feed before they require winding.[2]
- Ensure the feed does not exceed 30min.
- Once the feed is complete, wind the infant again.
- Ensure the child is comfortable. Ideally and if safe, allow the child to sit up for 20–30min after feeding and remain with them to reduce the risk of regurgitation/aspiration.[2]
- Discard any unused feed within 2h.
- Document the volume of the feed taken on a fluid balance chart.
- Document any possets/vomits and the estimated volume.
- Wash the bottle, teat, retaining ring, and lid in warm soapy water, rinse thoroughly and place in an appropriate sterilizing unit (see 📖 Care of infant feeding equipment, p. 440).

Practice tips

- The feed requirements of an average healthy infant during the first week of life are approximately 120mL/kg/day. Subsequent feed requirements rise to approximately 150mL/kg/day.

Pitfalls

- ❶ Infant formula feeds should not be warmed in a microwave as this can result in the development of 'hot spots'.[3]
- Formula milk does not contain the antibodies evident in human milk so may not confer the same health benefits associated with breast milk.
- Cow's milk should not be given as a main drink to children under 1yr.[4]
- Follow-on formula is not suitable for babies under 6 months.[4]
- ❶ Babies should not be left alone with a bottle. *Danger of choking.*
- ❶ Babies should not be fed, whilst lying flat as this increases the risk of vomiting and aspiration of both feed and vomit into the lungs.[2]

[1] Coyne I, Neill F, Timmins, F. (2010). *Clinical Skills in Children's Nursing.* Oxford University Press, Oxford.

[2] Trigg E, Mohammed TA. (2010). *Practices in Children's Nursing: Guidelines for Hospital and Community,* 3rd edn. Churchill Livingstone Elsevier, Edinburgh.

[3] Department of Health (2009). *Birth to Five.* Produced by COI for the Department of Health, London. Available at: 🔗 http://www.dh.gov.uk/publications.

[4] Department of Health (2010). *The Pregnancy Book.* Produced by COI for the Department of Health, London. Available at: 🔗 http://www.dh.gov.uk/publications.

Making up infant formula

Background

Infant formula is derived from processed, skimmed cow's milk. It is treated so that babies can digest it, and vitamins, minerals, vegetable oils, and fatty acids are added to ensure that infants receive all the nutrients they require.[1] Infant milk powder is not a sterile product and, consequently, can contain bacteria such as *Cronobacter sakazakii* (formerly *Enterobacter sakazakii*) and more rarely *Salmonella*.[1] Therefore, it is important that formula feeds are prepared carefully and safely to ensure that such bacteria are killed and so rendered unable to cause infection. ❶ Infections are rare, but can be potentially life threatening; hence, thorough sterilizing of all feeding equipment is also vitally important. (See 📖 Care of infant feeding equipment, p. 440.)

Equipment

- Clean, clear working environment.
- Correct powdered milk formula.
- Correct measuring scoop (usually the scoop enclosed with the milk product).
- Clean knife/sterile spatula.
- Clean, running, cold tap water.
- Kettle.
- Sterile bottle/teat.
- Apron (if in the hospital setting).

Procedure

- Ensure a clean, clear work surface is available.
- Wash and dry your hands thoroughly.
- Apply a plastic apron if in the hospital setting.
- Ensure that the correct powdered formula is available and labelled for the appropriate patient.
- Check the expiry date and the date that the powder was opened. Powdered formula milk should be discarded 28 days after opening. In the acute setting, the date the formula was opened must be clearly displayed on the outer packaging.
- Ensure that the correct measuring scoop is available. Only the scoop specified by the manufacturers and enclosed with the milk powder should be used. Use of the wrong scoop can lead to an inappropriate concentration of milk.
- Fill the kettle with fresh clean tap water and boil. Formula milk must be made up with water hot enough to kill any bacteria that may be present (at least 70°C—allow the boiled water to cool for no longer than 30min).
- If a cold water sterilizing system has been used shake off any excess solution and rinse the bottle, teat, retaining ring, and cap in cool boiled water.
- Assemble the bottle—ensure the teat and cap are placed on the upturned lid of the sterilizer as opposed to the work surface.[1]

- Pour the correct amount of water into the sterile bottle and allow to cool for up to 30min.
- Always add the water first to ensure the correct ratio of powder to water.
- Make up one feed at a time only (see 📖 Practice tips, p. 439).
- Fill the scoop with milk powder—level this off with the flat edge of a clean knife/leveler provided (use a sterile spatula in the hospital setting). Do not pack the milk powder firmly into the scoop.
- Following the manufacturer's instructions, add the correct number of scoops to the water.
- Screw the retaining ring and teat onto the bottle, taking care not to touch the teat. Apply the lid and shake the bottle until all the milk powder has been dissolved.
- Cool the milk quickly by holding it under cold running water—❶ Fluid at 70°C is still hot enough to burn/scald.
- Test the temperature of the milk by applying a few drops onto the underside of the wrist. The milk should feel warm, but not hot.
- Feed the infant immediately (see 📖 Infant feeding: formula feeding, p. 436).

Practice tips

- Bacteria multiply quickly at room temperature and can even multiply in some fridges, albeit more slowly. It is advisable to make up a new bottle for each feed.[1]
- It is not advisable to use water that has already been boiled or water that has been artificially softened to make up infant formula. If bottled water is used this must be boiled to ensure it is hot enough to kill any bacteria that may be present in the powder.
- ❶ Very young infants are most at risk. It is advisable to use sterile ready-made liquid formula for premature or low birth weight babies (1).

Pitfalls

- Failure to follow the manufacturer's instructions in relation to: the ratio of scoops to the volume of fluid/use of the wrong scoop/packing too much powder into the scoop; may lead to an incorrect concentration of milk which can make the child ill:
  - Too much powder can lead to constipation/dehydration.
  - Too little powder can result in the infant not receiving the required amount of nutrients.
- ❶ Care should be taken if using bottled mineral water as some brands are not suitable for infants due to their high Na content.

Associated reading

Coyne I, Neill F, Timmins F. (2010). *Clinical Skills in Children's Nursing*. Oxford University Press, Oxford.

[1] Department of Health (2009). *Birth to Five*. COI, London. Available at: 🔗 http://www.nhs.uk/birthtofive.

Care of infant feeding equipment

Background

Breast feeding is the healthiest way to feed a baby. Some women, however, are unable to, or choose not to, breast feed and instead use formula milk. Some women who breast feed may also express breast milk to give to their baby via a bottle, e.g. If a mother is going to be away from her baby for a period of time or is returning to work. In either case, it is important that all feeding equipment is properly cleaned and sterilized in order to help protect the baby against infection.

Equipment

- Hot soapy water.
- Bottle brush.
- Running cold water supply.
- Cold water sterilizing unit or Steam sterilizer.

Procedure

- Wash hands.
- Clean and rinse the bottle and teat in hot soapy water as quickly as possible following a feed, using a clean bottle brush.
- The bottle and teat should be thoroughly cleaned inside and out.
- Rinse all feeding equipment in cold running water before placing into the chosen sterilizer unit.

Cold water sterilizing

- Follow manufacturer's instructions to make up the sterilizing solution.
- The sterilizing solution should be changed every 24h.
- Leave all feeding equipment in the sterilizing solution for at least 30min before use.[1]
- Ensure all equipment remains completely submerged in the solution.
- Ensure that no air bubbles are evident in the bottles/teats.

Steam sterilizing

- Follow relevant manufacturer's instructions.
- Ensure all bottles and teats are placed carefully in the sterilizing unit.
- Position bottles, teats, retaining rings and bottle lids in the unit with the openings face down.
- Wash hands before removing any feeding equipment.

Practice tips

- Any equipment not used immediately should be re-sterilized before use.[1]
- If the bottles and teats are not going to be used straight away they should be fully assembled and the lid applied to ensure that the inside of the bottle and outside of the teat do not become contaminated.[2]
- All equipment used for feeding children under the age of 1yr needs to be sterilized.
- For some particularly vulnerable children sterilizing may need to continue for longer.
- By sterilizing all feeding equipment, washing your hands and keeping the preparation area clean the chance of a baby getting diarrhoea and vomiting will be reduced.[1]

Pitfalls

As it is impossible to destroy all the bacteria that may be present in infant formula a fresh bottle should be made up for each feed (see 📖 Making up infant formula, p. 438).

[1] Department of Health (2011) *Guide to bottle Feeding*. Available at: ℘ http://www.dh.gov.uk/prod_consum_dh/groups/dh_digitalassets/documents/digitalasset/dh_124526.pdf (accessed 11 November 2011).

[2] Department of Health (2005).*Guidance for Health Professionals on Safe Preparation, Storage and Handling of Powdered Infant Formula*. Available at: ℘ http://www.dh.gov.uk/prod_consum_dh/groups/dh_digitalassets/@dh/@en/documents/digitalasset/dh_063693.pdf (accessed 20 September 2010).

Weaning

Background

The introduction of complementary food to the diet (*weaning*) is a critical nutritional stage in the infant's life, and the optimal age has been much debated. The period from birth to 1yr is a time of nutritional vulnerability when attention to good nutrition is crucial to support rapid growth and development. Therefore, weaning is described as the process of gradually changing an infant's diet from milk alone to combining milk and solids. In 1994 the UK government recommended that the introduction of solid foods be delayed until 4–6 months. This was revised in 2003 to reflect updated WHO guidelines,[1] which recommended delaying the introduction of solids until the infant is 6 months.

Procedure

Ready prepared baby foods

- Check 'sell by' and 'best by' dates.
- Check that the seals on cans and jars have not been broken or damaged.
- Check labels for sugar and salt content.
- Check labels to ensure that 'sugar free' foods do not contain added sugar or sweeteners.

Introducing a range of drinks

- Breast milk.
- Formula milk.
- Follow-on-milks.
- Water.
- Fruit juices well diluted, after 6 months.

Vegetarian and vegan diets

- Key considerations should include composition of breast milk from vegetarian and vegan mothers. Composition is similar to non-vegetarian mothers with the exception of fat composition.
- Breast-fed vegan infants may require supplements of vitamin B12, and older infants may need zinc supplements and reliable sources of iron and vitamin B12.

Baby-led weaning

This is a method, which allows the infant to control the solid intake by self-feeding from the beginning of the weaning process. Baby-led weaning emphasizes the exploration of taste, texture, colour, and smell.

Successful weaning

- Allow plenty of time and use play as appropriate.
- Feed the child in a high chair or your lap.
- Remain in attendance with or near the child when they are eating due to risk of choking.
- Introduce new food and textures gradually.
- Persevere—if the infant refuses, take the food away and try again later.
- Proceed at the infant's pace and, remember, weaning can be messy.

Foods to avoid (NHS Choices 2009) include:

• Salt.
• Sugar.
• Honey.
• Nuts/seeds.
• Low fat/low calorie.
• High fibre.
• Certain types of fish, e.g. shark, swordfish, marlin due to high levels of mercury.
• Raw shellfish can increase the risk of food poisoning.
• Raw and lightly cooked eggs.

Practice tips

• Pureed or well mashed food is recognized as the '*bridge*' between liquid and solid food
• It is easy to monitor how much the infant is taking from a spoon.
  At 6 months the infant can take food off a spoon using their upper lip, rather than sucking from the spoon.
• For an example of weaning diets see 📖 Associated reading, p. 443.[2]

Pitfalls

• Solid foods should never be given before 4 months—the early introduction of solids has been associated with diarrhoea in infancy, greater risk of respiratory wheeze, and increased percentage body fat and weight in childhood.[1]
• Wheat-based foods containing gluten (wheat, flour, breakfast cereals, rusks, etc.) should be avoided up to 6 months of age as they are potential allergens.
• Tea and coffee are not suitable for babies and young children as they reduce iron absorption and, if sugar is added, may contribute to tooth decay.
• Herbal teas are not recommended because some are toxic for infants causing physiological problems, such as an increased heart rate.
• Avoid 'prop feeding' from a bottle as this may contribute to ear infections. Ideally, the infant should be in the upright position to prevent fluid moving between the oropharynx and Eustachian tube of the ear.

Associated reading

World Health Organization (WHO) (2001). *WHO: Fifty-Fourth World Assembly. Global Strategy for Infant and Young Children Feeding*. Available at: 🔗 http://apps.who.int/gb/archive/pdf-files/WHA54/ea54id4.pdf.

Wright CM, Parkinson KN, Drewett RF. (2004). Why are babies weaned early? Data From a prospective population based cohort study. *Arch Dis Childh* **89**, 813–16.

[1] Scott JA, Binns CW, Graham KI, Oddy WH. (2009). Predictors of early introduction of solids in infants: results of a cohort study. *Biomed Pediat*. Available at: 🔗 http://www.ncbi.nlm.nih.gov/pmc/articles/PMC2754451/?tool=pubmed (accessed 7 May 2010).

[2] Scanlon K, Sorrentino AL. (2006). Health problems during infancy. In: Glasper A, Richardson J. (eds) *A Textbook of Children and Young People's Nursing*. Elsevier, London.

Food allergy

Background

Allergy defined

A food allergy is a heightened reaction (known as sensitivity) to a particular food. This is an immune-mediated adverse reaction and is different from food intolerance, which is a non-immune-mediated adverse reaction. ❶ A severe reaction resulting in anaphylaxis is a life threatening condition. Rapid treatment is crucial in managing this emergency and preventing fatalities (📖 Management of food allergy/anaphylaxis treatment, p. 448). A child with asthma has an ↑ chance of suffering a severe reaction. Food allergies can have a profound impact on the child and family. Diagnosis with supportive long-term management between health professionals, the family, and the child can help alleviate the daily anxiety and help the child participate in normal childhood activities.

Common paediatric food allergies

- Cow's milk.
- Egg whites.
- Fish (especially cod and shellfish).
- Wheat.
- Tree nuts (especially peanuts).
- Soya bean.
- Fruit:
  - Allergy to fruits is less common than other allergens on the list; however, more cases are being discovered and are often associated with individuals who also have allergies to pollen.
  - More often than not the symptoms are mild in nature affecting the mouth and causing itching/rash/blisters where the fruit has touched the lips.
  - More severe reactions have been documented, but are rare.
  - The most common fruits are: apples, kiwi, peach, plums, and cherries. Cooking the fruit before consumption may reduce or even eliminate the reaction.

ImmunoCAP RAST allergy blood test (RAST test)

- This blood test measures the specific IgE in the serum.
- Specific IgE is a substance produced by the body when a person has an allergy.
- The results will take some time to come back from the laboratory and will be given to patients during their next outpatient appointment.

Skin test

- The skin prick test is a quick, reliable, and safe method to ascertain whether a child is allergic to common foods.
- It can be completed at an outpatient appointment and takes approximately 20min. (❶ Emergency drugs and equipment should be available).
- It involves placing a small drop of an allergen onto the child's arm and then 'pricking' the skin at a 90° angle (outer dermis only).

- After 15min the doctor will be able to read the results. A positive reaction shows a wheal (raised area) surrounded by redness (a flare) >3mm or more.
- Results can then be discussed with the child/adolescent and family.

Signs and symptoms of an allergic reaction

Mild to moderate reactions include:

- *GI:* nausea, vomiting, abdominal cramps, diarrhoea.
- *Skin and mucosal:* flushing, urticaria (itchiness), and angioedema.
- *Respiratory:* runny nose, sneezing.
- *Ocular:* red, swollen, watery, and itchy eyes.
- *Oral:* mouth ulceration, lip swelling, metallic taste in the mouth.

❶ Severe reaction = anaphylaxis

- *Respiratory:*
  - *Upper airway*—stridor, hoarseness, difficulty in swallowing, tongue swelling.
  - *Lower airway*—wheeze, cough, chest tightness, cyanosis.
- *Cardiovascular:* tachycardia, arrhythmia, shock, hypotension.
- Feelings of impending doom, anxiety, headache, loss of consciousness.

Practice tips

- Adolescents may experience food allergies during puberty, due to changes in hormones and the body's threshold. Once through puberty the body settles and the adolescent may not experience any further reactions.
- Anaphylaxis can be one or both severe reactions (respiratory and circulatory).
- For a reaction to be classed significant you need to have one severe reaction or two or more minor reactions.

Associated reading

🖰 http://www.allergyuk.org.

Food challenge/management of food allergy

Background

Children attend a day case admission for their food challenge test, upon the Consultants request. This usually follows an emergency admission to hospital/referral from their GP due to a previous allergic reaction. A detailed record of the child's medical and family history should already have been taken during an outpatient appointment. A RAST test and/or skin allergy test (📖 Food allergy, p. 444) should also have been done. This helps the consultant decide whether the food challenge is required/ the individual risk this poses for the child. Food challenges are conducted when other tests have been inconclusive or results indicate a child may have grown out of their allergy. Valid parental consent is required before the test can be done.

Procedure

Preparation for the food challenge

Parent and child

- The child should be nil by mouth (NBM) from midnight the evening before the test. If a mother is breast feeding please continue as normal.
- No antihistamine medications should be given for 72h prior to the challenge as this could mask a reaction.
- Parents should inform the hospital if their child has a wheeze, temperature, or diarrhoea or vomiting, or is generally unwell as the test will need to be rescheduled.
- Asthmatic children should bring their inhalers to the appointment.
- Parents should be prepared to remain with the child for the entire length of stay.
- Food and snacks that can be safely eaten by the child should be brought for after the test along with spare clothes in case the child vomits.

Health professionals

- Ensure valid consent has been obtained.
- Ensure emergency medication has been prescribed in accordance with drug policy and child's admission weight, e.g. chlorpheniramine, adrenaline, and hydrocortisone (📖 Anaphylaxis, p. 320).
- Ensure oxygen, suction, and resuscitation equipment is available (📖 Respiratory arrest and basic life support, p. 324).

During the procedure

- Welcome the child/parent to the ward, introduce yourself, and orientate them to their surroundings. Show them the bedside call button.
- Ensure the parent and child knows why they have come to hospital, and what to expect during the controlled food challenge.

- Complete nursing paperwork. Gain as much information as possible on previous allergic reactions. Document treatment previously required.
- ❶ Ensure all preparation instructions have been followed. It is unsafe to proceed otherwise and a new appointment will be required. If this occurs ensure verbal and written preparation instructions have been given prior to discharge. If there is a language barrier use language line/interpreter. Ensure this is documented in the notes and an interpreter booked for the next admission.
- Complete a full set of patient observations (📖 Vital signs examination, p. 6).
- Document the child's weight and measure their peak flow (📖 Recording peak flow, p. 354).
- Make a visual assessment, check the skin to ensure no rashes or swelling are present.
- Obtain an appropriate medical review to ensure that the child is fit and well enough to commence the test.
- Inform the medical team when the challenge is due to begin so they can be on the ward.
- Ensure emergency medication/equipment is within easy reach and medication is prescribed correctly.
- Once the test begins the child and parent cannot leave the ward, and must be nursed on the open ward in view of staff. Toys/games can be brought to the bedside.
- Commence the food challenge by rubbing a small piece of the food on the inside of the child's lower lip (on the oromucosal junction).
- Wait 15min, if there is no reaction; give the child a small piece of the challenge food to eat.
- Give incremental amounts of the challenge food at 15-min intervals. On each occasion double the dose. A good food test challenge is total 8g of food. However, hospital policies may vary.
- Monitor and record the child's vital signs every 15min.
- ❶ Stop the challenge promptly if there are any signs of an allergic reaction:
  - Administer the prescribed chlorpheniramine and inform the doctor immediately.
  - Proceed to emergency medication/treatment if anaphylaxis occurs (📖 Anaphylaxis, p. 320). The child will need to stay in hospital and be monitored overnight following adrenaline administration.
  - A doctor must review the child prior to discharge home.
  - Clearly document that the child has had a positive allergic reaction to the food.
- The challenge is complete when the child has eaten the total amount of the food challenge with no reaction.
- Monitor the child for a further 2.5h after the last dose of food to ensure there is no delayed reaction.
- Record and document vital signs again including a peak flow if age appropriate prior to discharge.

Negative tests
- Discharge advice is to continue to avoid the food until seen by the Consultant and dietician at the child's next outpatient appointment.
- Food can then be slowly introduced into the child's diet in accordance with medical advice.
- The child's GP, health visitor, and school nurse should be informed of the outcome of the food challenge test.

Positive tests
- Adrenaline auto-injector Pen training should be given and 2 adrenaline pens prescribed and given to the parent prior to discharge (📖 Management of food allergy/anaphylaxis treatment, p. 448).
- Refer to a dietician.
- The child's GP, health visitor, and school nurse should be informed of the outcome of the food challenge test.
- The medical notes should be returned to the referring consultant so a follow up outpatient appointment can be arranged.

Practice tips
- The hospital environment is alien to the child and disrupts their routine. Play and age appropriate language should be used to try to lessen the effect (see Chapter 6).
- Parents are often nervous about the challenge and may have lots of questions. Set time aside to listen and answer their questions. Give reassurance and support.
- Look at patient/staff ratio when allocating care. Some Trusts prefer to have food challenges nursed as one to one care. If your Trust policy allows you to have other patients, while conducting a food challenge please ensure they are low dependency.
- Routine IV cannulation is not usually required as the test is not designed to precipitate anaphylaxis.
- Adolescents will be managed differently, allowing them to take an active role in their admission, dependant on their maturity and level of comprehension.

Pitfalls
- ❶ High risk patients should not be food challenged.
- Remember that some cough and cold medication should be avoided prior to the test as it may contain antihistamines.

Management of food allergy/anaphylaxis treatment
Background
Children who are at risk of experiencing a moderate to severe allergic reaction will be prescribed two adrenaline auto-injector pens by their doctor. This device (shaped like a large pen) contains either a 150- or 300-microgram dose of adrenaline (depending on the age/weight of the child).
- The adrenaline pen should be used in the emergency treatment of sudden life-threatening allergic reactions (anaphylaxis).
- ❶ Anaphylaxis occurs within minutes of exposure to the allergen, and prompt emergency treatment is needed to prevent possible fatalities.

- Training will be required to enable the responsible adult to use the device safely.
- Please refer to local policy as to which auto-injector device is currently being used within your Trust as there is more than one on the market.
- Adolescents may be shown how to self-administer the adrenaline as part of their self-management programme.
- Upon request a close, responsible peer may also be trained who can support the adolescent and administer the adrenaline if needed.

Procedure
Management of food allergy
- Allergen avoidance.
- Dietetic support.
- Maintenance of normal feeding behaviour.
- Medication to be carried at all times.
- When eating out, the chef should be informed of the child's allergen.
- For nut/fish-based allergies, check that cooking oil is not nut/fish based.
- Medical alert bracelet (optional, but recommended).
- Yearly training and updating in the safe use of the appropriate device.
- The child should be encouraged to lead an active and normal life.
- When travelling abroad, check with the airline before travelling to ensure the device can be kept with the child on the flight.
- Adolescents should avoid drinking alcohol as this lowers the body's threshold and ↑ the risk of having a reaction.

Anaphylaxis and emergency treatment in the community
- Set aside an hour for the training and gain consent.
- Check the child/parent knows why they have been given an adrenaline auto-injector pen.
- Obtain a clear history of events following the child's allergic reaction. If old enough, ask the child how they felt during the reaction.
- Explain what adrenaline is and how it works.
- Incorporate play into the training and allow the parent/child to look at and handle a dummy Pen (the device without the needle).
- It is important for parents to see it and practice giving it to the child.
- Written information including pictures showing how to administer the device should be included in the training.
- The health professional when happy with the parent/young person's technique should sign them as competent. This should go in the child's notes, with copies to the health visitor, school nurse, and GP.

Principles for administering the adrenaline auto-injector device
- Despite there being several different devices on the market, guidance for use of the adrenaline pen is similar. (Please refer to your Trust policy to see which device is being currently used).
- The injection should be administered in the outer fleshy part of the thigh only; it is an intramuscular (IM) injection that ensures prompt absorption of the adrenaline.
- Place the centre of the adrenaline pen in the middle of the palm of your dominant hand, firmly grip the pen, fingers facing towards you with your thumb nearest the yellow safety cap.

- *Depending on the device used:*
  - Place the black tip end onto the fleshy part of outer thigh at 90° angle. (The needle will go through clothes, including jeans).
  - Remove the yellow safety cap with your other hand and press the top end.

Or:
  - Remove the safety cap.
  - Hold the pen approximately 10cm from the outer thigh (black tip pointing towards the thigh).
  - Jab into the fleshy part of the outer thigh at a 90° angle.
- You will hear a click once the spring activated plunger is released. This pushes the hidden needle into the thigh muscle and administers a dose of adrenaline.
- Hold the adrenaline Pen firmly in place for 10s then remove and massage the injection area for 10s.

Following administration of adrenaline
- When the adrenaline Pen has been used parents should promptly call 999 even if their child appears to improve:
  - They should clearly state their child has just been given their adrenaline Pen for anaphylaxis and remain with their child.
  - Sometimes the child will require another dose, which can be given 5–15min following the first dose. (However, the ambulance crew will decide and administer this).
- Put the adrenaline pen back in the plastic tube and give it to the ambulance crew for safe disposal and to prevent needle stick injuries.
- The adrenaline pen may only be used once.
- Following adrenaline administration an inpatient hospital stay for at least 24h will be required.

Practice tips
- The effects of adrenaline can last for up to an hour in the body. Following administration, the child may feel light headed and/or nauseous, and become tachycardic.
- Sit or lie the child down prior to administration to prevent falls. Always tell the child what you are about to do to prevent further shock/ distress. (This is why practice is so important.)
- One auto-injector device comes with a needle shield to prevent potential needle stick injuries (please refer to the manufacture guidelines).
- The shelf life and storage instructions will vary depending on the device used. (Please refer to the manufacture guidelines).
- Answer questions honestly. From experience, I can honestly say the injection is painful and the adrenaline stings when administered; however, put this into context. Giving the adrenaline pen is an emergency; life-saving action that is painful, but short lived and certainly preferable to the frightening or potentially fatal effects of anaphylaxis.
- Two adrenaline pens will be prescribed; one should be kept at the child's school. The school nurses/teachers must be trained to administer it.

- The parent must always have the second adrenaline pen with them when out with the child. At home it should be stored in an accessible place, but out of reach of children.
- ❶ If the device is used it should be replaced promptly. On discharge from hospital following an anaphylactic episode a replacement adrenaline pen should be prescribed.
- Professional advice should be sought if the child becomes afraid to have the adrenaline again following administration.
- Parents can sign up to a free text message alert system, which warns them when the adrenaline pen is due to expire. Information regarding how to access it should be included in the written information provided by the nurse conducting the initial training.
- For children who have experienced a severe allergic reaction, which affected their airway, the consultant may request additional training for parents in BLS. This will be provided by a qualified health professional alongside the adrenaline pen training. Separate parental competencies should be signed, and a copy put in the child's notes and sent to their GP, school nurse, or health visitor.
- It is advantageous if two responsible adults can undertake the adrenaline pen and BLS training. This provides a more robust safety plan and provides the parent with additional support in case they are unable to take the necessary actions required in an emergency.

Associated reading

Resuscitation Council UK (2010). *FAQS: Emergency Treatment of Anaphylactic Reactions. Guidelines for Health Care Providers*. Available at: ᔕ http://www.resus.org.uk/pages/faqAna.htm.

Genito-urinary system

History taking and assessment

Background
Problems with the urinary or reproductive systems can affect these systems and may also trigger problems in other body systems.

The functions of excretion and reproduction can be quite difficult to address with children and young people—they may cause embarrassment, laughter and/or self-consciousness. Even very young children are likely to be aware that these areas are generally not discussed publicly and may regard them as 'rude'.

The health professional needs to use a calm, matter-of-fact approach, while dealing sensitively with a child's discomfit (Box 16.1).

> ### Box 16.1 Dealing with a child's discomfit
> - Ensuring privacy and deepest respect for the dignity of the child/ young person are essential
> - Consider the sex of the professional undertaking history taking and/ or assessment. Will the child/young person be more comfortable with someone of their own sex?
> - Encourage parent to be present with a younger child, and give the older child/adolescent the choice of whether a parent is present or not

History
Urological
Information may be needed on the following:
- Urological abnormalities noted at birth.
- Urinary difficulties in the first 24h of life.
- Past urinary complaints.
- *Toilet training*: age initiated and completed.
- *Enuresis*: frequency, time of occurrence, control methods used.
- Unusual behaviours associated with urination, e.g. inappropriate places, refusing to use toilet.
- Child and/or parent concerns.

Genital
Information may be needed on the following:
- Reproductive abnormalities noted at birth.
- Past complaints.
- If a girl, has she had the cervical cancer vaccine?
- Any recent relevant accidents, e.g. falling off bike & causing trauma?
- Underlying health conditions, e.g. sickle cell can lead to priapism.
- Any discharge—could be sign of STD, abuse.
- Sexuality and sexual behaviours.
- *Sexual activity*:
  - Safe sex knowledge, practice, and birth control.
  - Child and/or parent concerns.
  - Menstrual history in girls.

Assessment

Assess the following:
- BP–often elevated with nephritis and nephrotic syndrome.
- Height, weight, and BMI.
  - Failure to thrive can be associated with urinary tract infection (UTI).
  - Increased weight can be associated with nephrotic syndrome.
- Ear position and formation–low-set or abnormal ears may be associated with renal disease.
- Urinalysis.
- Genital care/behavior.

It may be helpful to ask questions like:
- 'Do you have parts of your body that no one is supposed to look at, touch, kiss, or tickle? What do you call those body parts? Has anyone ever touched, tickled, kissed, or hurt those parts?
- Soiling post-toilet training.
- 'Is your child able to wipe him/herself after toileting without help?
- Do you perform some aspects of care during bath/shower?
- Follow local guidelines on examination of a child/young person in whom sexual abuse is suspected.

Practice tips

- Discussion of these issues may be difficult for the child. Involve parents as appropriate for the individual child in helping the child understand that it is necessary and acceptable.
- It may help to involve a play specialist and/or to use a doll to demonstrate certain things and ask the child to show you what they do or what it's like for them.
- Assessment involving the genitourinary system may highlight areas of concern in regard to sexual activity and possible or actual harm to the child. Ensure that you neither lead nor actively encourage or discourage disclosure. Document and report as per local policy. Offer support and reassurance to the child/young person.

Associated reading

Horner G. (2007). Genitourinary assessment: an integral part of a complete physical examination. *J Pediat Health Care* **21**(3), 162–70.

Urinalysis

Background

Urinalysis is used to:

- Screen for diseases, such as diabetes mellitus.
- Confirm or exclude conditions, such as urinary tract infection.
- Monitor the progress of an existing condition.

Dipstick urinalysis relies on the practitioner to perform the procedure in accordance with the manufacturer's instructions.

Automated colorimetric measurement devices are available for accurate reading of urine testing strips. Practitioners should be trained and assessed as competent in the use of these devices.

Equipment

- Clean urine specimen in disposable container or jug.
- Non-sterile gloves.
- Apron.
- Reagent strips.
- Patient record.
- Universal specimen container.

Procedure

- Check whether a specimen has been ordered for laboratory testing.
- Gather equipment on a clean, hard surface in a private environment.
- Check that reagent strips are in date and that strip container does not appear to be contaminated—replace if necessary.
- Wash hands and don non-sterile gloves.
- Dip urine testing strip into urine. Ensure all reagent areas are covered. Remove immediately. Remove excess urine by tapping the edge of the strip on the side of container.
- Hold the urine-testing strip alongside the container, without allowing the strip to come in contact with the container, so that you can compare the colour changes on the strip as they occur.
- Ensure that the different colour pads are read at the correct intervals as indicated by the manufacturer's guidelines.
- Once you have read the strip, obtain specimen if already ordered or if results would indicate the need for investigation.
- Dispose of equipment according to local policy.
- Wash hands.
- Document your findings in the patient's notes.
- Report any significant findings.

Practice tips

- Ensure that the strip you are using has all the necessary colour pads on it to test for the constituents you need to monitor.
- It is important to consider human error in the interpretation of subtle colour changes, which can lead to inaccurate results.
- When storing urine testing strips, follow the manufacturer's guidelines.
- When small amounts of albumin and globulin are present in the urine, the levels will often not be high enough to show on a reagent stick.
- When testing for urinary protein, use an early morning sample to ensure sufficient concentration.
- Consider the effect of menstrual blood on urinalysis results.

Associated reading

Dougherty L, Lister S. (eds) (2011). *The Royal Marsden Hospital Manual of Clinical Nursing Procedures*, 8th edn. Wiley-Blackwell., Oxford.

Trigg E, Mohammed TA. (2006). *Practices in Children's Nursing: Guidelines for Hospital and Community* Churchill Livingstone, Oxford.

Obtaining a suprapubic aspirate

Background

Performed to obtain a *sterile* specimen of urine (most frequently in an infant) directly from the bladder, to exclude a urinary tract infection (UTI) in a severely ill infant or young child. This will be part of the full septic screen and is often undertaken before a lumbar puncture and is an aseptic procedure. Performed by an experienced doctor or nurse practitioner.

Equipment

- Pain relief.
- Sterile gloves.
- 5- or 10-mL syringe and large bore (22G) injection needle.
- Sterile towel.
- Local anaesthetic agent and equipment to deliver.
- Urine sample bottle and specimen request form.
- Additional sterile container/bowl.
- Chlorhexidine solution (or cleansing solution as per local policy).
- Small adhesive plaster.
- Suitable distraction aids or play specialist.

Procedure

- Undertake comprehensive nursing and medical assessment.
- This will include ascertaining last time the infant had a wet nappy, as bladder needs to be full. Ultra sound may be used to identify a full bladder.
- Consult with child and parents, explaining procedure.
- Gain informed consent.
- Consider local anaesthetic as appropriate.
- Gather and prepare all equipment in treatment room or private area.
- Position child in supine position, place infant's legs in 'frog leg position' if requested.
- Consider privacy and dignity needs.
- Provide distraction if appropriate.

The person undertaking the procedure will:
- Prepare the bottle by labelling and signing pathology request form.
- Wash hands and apply sterile gloves.
- Prepare the skin.
- Towel the sterile field.
- Assemble syringe and needle.
- Clean the skin as per local policy.
- Undertake the procedure inserting the needle at a 90° angle into the abdomen centrally approximately 1–2cm above the symphysis pubis and maintaining negative pressure to the syringe until urine appears.
- Once specimen obtained will remove needle while applying pressure to exit point for 1–2min.

Ask the nurse

- To present the urine specimen bottle, so the urine can be transferred into the sterile bottle.
- To apply plaster to site if appropriate, after checking for allergies.
- Ensure specimen is correctly dispatched to microbiology as soon as possible preferably immediately.
- Complete nursing documentation.
- Look for, and advise parents regarding, potential complications. Perforated bowel can occur—perhaps indicated by increased abdominal pain, change in vital signs. Fresh blood may be present in urine following procedure. Document, report, and seek medical review as condition indicates.

Practice tips

- Clear explanation to parent can help reduce their anxiety,
- An additional member of staff to support parent can be helpful.
- Use care and discretion when preparing and wielding the needle—its size can be very daunting to the child and observing parent.
- Have sterile pot/bowl handy for clean catch specimen as child may urinate as their abdomen is pressed to palpate bladder.

Associated reading

Lissauer T, Clayden G. (2001). *Illustrated Textbook of Paediatrics*, 2nd edn Mosby, London.

Urine collection using urine pad or bag

Background
Bacterial contamination can easily occur when urine samples are collected. It can be particularly difficult to obtain a non-contaminated specimen from babies and young children who have not yet been toilet-trained. Use of a urine collection pad or bag may be an appropriate method of specimen collection from these individuals.

Equipment
- Sterile urine collection pad or bag.
- Usual skin cleanser, clean disposable wipes.
- Clean nappy or pants.
- Sterile 5- or 10-mL syringe and needle.
- Alcohol wipe.
- Sterile specimen container, labelled with child's details.
- Sterile pot/bowel to attempt clean catch specimen.

Procedure
- Ensure that you are familiar with and adhere to local policy regarding choice of collection method.
- Explain procedure appropriately to child and parent and gain consent.
- Ensure privacy.
- Wash hands.
- Clean the urethral/perineal area and allow to dry.
- Attempt to collect a clean catch specimen by sitting baby/toddler on parent or carer's lap with sterile bowel placed strategically under their urethra. Maintain their dignity using a towel; protect carer's lap with towels.
- If this fails either
  - Place urine collection pad inside clean nappy or pants (follow manufacturer's guidelines).
  - Or place urine collection bag in place, with collection hole adjacent to urethra (in boys, penis should be inserted into bag). (Follow manufacturer's guidelines.)
- Check frequently whether child has passed urine and collect sample as soon as possible.
- Wash hands.
- Remove bag and take away into utility area.
- Either:
  - Aspirate urine from pad with sterile syringe and inject into sterile container, taking care to avoid touching the sides with the syringe.
  - Or clean base of bag with alcohol-based wipe and allow to dry. Aspirate urine by inserting sterile needle and syringe into cleaned area of bag and drawing bag. Inject syringe content straight into sterile container, taking care to avoid touching the sides.
- Dispose of equipment according to local policy.
- Ensure child is clean and comfortable.
- Ensure specimen is correctly labelled and sent to the laboratory with completed specimen request form which includes detail of collection method.
- Document and report procedure as appropriate.

Practice tips

- Always follow local policy and product manufacturer's guidelines.
- *Always* use products which have been manufactured specifically for urine collection and *do not* use cotton-wool balls, gauze, or sanitary towels as an alternative.
- If using a collection pad, it is recommended that the pad is changed every 30–45min to reduce the risk of contamination.
- Use of an enuresis wetting alarm can be considered to detect quickly when the child has micturated.

Pitfalls

- Urine collection bags and pads are more susceptible to contamination than the clean catch method, due to the close and prolonged contact with the skin around the anogenital area.

Associated reading

Alam MT, Coulter JB, Pacheco J, et al. (2005). Comparison of urine contamination rates using three different methods of collection: clean-catch, cotton wool pad and urine bag. *Ann Trop Paediat* **25**, 29–34.

Rogers J, Saunders C. (2008). Urine collection in infants and children. *Nursing Times*. **104**, 40–2.

Types and sizes of urinary catheter

Background

Urinary catheters can be used to relieve obstruction of the urinary tract, to facilitate post-operative repair, to assist in achieving urinary continence where bladder control is weak or absent, and to measure urinary output.

In determining the most appropriate type of catheter for use, consider why and for how long it will be *in situ*.

There are two types of catheters:
- In-dwelling catheter.
- Intermittent catheters.

In-dwelling catheters are held in place via a balloon. These can be used for short- and long-term usage.

❶ The smallest size of catheter that will allow effective bladder drainage should be selected (Table 16.1). Use of a catheter that is too large may irritate the trigone muscle at the base of the bladder, causing spasm, pain, and by-passing.

In-dwelling catheters

Indications for use
- Acute/chronic urinary retention.
- Instillation of drugs.
- Monitoring urine output.
- Pre/post-operatively.
- Bladder washouts.
- Investigations, e.g. urodynamic studies.
- Maintaining urethral patency.
- Incontinence.

Lifespan
- Short-term in-dwelling catheters can usually remain in place for up to 7 days.
- Long-term in-dwelling catheters remain in place for 12 weeks, unless an infection indicates more frequent changes. (Usually Hydrogel® coated or 100% silicone.)

Pitfalls
- Urine infections.
- Trauma to the urethra.
- Leakage.
- Encrustation.
- Biofilm formation.

Intermittent catheters

Indications for use

- Retention of residual urine.
- Post-operative retention.
- Patency of the urethra.
- Draining residual urine.
- Continence management.
- Intermittent catheters are single use, which involves passing the small tube into the bladder, allowing urine to drain, and then removing the tube.

Pitfalls

- Urine infections.
- Trauma.
- Bleeding.
- Formation of a false passage.
- N.B. The rate of infections and trauma is reduced compared to that of in-dwelling catheters.

Suprapubic catheters

Suprapubic catheters can be used for short- and long-term use. Patients experiencing problems related to urethral catheters or who have a long-term disability may require a suprapubic.

Table 16.1 General sizing guideline

Size 6Ch	Up to 2yrs
Size 8Ch	2–10yrs
Size 10Ch	10–14yrs
Size 14Ch	14yrs upwards

Catheter valves

A valve can be used, instead of a drainage bag, for children with a long-term catheter.

The catheter valve can be released several times a day when the child feels that the bladder is full and needs to be emptied. It is therefore necessary to carefully assess the child and his or her bladder function before selecting a catheter valve.

Catheter valves should be changed every 5–7 days.

A catheter valve is contraindicated for patients with reduced bladder capacity, absence of bladder sensation, limited cognitive ability/development, as well as those who do not have the manual dexterity to operate it.

Associated reading

Robinson J. (2006). Selecting a urinary catheter and drainage system. *Br J Nurs* **15**(19), 1045–50.
Rhodes C. (2009). *Nottingham Children's and Young Peoples Hospital Nursing Procedure. Catheterization Package*, 1–22.
Wyndale J, Maes D. (1990). Clean intermittent self catheterization, a 12 year follow up. *J Urol* **143**, 906–8.

Female catheterization

Background

Girls may be catheterized to relieve urinary retention, after urological and gynaecological surgery, during investigations such as urodynamic studies, and for the instillation of intravesical medications. Catheterization may also help with short- and long-term management of urinary incontinence.

The type of catheter used, a Foley catheter, is designed to be retained in the bladder. It has a balloon for inflation with sterile water, which will anchor it in the bladder.

Equipment

- Sterile catheterization pack.
- Suitably sized and type of catheter + a spare (see Table 16.1 for general sizing guide).
- Two pairs of sterile gloves.
- Cleansing fluid, as in local policy.
- Syringe and sterile water for non-filled catheters.
- Lubricant gel containing local anaesthetic (NB needs prescription).
- Catheter drainage bag.
- Universal container labelled with child's details.
- Hydrocolloid dressing and tape.
- Good lighting.
- Protective material for bedding.
- Blanket or other covering for child.
- Suitable assistance both for positioning the child, providing support, distraction, and the procedure itself. A parent will be very helpful to support and distract the child, but consider whether they wish/feel able to assist with this procedure.

Procedure

- Provide full and appropriate explanation to child and parent, and gain consent for procedure.
- Consider the need for pre-procedural analgesia and ensure it is prescribed and administered in time for appropriate effect. Use distraction and involve the play specialist.
- Check whether the child has a known allergy to latex.
- Determine type and size of catheter to be inserted (selecting a latex-free type where needed—the only types of catheter that are latex-free are PVC and 100% silicone).
- Ensure local anaesthetic gel has been prescribed and specimen request card completed (if required).
- Gather equipment and helpers.
- Ensure that suitable play/distraction is in place for the child.
- Ensure privacy and that lighting is adequate for procedure.
- Help the girl to position herself, or move her to a position on her back without underwear, with knees bent, hips flexed, and legs apart.
- Protect bed linen by placing a disposable pad under the child's bottom. Cover her with a blanket.
- Wash hands.

- Prepare the sterile field and equipment.
- Uncover the child.
- Wash hands again and don sterile gloves.
- Cover child's thighs with sterile towels.
- Separate the labia minora using a swab, to view the urethral meatus.
- Cleanse the labia and urethral meatus (with cleansing agent, as per local policy) with downward strokes using single swabs, to lower the risk of contaminating the urethral meatus with bowel flora.
- Gently insert the nozzle of the anaesthetic applicator into the urethral meatus and slowly instill the gel into the urethra. (2–3mL lidocaine in the younger child, up to 10mL in the older child.)
- Wait 3–5min, then wipe away excess gel.
- Also apply sterile lubricant gel to the tip of the catheter.
- Dispose of gloves, wash, dry hands, and put on new sterile gloves.
- Place a containing vessel between the child's legs. Holding the catheter in the dominant hand, gently feed it into the urethral orifice.
- Angling it slightly upwards and backwards, pass it into the bladder.
- When urine starts to flow down the catheter, advance another 2–4cm.
- Slowly inflate the balloon with the amount of sterile water specified by manufacturer.
- Secure to upper thigh or abdomen ensuring there is a small loop to avoid tension when child moves. Apply hydrocolloid dressing to the child's leg to protect skin from adhesive tape.
- Attach a catheter drainage bag.
- Make the child comfortable.
- Send some of urine drained during procedure for laboratory testing, if required.
- Dispose of equipment according to local policy.
- Wash your hands.
- In the patient's notes, record the date, the type, and size of catheter, and the amount of water in the balloon.
- Discuss and agree the plan of care with child and parent.

Practice tips

- Be aware that this can be an uncomfortable procedure and that the child may find it traumatic and may also find it difficult to maintain the required position—consider analgesia and sedation.
- Take time to prepare the child—use of a doll to demonstrate the procedure may be useful.
- The intimate touch required for this procedure should be considered—the child may be fearful and confused as she will understand that such touch should not occur. Involve parents in helping the child understand that, in this instance, it is necessary and acceptable.
- If you accidently place the catheter in the vagina, leave it in place and put another in the urethra. Remove the first catheter once urine starts to flow.
- The child should not feel any pain during inflation of the balloon; if she does, the balloon may be in the urethra. Deflate the balloon and advance the catheter a few more centimetres, then try again.

- If the child complains of undue pain or discomfort; if you notice bleeding other than that which might be experienced in minor trauma; or if you continue to feel resistance to passage of the catheter and cannot pass this into the bladder, stop the procedure and seek medical advice.
- Most catheter packaging comes with a sticky label which contains all the necessary information (catheter material, size, lot number, expiry date, and balloon size).
- Nasogastric (NG) tubes must not be used as urinary catheters!

Associated reading

Dougherty L, Lister S. (eds) (2008). *The Royal Marsden Hospital Manual of Clinical Nursing Procedures.* 7th edn. Wiley-Blackwell, Oxford.

Skills for Health. (2008). *CC05. Insert, Secure and Monitor Urethral Catheters.* Skills for Health, London. Available at: ℘ http://www.skillsforhealth.org.uk.

Male catheterization

Background

Boys may be catheterized to relieve urinary retention, after urological and gynaecological surgery, during investigations such as urodynamic studies, and for the instillation of intravesical medications. Catheterization may also help with short- and long-term management of urinary incontinence.

The type of catheter used, a Foley catheter, is designed to be retained in the bladder. It has a balloon for inflation with sterile water, which will anchor it in the bladder.

Equipment

- Sterile catheterization pack.
- Suitably sized and type of catheter + a spare (see Table 16.1 for general sizing guide).
- Two pairs of sterile gloves.
- Cleansing fluid, as in local policy.
- Syringe and sterile water for non-filled catheters.
- Lubricant gel containing local anaesthetic (N.B. needs prescription).
- Catheter drainage bag.
- Universal container labelled with child's details.
- Hydrocolloid dressing and tape.
- Good lighting.
- Protective material for bedding.
- Blanket/other covering for child.
- Suitable assistance both for positioning the child, providing support, and distraction, and the procedure itself. A parent will be very helpful to support, and distract the child, but consider whether they wish/feel able to assist with this procedure.

Procedure

- Provide full and appropriate explanation to child and parent, and gain consent for procedure.
- Consider the need for pre-procedural analgesia and ensure it is prescribed and administered in time for appropriate effect. Use distraction and involve the play specialist.
- Check whether the child has a known allergy to latex.
- Determine type and size of catheter to be inserted (selecting a latex-free type where needed (the only types of catheter that are latex-free are PVC and 100% silicone).
- Ensure local anaesthetic gel has been prescribed and specimen request card completed (if required).
- Gather equipment and helpers.
- Ensure that suitable play/distraction is in place for the child.
- Ensure privacy and that lighting is adequate for procedure.
- Help the boy to position himself, or move him to a supine position, with legs extended and without underwear.
- Protect the bed linen by placing a disposable pad under the child's bottom. Cover him with a blanket.
- Wash hands.

- Prepare the sterile field and equipment.
- Uncover the child.
- Wash hands again and don sterile gloves.
- Placing sterile towels over the child's genital area surrounding the penis.
- In a post-pubertal boy, retract the foreskin. It is important not to fully retract the foreskin, as it may be difficult to reduce.
- Clean the top of the meatus, passing over the glans in one movement, and then discard swab.
- Using another swab, clean the underside of the meatus. Discard swab.
- Place a few drops of anaesthetic gel on the urethral meatus. Insert the nozzle of the syringe into the meatal opening and instill gel into the urethra. 2–3mL lidocaine in the younger and up to 10mL in older child.
- Hold the glans penis closed to stop the gel from seeping out.
- Using a dry swab, wipe the underside of the penile shaft several times from top to bottom, to move the gel towards the prostatic urethra.
- Wait 3–5min for the anaesthetic gel to take effect.
- Also apply sterile lubricant gel to the tip of the catheter.
- Dispose of gloves, wash, and dry hands, and put on new sterile gloves.
- Place a containing vessel between the child's legs. Holding the catheter in the dominant hand, gently feed it into the urethral orifice.
- With a smooth, slow action, pass the catheter through the urethra, and into the bladder. As you reach the external sphincter, there is usually a feeling of resistance; at this point, if the child is able, ask him to cough or bear down as if he wanted to pass urine, while continuing to pass the catheter into the bladder.
- When urine starts to flow down the catheter, advance another 2–4cm.
- Slowly inflate the balloon with the amount of sterile water specified by manufacturer.
- Secure to upper thigh or abdomen ensuring there is a small loop to avoid tension when child moves. Apply hydrocolloid dressing to the child's leg to protect skin from adhesive tape.
- Attach a catheter drainage bag.
- Make the child comfortable.
- Send some of urine drained during procedure for laboratory testing, if required.
- Dispose of equipment according to local policy.
- Wash your hands.
- In the patient's notes, record the date, the type, and size of catheter, and the amount of water in the balloon.
- Discuss and agree the plan of care with child and parent.

Practice tips

(See 📖 Female catheterization, p. 464.)

Associated reading

(See 📖 Female catheterization, p. 464.)

Intermittent catheterization

Background

Intermittent catheterization is frequently used with children and young people who experience incomplete bladder emptying. Parent and child can be taught to undertake this procedure provided they have the manual dexterity, cognitive ability, motivation, and appropriate bladder capacity.

❶ Child and/or parent undertaking this procedure will need careful preparation, support, and should not carry it out independently until they are confident and competent.

When performed at home by child/parents this is a 'clean' procedure, health care professionals (HCPs), whether in hospital or community, must use aseptic technique to minimize the risk of infection.

Intermittent self-catheterization is also a technique used in the management of recurrent urethral strictures, where self-dilatation is used to keep the urethra patent and to prevent recurrence of strictures.

The tube is removed immediately after drainage is complete. This method of periodic bladder drainage allows the bladder to fill and empty, thus mimicking normal bladder function. Intermittent self-catheterization also enables the child to gain control of their bladder, and gives them the opportunity to become self-caring and achieve a better body image.

Equipment

- Suitably sized intermittent use packaged catheter. The smallest effective catheter is generally used, generally between 6Ch and 10Ch for children).
- Lubricating gel without local anaesthetic (when using a non-coated catheter).
- Sterile water in sachet.
- Soap.
- Towel.
- Sterile gloves (if required).
- Mirror (if required for self-catheterization).
- Clean wash cloth.
- Receiver, jug, or toilet.

Procedure

- If procedure to be carried out by health professional, provide appropriate explanation to child and parent, and gain consent.
- Gather equipment.
- Wash meatal orifice with soap and water.
- Wash hands.
- If using a coated catheter with an integral sachet of sterile water, squeeze the sachet at the top of the catheter and allow the water to cover the catheter.
- If there is no integral sachet of sterile water, water will need to be added to activate the lubricant. Open the catheter packaging from the funnel end by about 5cm; then, using water from the mains cold tap, fill the catheter packet to half full.

- Leave it to soak for 30s.
- Wash hands.
- If child is undertaking this procedure it may not be deemed necessary for them to don gloves, as this is a 'clean' procedure—check local policy.
- If practitioner or parent is undertaking procedure they should don sterile gloves.
- Adopt optimum position to find meatal opening—this may be sitting, lying, or standing.
- If using a non-coated catheter, a lubricant gel may be applied to the urethra before insertion. (If using a coated catheter, no gel is required because the coating becomes activated on contact with water).
- Release a drop of gel to coat the nozzle of the applicator to allow for ease of insertion into the urethra.
- Insert the applicator into the urethra and apply steady pressure to the accordion syringe.
- Maintain pressure to the accordion syringe as the applicator is removed from the urethra.
- Insert catheter into the meatal opening smoothly, through the urethra and into the bladder.
- Once urine begins to drain, hold funnel end of catheter over receiver, jug, or toilet.
- Remove catheter once flow has stopped.
- Place a finger over the funnel end of the catheter as it is about to leave the urethra, to prevent urine spilling onto clothing, etc.
- Dispose of equipment appropriately.
- Wash hands.
- Complete records as required.

Practice tips

- The use of lidocaine gel is not encouraged in recurrent use of catheters owing to the risk of overdose.
- It may be helpful for the child/young person to use a mirror to help them identify the meatal opening and urethra.
- Depending on the type of catheter, its surface may remain clear or appear frosted once it has been wetted.
- If the child/young person is undertaking this procedure on their own they will need to secure the package, once opened, in an upright position. This can be done by sticking the packet to a smooth, dry surface, such as a bathroom tile, after peeling the label off.
- In the acute setting, single-use catheters are used to reduce the risk of infection, but reusable catheters are commonly used in the community.
- If the patient is using a reusable catheter at home, he or she needs to wash the catheter through with running water and store it in a dry plastic bag, using a clean bag on each occasion.
- Catheters with an integral coating are designed for single use only and must be disposed of after use.
- Reusable catheters, without coating, can be used for up to seven days before being discarded.

- NG tubes must not be used as urinary catheters!
- Child and family should receive information on what to look out for, e.g. signs of infection, trauma, etc. who to contact in case of problems and queries, equipment ordering and supply.
- Consider promoting contacts with other families with similar care needs if agreed by both parties.

Associated reading

Bennett E. (2002). Intermittent self-catheterization and the female patient. *Nurs Stand* **17**(7), 37–42.

Skills for Health. (2008). *CC06: Enable individuals to carry out intermittent catheterization.* Skills for Health, London. Available at: ℬ http://www.skillsforhealth.org.uk.

Catheter care

Background

In-dwelling urinary catheters should only be used after alternative methods of managing urinary problems have been considered.

It is essential that children who have had an in-dwelling catheter inserted are given adequate and appropriate information on why they need it, and how it is to be cared for.

They and their families can be educated and supported to undertake care themselves as and when they are able and willing to do this, to promote independence and a sense of control.

Personal hygiene for a child with a catheter

Procedure

• Wash hands and don non-sterile gloves.
• Use mild soap and water with a single use disposable cloth, or clean personal wash cloth kept solely for this purpose, to clean around the catheter site.
• When cleaning the urethral orifice:
  • Clean away from the opening to avoid contaminating it.
  • Make sure that you clean from front to back in girls.
• Remove and dispose of cloths and gloves according to local policy.
• Daily washing is recommended but wash more frequently if there is any discharge.
• Document and report condition of skin around entry site and characteristics of any discharge.

Emptying a catheter bag

Procedure

• Explain procedure to child and parent appropriately and gain consent.
• Wash hands.
• Don non-sterile gloves.
• Ask child to sit in comfortable position.
• Hold valve over a clean disposable container or jug.
• Clean valve with alcohol wipe and allow to dry.
• Open valve, and empty the bag, ensuring that the valve does not touch the container.
• When all urine has drained, close valve.
• Clean outlet port according to local policy and allow it to dry.
• Cover the jug with clean disposable paper cover.
• Transport jug carefully to toilet, or dirty utility room, and dispose of urine.
• Remove and dispose of gloves according to local policy.
• Ensure that child is comfortable and that catheter is well secured to prevent tension and/or contamination.
• Ensure that bag is positioned appropriately below the level of the bladder to reduce the risk of backflow, using bag holder, straps, etc. well away from the floor or other potential contaminant.
• Document amount and characteristics of urine in fluid balance record and nursing notes.
• Report any concerns and consider requesting order for and obtaining catheter specimen for laboratory analysis if necessary.
• Catheter bags should be changed every 5–7days.

Leg bags

- If a leg bag is the most appropriate urinary drainage system for the child, consider the following:
  - The length of the tubing (short, medium, or long).
  - The volume of urine to be contained (350, 500, or 750mL).
  - The outlet tap, which needs to be easy to open for the user/carer.
- Most leg bags have an integral sampling port to enable a urine sample to be taken.
- The leg bags worn by most patients hold 350, 500, or 750mL, although larger sizes can also be obtained.
- Specially designed larger-capacity leg bags are available for wheelchair users.
- If a large-capacity bag is preferred for use overnight, 2L bags (not worn on the body) are available.
- Bags are also now available that are worn roughly in the position of the bladder, with an anti-reflux valve that prevents urine flowing back into the bag.
- There are several ways of fixing the drainage bag to the leg, which help to support the bag and prevent traction on the catheter. These include:
  - Open-weave 'net' sleeves to fit the thigh or calf.
  - Leg straps and garments.
- All leg bags must be changed every 5–7days.

Catheter removal

Equipment

- 10-mL luer slip syringe.
- Non-sterile gloves.
- Cleaning solution—as per local policy.
- Gauze.
- Receiver.
- Clinical disposal bag.

Procedure

- Explain procedure as appropriate to child and parent, and gain consent.
- Gather all equipment.
- Check the catheter to determine how much water was used to inflate the balloon.
- Ensure the child is comfortable and positioned supine.
- Wash hands and don non sterile gloves.
- Ensure container/receiver is next to the child to ensure minimal spillage.
- Clean around exit site if necessary as per local policy.
- Attach the syringe to the outlet and deflate the balloon, allow all water from the balloon to drain back naturally into receiver.
- Slowly remove the catheter.
- Clean child's genital area, observing for soreness, inflammation.
- Dispose of catheter and all equipment as per local policy.
- Wash hands.
- Document removal and condition of genital area in child's health record.
- Report any concerns.

Practice tips

- Encourage adequate fluid intake (subject to any prescribed fluid restriction) in a catheterized child.
- Cranberry juice *may* reduce the risk of urinary tract infection.
- Teach the child and family, where appropriate and they wish it, to care for the catheter. This will promote independence and reduce the risk of cross-contamination.
- Bathing or showering is possible with the catheter in situ.
- Detecting pH changes through urinalysis may help to identify risk of catheter blockage or urinary tract infection.
- Ensure that catheter is secured to upper thigh or abdomen ensuring there is a small loop to avoid tension when child moves.
- Ensure that bag is always positioned appropriately, using bag holder, straps, etc. as appropriate, well away from the floor, or other potential contaminant

Associated reading

Dougherty L, Lister S. (eds) (2008). *The Royal Marsden Hospital Manual of Clinical Nursing Procedures*, 7th edn. Wiley-Blackwell, Oxford.

Bladder washouts

Background

- If a catheter ceases to drain or is not draining adequate amounts a blockage may be suspected. In the case of blockage a flush or bladder washout may need to be performed. Reasons for blockage include;
  - Sediment in the urine.
  - Pus.
  - Blood clots.
  - Debris.
- It is important to exclude other reasons why the catheter may not draining adequately before flushing, these may be:
  - Constipation.
  - Patient position.
  - Bladder spasms.
  - Kinked catheter.
- Bladder washouts are particularly useful in patients who have had a Mitrofonoff procedure and produce large amounts of mucous.
- The frequency and volume of the washouts will be directed by the Urologist.
- Daily washouts should only be carried out for a limited period of 1–2 weeks unless directed by a doctor in long term catheter patients.

Equipment

- 1 x sterile field.
- 50mL bladder syringe.
- Normal saline sachet.
- Receiver.
- New drainage bag.
- Non-sterile gloves.
- Alcoholic chlorhexidine gluconate bp 2% and isopropyl alcohol 70%.
- Wipe.

Procedure

- Prepare the patient and carer for the procedure by providing a full explanation and gaining consent.
- Use distraction techniques as appropriate.
- Ensure the patient is lying down in a clean area.
- Wash hands thoroughly.
- Place sterile field under catheter and drainage bag.
- Wearing gloves wipe round the connection of the catheter and drainage bag and disconnect.
- Draw up 30–50mL of saline into the bladder syringe.
- Attach the bladder syringe to the catheter and instill the saline into the bladder.
- Allow the saline to free drain into sterile receptacle.
- Repeat this process if there is visible mucous, or debris until clear, and urine draining.
- Connect new catheter bag.
- Discard of waste according to local policy.

Practice tips
- An aseptic technique does not need to be carried out when instilling catheter flushes. Increased fluid intake will not prevent blockages but will result in dilute urine output, also reducing the risk of constipation.
- Always refer to local policy.

Associated reading

Pomfret I, Bayait F, Mackenzie R, et al. (2004). Using bladder instillations to manage in-dwelling catheters. Br J Nurs 13(5), 261–7.

Principles of haemodialysis

Background

Haemodialysis is a form of extracorporeal renal replacement therapy mainly carried out in the hospital setting for acute and chronic conditions. The treatment was pioneered in the early 20th century but became a viable option as an ongoing therapy around the 1960s. Since this time the principles of haemodialysis have remained the same, but the technology involved in the procedure has greatly improved.

Equipment

- Access for haemodialysis can be short- or long-term in the form of a central venous line which can be placed under sedation for acute therapies or surgically for chronic or longer term treatments.
- An arteriovenous fistula can be used in patients who require long term access and is formed by connecting an artery and vein together. This allows a section of the vein to become engorged and therefore large enough to insert wide bore needles designed to provide adequate blood flow from, and back to, the patient.
- Haemodialysis machines are highly technical and require programming for each individual patient's needs for every session.
- The calculated fluid removal and electrolyte balance can be tailored to the requirements of the child by making changes to the programme or dialysate fluid.
- The machines are able to detect sensitive changes in the pressure created from blood flow and within the dialyser.

Procedure

- Adequate venous access is required in order to remove and return blood from the patient at the appropriate and calculated flow rate (6–8mL/kg/min).
- Haemodialysis uses the principles of diffusion for solute removal, and osmosis, and ultrafiltration to remove excess water.
- These processes are achieved by passing the patients' blood through a dialyser, which has a counter current of dialysate fluid flowing on the opposite side of the semi-permeable membrane.
- During this phase the blood is 'cleaned' before being returned and the waste products are taken away by the dialysate.
- There are no set criteria or time limits for haemodialysis treatments and the therapy needs to be tailored to the patients' requirements.
- Standard chronic haemodialysis has historically been 4h, three times a week, but this may not always meet the child's needs if more fluid removal is necessary or they do not tolerate the treatment very well.
- Shorter, more frequent sessions are now considered to be more appropriate and better suited for patients, especially younger children.
- Haemodialysis can be performed in the home setting but is more common within the adult population. This is due to a number of factors including length of time to transplantation and potential instability of younger children during treatments.

Pitfalls

The main potential problems seen in haemodialysis are those of hypotension, infection, and clotting.

- *Hypotension* is generally seen when the patient is having fluid removed during their treatment. Fluid being removed from the patients circulating blood volume faster than the body can shift excess fluid back in is the main reason for this to happen and it is usually short lived. Close monitoring of blood pressure (BP) before, during, and after the haemodialysis session is paramount to the child's safety and can help to avoid the occurrence of hypotension.
- *Infections* in haemodialysis patients are mainly due to contamination in the central venous line or exit site. These infections are usually identified and treated quickly due to the frequency the child attends the dialysis unit.
- *Clotting* of the blood in the circuit during treatment can result in the patient loosing up to 10% of their blood volume. To avoid this problem anticoagulants are used, but need close monitoring to avoid any unwanted effects for the patient.

Associated reading

Smith E. (2004). Assessment and management of the child requiring chronic haemodialysis. *Paediat Nurs* **16**(7), 37–41.

Principles of peritoneal dialysis

Background

Peritoneal dialysis (PD) is an effective renal replacement therapy which can be carried out in the hospital or home setting for acute and chronic conditions.

Equipment

- Standard dialysis fluid is a sterile water based solution with a buffer (bicarbonate and/or lactate), Na, Ca, Mg, Cl, and glucose. The concentration of glucose (usually 3 different strengths) determines the amount of fluid removal during the therapy. Higher strengths of glucose in the fluid remove more excess fluid from the blood.
- PD machines have been developed to be portable and easy to use.
  - They have been designed to deliver accurate amounts of fluid to patients ranging from small infants to large adults.
  - The machines are fully automated and, once connected the patient can sleep whilst the therapy is in progress.
  - They require programming for the patient's specific prescription, which can be done manually, or by a memory card, which is downloadable to examine the patient's therapy.
  - The dialysis fluid is heated by the machine to body temperature to avoid any discomfort.

Procedure

- PD works by instilling dialysis fluid into the peritoneal cavity through a surgically implanted catheter.
- Whilst dwelling in the peritoneum, for the prescribed amount of time, the fluid uses the natural processes of osmosis and diffusion to remove excess water, and toxins from the blood using the semi-permeable characteristics of the peritoneal membrane to act as a filter.
- Fill volumes are calculated using the child's body surface area (800–1200mL/m^2) and dwell times are assessed in line with blood results, residual renal function and urine output.
- The therapy can be done manually by means of a twin bag system using gravity to empty and fill the peritoneum with dialysis fluid. This method of PD is called continuous ambulatory peritoneal dialysis (CAPD) and is performed in the home/community setting with usually 4 exchanges being required per day.
- The most common method of PD in children uses an automated machine and is carried out overnight to avoid interruption to school and social life.
- This method, termed continuous cycling peritoneal dialysis (CCPD), uses a large amount of dialysis fluid to perform more fills with shorter dwell times throughout the night and a long 'day dwell' during the daytime.

Pitfalls

The main problems seen with peritoneal dialysis are peritonitis and exit site/tunnel infections.

- Peritonitis is an inflammation of the peritoneum caused by infection. It is characterized by cloudy dialysis drain fluid, abdominal pain, and temperature.
  - The cause of the infection sometimes remains unknown but can usually be attributed to disconnection, line splits, or poor technique.
  - Peritonitis needs to be treated quickly and effectively in order to minimize the potential damage it can cause to the peritoneum.
  - Treatment can be targeted directly at the infection with the use of intraperitoneal antibiotics. Infections cultured as fungal will require removal of the catheter and more than likely a period of time on haemodialysis before re-insertion.
- Exit site infections are characterized by inflammation, redness, pain, and/or oozing from the area where the catheter leaves the body.
  - The exit site should be covered with a plain sterile dressing, and the catheter anchored by a tube holder, or tape to avoid movement, or pulling.
  - Poor management of the exit site or younger children touching this area can cause infection to be introduced.
  - A course of oral antibiotics and/or a topical ointment are usually sufficient to treat most infections.
  - If left untreated or if particularly virulent, the infection may track along the tunnel where the catheter is placed.
  - The main concern for this progression is that the infection may enter the peritoneum and cause peritonitis.
  - Tunnel infections may require admission for intravenous antibiotics and sometimes catheter removal.

Associated reading

Metheny NM. (2011). *Fluids and electrolytes balance: nursing considerations*, 5th ed. Bartlett Learning.

Haemofiltration

Background

Haemofiltration is a form of renal replacement therapy (RRT). It is generally provided within the critical care environment as a continuous therapy. The main advantage of this therapy over intermittent haemodialysis is that it is a slower, gentler treatment for fluid, and solute removal, and is therefore better tolerated in the haemodynamically unstable patient.

Haemofiltration requires a double lumen venous catheter to be inserted into either the internal jugular, subclavian or femoral vein. This access will generally be an acute, short term catheter which can be inserted quickly within the critical care environment in a patient who is sedated and ventilated (see Fig 16.1). It is therefore often referred to as continuous veno-venous haemofiltration (CVVH).

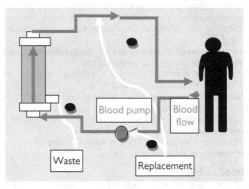

Fig 16.1 Haemofiltration.

Aims of therapy

As with all RRT the aims of therapy would be one or more of the following;

• Fluid removal.
• Normalize acid base balance.
• Waste product removal.
• Normalize electrolyte abnormalities.

The extent to which therapy delivers all of these aims will be dictated by the patient's clinical status and the rationale for commencing treatment.

How it works
- Utilizes an extracorporeal circuit and haemofilter.
- Haemofilter consists of semi-permeable membranes, which allows fluid and small-moderate sized solutes to pass across.
- The patient's blood flows through the circuit due to pressure exerted by the blood pump incorporated into the machine.
- Large volumes of fluid can be removed to enable solute removal (waste).
- This fluid is then replaced by a physiological solution (replacement) pre- or post-filter, or a combination of the two.
- Fluid removal can be programmed, based on a thorough assessment of the patient's fluid status.

Clinical indications
- Hypervolaemia.
- Acute renal failure.
- Inborn errors of metabolism.
- Drug ingestion/poisoning.
- Optimizing nutritional requirements in fluid restricted patients'.
- Sepsis:
  - The rationale for using for haemofiltration for sepsis is still under debate.
  - It is thought that it removes some of the inflammatory mediators.

Pitfalls
Cardiovascular instability on initiation
- ↑ risk in inotrope dependent patients due to dilution of inotropes.
- ↑ risk in low body weight patients due to % of circulating volume in extracorporeal circuit.

Hypothermia
- Very efficient method of cooling.
- Most modern machines have fluid warming device.

Clotting of circuit
Anticoagulation administered into the circuit to overcome such problems.

Bleeding
If anticoagulation is not correctly monitored and titrated there is risk of bleeding in the patient.

Infection risk
Associated with poor infection control measures when handling the circuit or vascular catheter.

Electrolyte disturbances
- The physiological replacement solution can be bicarbonate or lactate based.
- Initiating treatment will impact upon serum levels (e.g. K, Na, glucose).
- Hypophosphatemia is a significant risk as no commercially available solution exists with phosphate added.

Specialist service
- CVVH is a therapy provided fairly infrequently within the paediatric population.
- Requires nursing staff with specialist skills and knowledge to provide safe and efficient service.
- More complex than other treatments such as PD.
- Need specialist equipment suitable for use within the paediatric population.
- Modern paediatric machines have more sensitive volumetric control so are more accurate when dealing with lower body weight patients. In addition to being able to provide purely CVVH modern machines have other therapy options.

Continuous veno-venous haemodiafiltration (CVVHDF)
See Fig 16.2.
- Commonly used therapy in paediatric centres around the UK.
- In addition to ultrafiltration and convection utilized in CVVH there is an addition of dialysate flow, creating a diffusive element to therapy.
  - Diffusion—solutes move from high concentration to low concentration until equilibrium met.
  - Created due to countercurrent flow of blood and dialysate fluid.
- Good for improved clearance of smaller solutes.

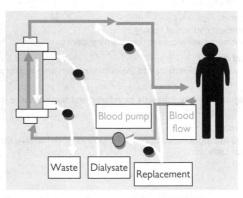

Fig 16.2 Continuous veno-venous haemodiafiltration (CVVHDF).

Associated reading

Metheny NM. (2011). *Fluids and electrolytes balance: nursing considerations*, 5th ed. Bartlett Learning.

Musculoskeletal system

History taking

Background

Obtaining an accurate health history is part one of the data gathering process in learning and understanding the child's problem. The nurse is often the first health professional that the child and family come into contact with. The objective is to gather subjective data, evaluate the given information and combine it with the physical assessment to make clinical decisions, formulating a nursing diagnosis. Effective communication using verbal and non-verbal skills, will establish a rapport and a relationship that will affect the success of the health history interview.

Before beginning the interview:
- Introduce yourself.
- Confirm the parents' and child's use of the English language.
- Consider the need for an interpreter.
- Review child's medical notes.

Presenting complaint

- Get the child and parents to tell you the health problem.
- Good listening and questioning skills are required.
- The aim is to achieve a good description of what the problem is (Box 17.1 provides a useful mnemonic).
- Question the child using appropriate age- related speech. use open-ended questions such as 'Tell me about . . .', 'What happened?' 'Where does it hurt?'
- Find out from the child and parents:
  - What the problem is.
  - When the problem started.
  - How did it start—was there a preceding illness or trauma?
  - What are the characteristics of the problem, e.g. what does it feel like—is there sharp/dull pain? Are the symptoms constant or intermittent? Do they have a problem walking, such as a limp?
  - What makes it worse/better—analgesia/rest?
- Use play as a communication tool.
- Take time to gain the child's trust.
- Ensure the environment is non-threatening.
- Give older children the opportunity to answer for themselves. Get to know your patient—are they at school or in college? What hobbies do they have? Are they still able to participate in these?
- Listen to the parents. Mothers especially have accurate intuition in relation to their child's presenting symptoms.
- Use eye contact and show interest.
- Clarify and summarize the information given by the parents.

❶The nurse needs to be aware of an inconsistent history for the presenting problem.

Example: a fractured femur in a non-ambulant child may be a case of child abuse.

Box 17.1 A useful mnemonic to guide you through the health history interview is:

OLD CART[1]
- *O*nset: of symptoms
- *L*ocation: where the problem is
- *D*uration: how long do the symptoms last?
- *C*haracteristics: description of what the symptoms feel like
- *A*ssociated factors: any other related symptoms?
- *R*elieving/Aggravating factors: what makes symptoms worse/better
- *T*reatment: has the child had any treatment so far?

Past history

- Determine whether there is anything in the child's past medical history that might have an influence on, or determine the current problem.

Example: episodes of pain/limp that were disregarded as not being important at the time, in a child who now presents with persistent pain on weight bearing; this might be a diagnosis of Perthes disease or osteomyelitis.
- Consider birth history, prematurity, type of delivery.
- Review the child's past medical history, such as developmental milestones. For example, when did the child first walk? Is the child on any current medication? Are they up to date with their immunizations? (This is important to know, if bone or joint infection is suspected).
- Does the child have any allergies, e.g. antibiotics, skin tape.
- A review of recent travel may be useful. There may be a link with suspected bone or joint infection, and the child's return from travel abroad, e.g. African/Asian countries.
- A review of the child's diet may indicate deficiency, e.g. Vitamin D (which may also result from lack of sunshine/use of sun creams).

Family history

- Is there anyone in the family who has had an orthopaedic related illness/problem? This should be specifically related to childhood musculoskeletal problems and not those associated with the older person, e.g. osteoarthritis.

Example: developmental dysplasia of the hip.

Musculoskeletal assessment

- Explain the examination to the child and parents, and obtain verbal consent. Ensure the child has a full understanding of the procedure.
- A useful approach to musculoskeletal assessment is to follow the framework of:
  - Look.
  - Feel.
  - Move.

The nurse's physical assessment is dependent on the child's presenting problem. Consider the suggestions listed here in your assessment. Examples of assessment strategies are given.

Look
- Identify characteristics of the presenting problem, e.g. observe the child's gait and posture looking for asymmetry.

Example: hip pain—the child will limp. Unequal leg lengths will cause a non-painful limp.

Or
- Observing for skin discolouration or pressure ulcers. Limb swelling and/or redness.

Example: pin site infection.

Feel
- Examine and palpate the problem area—is there tenderness or an increase in size? Is there warmth or tenderness?

Example: osteomylelitis.
- Check pulses, capillary refill time, and sensation.

Example: neurovascular assessment.

Move
- Check for active range of movement, asking the child to move their limbs and if a gait problem, observe the child walking. Assess for normal range of movement of their joints. Assess active, passive and resisted movement.
- Question if joint movement is restricted whether this is normal for that child, e.g. a child with cerebral palsy. If movement exceeds normal, is the child hypermobile?
- Is movement painful?

Example: reduced hip movement in a child with irritable hip.

Practice tips
- Musculoskeletal assessment is most likely to be focused on a problem area, as opposed to a general review of whole body. However, remember to assess the joint above and below the problem area for normality.
- Consider what the normal range of motion for each joint is.
- Compare affected side with the movement of the normal side.
- Use an appropriate pain assessment tool, e.g. FACES, FLACC, VAS.
- Infants can be examined on a parents lap.
- For a thorough examination exposure of the 'problem' area is necessary.
- Be sensitive to the older child who may be reluctant to remove clothing.
- Observe the child's facial expression throughout the examination. This helps in identifying non-vocalized pain.
- Height, weight, and baseline observations may be useful, e.g. weight for drug calculations, temperature if infection is suspected.

Orthopaedic examination may include further tests and arranging for investigations to determine a diagnosis. These may include testing for normal reflexes and muscle strength and arranging for appropriate radiological investigations such as X rays or MRI.

Assessment of X-rays

- Are the bones or normal shape, and size? Are they in correct alignment? Is the physis (growth plate) affected?
- Are the components of the joint in correct position?

Example: slipped capital femoral epiphysis (the femoral head has slipped off the physis or growth plate).

- Is new bone growth evident or is there abnormal bone growth?

Example: avascular necrosis in Perthes disease.

Assessment of bloods

- Are these within normal reference range?
- A raised white count and CRP indicates infection.

Associated reading

Cash S. (2007). Principles of Physical Assessment. In: Glasper EA, McEwing G, Richardson J. (eds). *Oxford Handbook of Children's and Young People' Nursing*. Oxford University Press, Oxford.

Douglas G, Nicol F, Robertson C. (2005). *Macleod's Clinical Examination*, 11th edn. Churchill Livingstone, Edinburgh.

Hunter D. (2010). Triage nurse X ray protocols for hand and wrist injuries. *Emerg Nurse* **17**(9), 20–4.

[1] Rushforth H. (2009). *Assessment Made Incredibly Easy*. Lippincott Williams & Wilkins. London.

Neurovascular assessment

Background

Neurovascular observations are an essential element of orthopaedic nursing and should form the basis of the assessment of a child with an Orthopaedic condition or injury. Early detection of the warning signs of compartment syndrome is crucial and must be acted upon immediately in order that this extremely serious and limb-threatening condition is avoided.

Assessment

- Explain the process to the child and family
- A thorough assessment of the following should be made:
  - *Colour*—the digits should be pink. Any alteration in colour, i.e. bluish tinge, purple or white digits is indicative of inadequate blood supply. Consider natural skin colour and how this may affect assessment.
  - *Warmth*—the digits should be warm. Compare with the contralateral side and consider other reasons for cool digits, i.e. lengthy surgery or the presence of a wet plaster.
  - *Sensation*—the child should be able to feel touch in all digits and should not be experiencing numbness or tingling.
  - *Movement*—the child should be able to flex, extend, and abduct their fingers and/or toes. They should also have thumb–finger opposition. Passive movements must also be assessed.
  - *Capillary refill*—when the child's nail bed is pressed down for 5s the colour should return in less than 2s.
  - *Pulses*—if accessible the pulses should be strong and equal to the other side.
  - *Pain*—should be controlled with analgesia. It should be located at the fracture site and should not be out of proportion to the injury. Use appropriate pain tool for assessment.
  - *Swelling*—to be expected following an orthopaedic injury or surgery. The affected skin should not be taut or shiny.

Practice tips

- The affected limb must never be elevated above the level of the heart.
- Check that plaster of Paris (POP) and bandages are not too tight.
- If altered neurovascular observations are detected, elevate the limb, consider splitting the POP or bandages to skin, and throughout their full length (seek advice first unless stated in notes) and contact orthopaedic registrar for review.
- When splitting is ordered, always split POP or bandages to skin, and throughout their full length.
- Involve play specialist with distraction techniques and games that will get child to move digits even when fearful of pain.

- Encourage the child to actively flex and extend the affected digits several times an hour.
- The child may be frightened to move their fingers or toes for fear of it being painful—encouragement will be needed.
- Always consider other causes of altered observations, but seek advice urgently if symptoms persist or worsen.

Pitfalls

- It is difficult to assess the neurovascular status of a pre-verbal child.
- The affected limb must never be elevated above the level of the heart.

Associated reading

Judge NL. (2007). Neurovascular assessment. *Nursing Standard* **21**(45), 39–44.

Recognition of compartment syndrome

Background

Muscles are divided into compartments by deep fascia. In limbs, each compartment consists of muscle, nerves, blood vessels, and bone. The fascia, which surrounds the muscle compartment is inelastic and will not expand to allow for swelling or increased compartment contents.

- Compartment syndrome occurs when pressure within the muscle compartment is raised due to injury to the muscle that surrounds the compartment and/or haemorrhage.
- Soft tissue injury will cause a localized inflammatory response and oedema, which increases the compartment pressure.
- Haemorrhage occurs as a result of a fracture or soft tissue injury and will cause bleeding within the muscle compartment. This increases compartment contents and therefore elevates pressure.
- The presence of bandages or a POP may exacerbate the situation—their constrictive nature will prevent skin expansion to accommodate swelling. Internal pressure develops and further compromises the functioning of nerves and blood vessels.
- Compromised blood vessels and nerves are unable to function correctly and venous outflow and return will be obstructed.
- Eventually blood vessels will collapse causing further oedema, increased venous pressure and ongoing elevation of the soft tissue pressures.
- If left untreated, irreversible muscle necrosis may occur. This can result in permanent deformity and, rarely, may necessitate limb amputation.
- Compartment syndrome can occur in any muscle compartment, but most commonly occurs in the lower leg and forearm.

Procedure

Explain need for regular observation appropriately to child and family and gain consent.

Observe regularly (determine frequency in consultation with medical team) for:

- *Pain:* out of proportion to the injury, not located at the fracture site, and present on passive extension of the digits. The pain will be deep, unremitting, poorly localized, and will limit finger/toe movements due to inadequate oxygenation of muscle tissues, resulting in muscle ischaemia and necrosis.
- *Paraesthesia:* peripheral nerves can be affected within muscle compartments as increased tissue pressure will cause muscle and nerve ischaemia. Altered sensation will be present in some or all of the digits on the affected limb. Nerve damage sustained at the time of injury may also cause altered sensation in the digits of the affected limb.
- *Paralysis:* voluntary function in muscles may be lost as the muscles become weak due to evolving ischaemia. Loss of function may be irreversible. However, this can also be caused by nerve damage sustained at the time of injury.

- *Pulselessness*: the presence of a peripheral pulse is not a reliable indicator that compartment syndrome is not present as arteriole spasm or collapse, and subsequent loss of pulse is a late and very ominous sign.
- *Pallor Digits*: may become dusky as the blood supply is reduced to the peripheries. They may also be a deep red/purple colour (engorged) as venous return will be compromised by the increased tissue pressure. Digits may also be cool.
- *Capillary refill time/swelling*: capillary refill time may be reduced due to poor blood supply and compression of arterioles. Swelling and the presence of tense, shiny, or stretched skin are indicative of severe swelling and skin integrity may be threatened.
  - ❶ If compartment syndrome is suspected, urgent review by orthopaedic registrar or consultant must be sought.
  - Elevate the affected limb, and split POP or constricting bandages to skin and throughout their full length following discussion with the orthopaedic doctors.
  - Ensure that pain is regularly assessed using an appropriate pain assessment tool. Utilize pharmacological pain relief as prescribed in conjunction with distraction, guided imagery, etc., as appropriate to manage child's pain effectively.
  - Fasciotomy may be required. This will be carried out in theatre as an emergency procedure and involves the operative splitting of the fascia along the compartment length, decompressing the compartment, and allowing for expansion of the swollen muscle.

Practice tips

- Compartment syndrome can develop up to 3 days following injury or surgery.
- The affected limb must not be elevated above the level of the heart.
- Bandages and POP must always be split to skin, and throughout their full length.
- Deep, unremitting pain that is not relieved by analgesia and pain on passive movement of the affected digits is the most reliable indicator of an evolving compartment syndrome.
- If a fasciotomy is performed the patient should receive intravenous antibiotics until the wounds have been closed.

Associated reading

Wright E. (2009). Neurovascular impairment and compartment syndrome. *Paediatric Nursing*, **21**(3), 26–9.

Broad arm sling

Background

A broad arm sling will be used to immobilize an injured limb.
Common uses include:

- Fracture of the collar bone, shoulder, humerus, elbow, forearm, wrist, or fingers.
- After reduction of a dislocated shoulder or elbow.
- Infections of the arm.
- Support an above the elbow plaster/injured arm.

Equipment

- Triangular bandage.
- Adhesive tape.

Procedure

- Explain procedure appropriately to child and parent and gain consent.
- Undertake pain assessment with appropriate tool and provide analgesia and/or distraction techniques as indicated.
- Make sure the patient's arm is supported.
- Place the bandage under the injured arm with the point to the elbow.
- Pull the end behind the patient's neck to the opposite shoulder (see Fig. 17.1a).
- Fold the lower end of the bandage up and over the injured arm and bring to meet the other end at the shoulder (see Fig. 17.1b).
- Tie the ends in a reef knot on the injured side.
- Secure the point by either twisting until the fabric fits the elbow snugly (see Fig. 17.1c), or by folding the point forwards and securing with adhesive tape (see Fig. 17.1d).
- Check circulation in the fingers and recheck every 10min and if necessary loosen the sling.
- Advise child/young person/parent/carer to:
  - Exercise the uninjured joints to avoid them becoming stiff.
  - Remove the sling at night.
  - Wear the sling as long as indicated.
  - Take arm out of the sling and exercise (if directed by doctor or physiotherapist) to prevent the shoulder, elbow, and fingers becoming stiff.
  - Rotate the upper arm and shoulder as tolerated.
  - Wiggle fingers.
- Ensure that discharge/home care information is appropriate and clear—consider written and pictorial advice to take home.
- Liaise as required with school and community services.

Practice tips

- Tuck both free ends of the bandage under the knot to pad it.
- Use a reef knot as it lies flat.

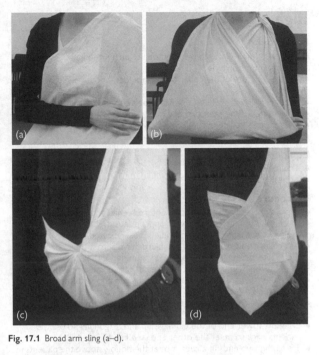

Fig. 17.1 Broad arm sling (a–d).

Associated reading

St John Ambulance et al. (2009). *First Aid Manual*, 9th edn. Dorling Kindersley, London.

High arm sling

Background

A high arm sling will be used to immobilize an injured limb.
Common uses include:

- Care of fracture of the collar bone, shoulder, humerus, elbow, forearm, wrist, or fingers.
- Support following reduction of a dislocated shoulder or elbow.
- Preventing/halting haemorrhage (alongside pressure dressing).
- Decreasing swelling of the forearm, wrist, or hand.
- Elevation of the child's arm.

Equipment

- Triangular bandage.
- Adhesive tape.

Procedure

- Explain procedure and gain consent from child and parent.
- Undertake pain assessment with appropriate tool, and provide analgesia and/or distraction techniques as indicated.
- Ask child, if able, to support the injured arm across their chest with their fingers resting on the opposite shoulder. If they are unable to do so enlist the help of parent/carer/health care professional (HCP).
- Place the triangular bandage over the injured arm with the point going just beyond the elbow (see Fig. 17.2a).
- Tuck the base of the bandage under the injured arm carefully (see Fig. 17.2b).
- Bring the lower end of the bandage up and diagonally across the patients back to meet the other end (see Fig. 17.2c).
- Tie to the two ends in a reef knot at the hollow above the patients collar bone.
- The either twist the point until it fits closely around the patients elbow (see Fig. 17.2d) or tuck the point in just above the elbow and secure with adhesive tape (see Fig. 17.2e).
- Regularly check the circulation and if necessary loosen the bandage.
- Make sure a parent/carer has been shown how to re-apply the sling.
- Advise child/young person/parent/carer to:
  - Exercise the uninjured joints to avoid them becoming stiff.
  - Remove the sling at night.
  - Wear the sling as long as indicated.
  - Take arm out of the sling and exercise (if directed by doctor or physiotherapist) to prevent the shoulder, elbow, and fingers becoming stiff.
  - Rotate the upper arm and shoulder as tolerated.
  - Wiggle fingers.
- Ensure that discharge/home care information is appropriate and clear—consider written and pictorial advice to take home.
- Liaise as required with school and community services.

Practice tips

- Tuck both free ends of the bandage under the knot to pad it.
- Use a reef knot as it lies flat.

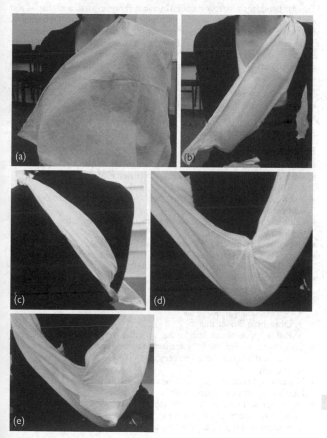

Fig. 17.2 High arm sling (a–e).

Associated reading

St John Ambulance et al. (2009). *First Aid Manual*, 9th edn. Dorling Kindersley, London.

Applying tubular bandage

Background

Tubular bandages are now supplied in a vast range of sizes and shapes and are largely replacing traditional bandages for support for minor limb trauma. Examples of lightweight tubular supporting products include Tubiton®, Tubinette®, Tubegauze®, and Tubifast®, which is elasticated. Tubular net bandages are versatile and easy to apply and remove (Netelast®, Setonet® are examples). Tubigrip® provides more powerful support, but negligible compression when used alone.

Selecting the correct size:
• Measure round the affected joint/limb at the widest point.
• Check the size guide.

Select the appropriate pack.

Procedure

• Provide appropriate information to child and family, and gain consent.
• Consider administration of analgesia in advance of procedure to achieve pain control.
• Involve other personnel, e.g. play specialist, as appropriate to provide support and distraction.
• Cut the correct size tubular bandage into a length twice the length of the limb to be bandaged.
• Use an applicator 'cage' if the correct size is available.
• For ankle, lower leg, elbow, knee, and thigh: pull bandage into limb like a stocking. Double bandage back over limb.
• For wrist and lower arm:
  • Make two small cuts in bandage for thumb.
  • Pull bandage over arm and push thumb through hole A.
  • Start doubling bandage back.
  • Draw hole B over thumb.
  • Pull top layer about 3cm further up the arm than the bottom layer.
• Check with medical staff/physiotherapist when bandage should be in place and when it should be removed—advise child and family accordingly.
• Monitor and record neurovascular status regularly (see 📖 Neurovascular assessment, p. 490).
• Encourage and support child and family in following any exercise regime ordered by physiotherapist.
• Document and report as appropriate.

Practice tips

• Do not fold over excess material or use with more than double thickness, as this will provide too much compression.

Applying a cervical collar

Background

A cervical collar may be used for palliative treatment of conditions, such as muscle spasm or to provide support after cervical fusion. It may also be used to augment splinting devices, when spinal injury is suspected.

Equipment

- Tape measure.
- Blunt scissors.
- Appropriate-sized cervical collar (selected following measurement).
- Sand bags.
- Wide adhesive tape.
- Manufacturer's guidelines for sizing and application.

Procedure

- Provide full explanation to child and parent and gain consent.
- Align the cervical spine through a manual stabilization if possible.
- The head should be immobilized throughout the procedure. One practitioner should stand behind the child with their hands on the child's head—thumbs on the forehead and fingers spread widely around head on each side. Lean forward into elbows on bed (or other surface) to maintain stability.
- The second practitioner should remove clothing from child's neck. Observe condition—look for bruising, swelling, etc.
- Remove other clothing, jewellery, etc., as appropriate.
- Measure to determine the correct collar size: for height, measure from the bottom of the chin to the top of the sternum. Measure around the neck for circumference.
- Select the appropriate collar by applying the patient's measurements to the manufacturer's size chart.
- Review the manufacturer's directions for applying the device.
- Slide the collar up from the chest to the chin until it is placed centrally.
- Wrap collar around child's neck—the chin support should fit snugly and the base should sit at the centre of the sternum.
- Secure with Velcro strap.
- Place sandbags each side of the child's head if necessary.
- Consider applying tape to trolley or bed, passing over the child's forehead and then applying to other side of trolley/bed to provide more stability. Ensure that tension is even and that child's head is straight.
- Document as appropriate—include collar size in record.

Practice tips

- Regularly check the skin under the collar and give skin care as appropriate to prevent breakdown.
- Always communicate with your partner holding manual cervical immobilization and checking for proper alignment to achieve optimum results.

Pitfalls

- A cervical collar will only stabilize the top 7 vertebrae, C1–C7. Other immobilizing devices, such as a backboard must be used to stabilize the remainder of the spinal column.
- Be aware that the collar may clamp the jaw shut and cause a child to choke if they vomit.
- In some cases, the collar may increase pressure in the intracranial region.

Applying a collar and cuff

Background

A collar and cuff is commonly used to provide a balanced arm sling, holding the arm in a position that enables gravity to apply some traction, and/or when the pressure of a full sling's fabric will exacerbate pain and discomfort.

Equipment

- Collar and cuff material and tie wrap.
- Blunt scissors.
- Waterproof adhesive tape.

Procedure

- Provide full and appropriate explanation to child and parent, and gain consent.
- Consider administration of analgesia in advance of procedure to achieve pain control.
- Gain clear instruction regarding required angle and position of arm.
- Remove clothing and jewellery from affected arm and neck.
- If collar and cuff will have to remain *in situ* at all times, ensure that it is applied underneath clothing.
- Provide support to the elbow of the affected arm—this may be done by the child themselves, parent, or second practitioner.
- Using one long piece of collar and cuff material, form a loop that will fit over child's head, with another loop around the affected wrist.
- Ensuring that affected arm will be held in the required position, cinch the 2 loops where they cross over with the tie wrap at the central chest point.
- Cut off any excess collar and cuff material and cover the raw ends next to the tie wrap with waterproof adhesive tape.
- Check neurovascular status.
- Advise child and carer:
  - How long child will need it and when/if it can be removed.
  - To observe neurovascular status—what to do if they have any concerns.
  - What physical activity can/should be undertaken while it's in place.
  - Regular exercise of fingers will help the circulation and decrease swelling.

Practice tips

- Cover with plastic food wrap to keep dry/clean when washing or engaged in 'messy' activity.
- To wash the child's chest and under the affected arm, ask the child to lean forward, allowing the arm to hang free without causing discomfort. Gentle pressure either side of the elbow fold will enable the skin to be washed and dried.

Splints

Background

Splints fall into two categories: dynamic and fixed.
- Dynamic splints control the range of movement, and/or promote the soft tissue development and healing.
- Fixed splint is a rigid device to support, control, and/or correct a limb.

Splints are used in children's orthopaedics to:
- Immobilize and rest a limb, i.e. after trauma.
- Control and restrict movement, e.g. stabilizing knee joint after surgery.
- Prevent limb deformities occurring, i.e. foot drop.
- Support and maintain corrected position of limbs, i.e. post-gastrocnemius lengthening surgery.
- Pain relief by altering physical dynamics, i.e. gel heel cups in Sever's disease.

Removable wrist and futura splints

These splints are commonly used for the management of buckle fractures of the distal radius. Buckle fractures are unique to children. A buckle fracture is an incomplete fracture that occurs because children have a thicker periosteum. When the bone sustains a force great enough to break it, the bone 'buckles' rather than fully fractures. The fracture is stable and a splint is required for pain relief.

Removable wrist splints can also be used for wrist soft tissue injuries.

Application procedure
- Provide appropriate information to child and carer and gain consent.
- Select a correctly sized, right- or left-handed, splint for the child.
- Place on the wrist and secure using the Velcro straps or ties.
- Do not secure too tightly. Check for neurovascular deficit.
- Advise carer (and child/young person if appropriate) that the splint may be removed for hygiene purposes.
- Advise (following consultation with medical personnel) whether the splint should be worn at night.

Mallet splint

Used to immobilize a digit when there is an avulsion fracture of the extensor tendon (see Fig. 17.3) In this injury, a small fragment of bone that is attached to the tendon has been pulled off. It is necessary to keep the finger in extension, to keep the muscle and its tendon relaxed, keeping the fracture fragment in close proximity to the injury site to allow healing.

Application procedure
- Provide appropriate information to child and carer, and gain consent.
- Select a correctly sized splint. Try on the same opposing digit that is uninjured for sizing.
- Keep the finger flat on a hard surface.
- Place the splint over the finger and secure at the base with tape.
- Advise that splint should only be removed once daily to wash finger.
- Finger must be rested on a flat hard surface before splint is removed.
- The finger is washed in this position and the splint reapplied.
- The finger must not be bent whilst the splint is removed.

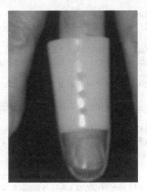

Fig. 17.3 Mallet splint.

Thomas splint

This splint is used to stabilize a fractured femur (see Fig. 17.4). The splint is unique in that it provides fixed traction and allows the patient with a fractured femur to be safely moved.

Equipment
- Thomas splint (correct size).
- Slings.
- Gamgee®.
- Adhesive skin traction kit—correct size.
- 6 bandages—appropriate size.
- Tape.
- Scissors.
- 2 tongue depressors—to act as windlass.

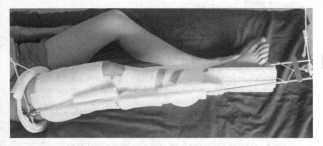

Fig. 17.4 Thomas splint.

Application procedure

❶ This splint should only be applied by healthcare professionals with the appropriate training.

• Provide appropriate information to child and carer, and gain consent.
• Check for allergies, reconsider tape and/or other equipment if needed.
• Gather equipment.
• Measure the affected limb for length and obliquely across the upper thigh.
• A correctly sized splint should be selected and adjusted to the correct measurements.
• The splint should then be prepared. First, the slings should be applied and then a layer of Gamgee® placed on the top.
• One member of staff should apply manual traction to the injured limb. This involves moving the fracture. Great care must be taken to observe for neurovascular deficit during this process. The manual traction remains in place until the Thomas splint is successfully applied.
• The other staff member applies the adhesive skin traction to the limb. It is important this is done smoothly to prevent pressure sores developing. This is further secured to the leg by bandaging in a figure of eight.
• Without releasing the manual traction the Thomas splint is then applied to the limb.
• The skin traction cords are then tied to the frame. The windlass is inserted and then spun as tightly as it will go.
• Fixed traction is achieved and the manual traction can be released.
• Bandage over the whole splint for additional security. The patient can be safely transferred.
• At this stage a repeat X-ray should be obtained to check the position of the limb.
• At all times the neurovascular status of the limb should be known.
• In most hospitals the Thomas splint is then supported by a system of traction cord, weights, and pulleys. This makes the splint less heavy and allows the patient to move around the bed reducing the risk of pressure sores.

Practice tips

• Check the traction equipment daily. Knots can loosen and traction cord fray.
• Protect knots in traction cord by covering with waterproof tape.
• Assess child regularly for complications of bed rest and perform the necessary nursing interventions to prevent these. Regular neurovascular assessment for the early detection of compartment syndrome is essential.
• Check for blistering under bandages—may be allergy/fracture blisters.
• Check for pressure sores on bony prominences and around ring of Thomas splint.
• Consider pressure relieving mattress or polymer gel pads.
• Encourage the child to decorate their bed, traction poles, etc.

International range of movement brace

This brace is used to stabilize and support the knee joint either after knee surgery or injury. The international range of movement brace (IROM) can be locked in extension or flexion; or the amount of knee flexion can be controlled. For example, following a Fulkerson's osteotomy, the IROM is initially locked in extension, then the range of movement is gradually increased to 30°, 60°, and 90° through rehabilitation.

Application procedure

• Provide appropriate information to child and carer, and gain consent.
• The patient should be laid down.
• Select the correct size IROM.
• Undo all the Velcro fastenings and foam wraps.
• Set the knee flexion parameters on the dials.
• Without flexing the patient's knee place the IROM under the patient's leg.
• The top foam should cover all of the thigh and the lower foam cover the lower leg.
• Wrap the foam around the leg and secure with the Velcro fastenings.
• Make sure the knee hinges are parallel with the knee joint.
• Advise that usually the brace has to remain on at all times. If the doctor allows the brace to be removed for hygiene purposes then it must be removed with the patient lying down. After the leg has been washed the brace should be reapplied as previously described.

Functional foot orthoses

Correct or maintain correction of limb deformity (see Fig. 17.5). For example, children with special needs that have hypotonia, the ankle–foot orthosis (AFO) enables them to lift/control their foot and be able to walk. In this instance, the splint is worn as a daytime splint. For post-surgical correction of tight gastrocnemius the splint is worn at night to prevent the muscle tightening during sleep.

Application procedure

• Some splints are ready made. In this instance, a correctly sized splint should be selected. For day time wear it is worn over a sock and within a shoe.
• Night-time splints are worn next to the skin or over special socks.
• If a correctly fitting splint is not readily available then the orthotist will take a cast moulding of the child's leg/foot and make an individual AFO.
• Observe the skin for pressure sores, especially in children with special needs who may have altered sensation of their limbs.

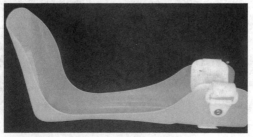

Fig. 17.5 Functional foot splint.

Boots on a bar

To maintain correction of talipes equinos varus treated with the Ponseti technique (see Fig. 17.6). Talipes is a 3-D foot deformity that is corrected by serial casting, and then an Achilles tenotomy. The corrected position needs to be maintained by the boots on a bar for 4yrs. Initially, the boots on a bar is worn for 23h/day for 3 months and thereafter at night time only.

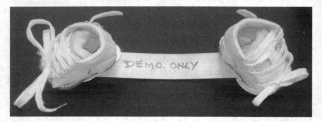

Fig. 17.6 Boots on bar.

Application procedure

• The shoes are measured and applied by the orthotist.
• The shoe needs to fit correctly as with any shoe wear. Pertinently, the child's heel must sit fully in the boot. The boot is usually set at 70° of abduction on the bar.
• Socks should not be worn with the boots on a bar as they make it easier for the child to pull the foot free of the boot.
• Careful observation of the skin is needed.
• Neurovascular assessment is recommended.

Piedro boots

Support and stabilize the feet. Piedros are often used for children with talipes or special needs, and various associated foot disorders. Piedros are an ankle boot with strong ankle supports (see Fig. 17.7).

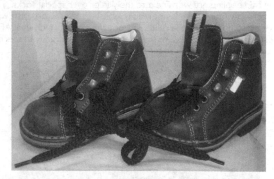

Fig. 17.7 Piedro boots.

Application procedure
- The shoes are measured and applied by the orthotist.
- The shoe needs to fit correctly as with any shoe wear.
- Piedros are a lace up boot and are worn in the same way as conventional shoe wear. Velcro® fastening is also available.
- Check the skin integrity.

Air cast walker

Supports a limb after injury or surgery whilst allowing weight bearing (see Fig. 17.8).

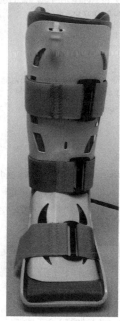

Fig. 17.8 Air cast walker.

Application procedure
- Choose a correctly fitting air cast walker.
- An inner sock is applied to the leg.
- The leg placed in the appliance and the tongue placed in.
- Secure with the Velcro® straps.
- Inflate.
- The patient may weight bear normally whilst wearing this appliance.
- Skin integrity should be checked, as should neurovascular assessment.

Associated reading

Benson M, Fixsen J, Macnicol MF, et al (Eds) (2010) *Children's Orthopaedics and Fractures*, 3rd edn. Springer, London.

Casts

Background

A cast is a rigid shell that must be well fitting when applied, to support the architecture of the body and underlying soft tissues of a limb or body. Plaster or resin-based casts are commonly used to immobilize limbs following trauma or orthopaedic surgery. Casts made of polyester or fibreglass casting tape are lightweight, watertight, and durable, and are available in a variety of colours and are one-fifth the weight of the POP cast. POP is an easy splinting material and the material of choice for new fractures, post operatively and where swelling and bleeding may occur.

The purpose of casting is to:

• Rest and protect the limb or part.
• Restore bony alignment.
• Limit movement.
• Restore function.
• Prevent or limit further soft tissue and neurovascular damage.
• Reduce pain, swelling, and muscle spasm.

❶ Casts should only be applied by suitably trained and competent practitioners.

Equipment

• Trolley.
• Elbow or knee rests.
• POP or fibreglass casting tape, and POP slabs and plaster strips to finish if required.
• Felt padding.
• Plastic sheeting, aprons, gloves, and plastic-covered pillows/cushions.
• Soft padding and stockinet.
• Plaster scissors.
• Bucket or bowl of water at 20–25°C.
• Wash bowl for child.
• Rubbish bag.
• Documentation.
• Instruction leaflets.

Application of a cast

• Application should be according to local policy guidelines and evidence base.
• Involve parent/carer or trusted adult, and written consent or assent may be required according to local policy.
• Appropriate numbers of suitably qualified staff should be available throughout the procedure to support the child and family.
• Use play therapy or distraction techniques.
• Age appropriate language to explain the procedure to the child or young person and carer and gain consent.
• Remove all jewellery and clothing on the affected limb.
• Protect the child's clothing as plaster application can be messy.

- Analgesia should be prescribed and administered to reduce anxiety, relieve pain, and increase compliance.
- The limb is prepared with stockinet and/or wool padding.
- The cast bandage is soaked in the warm water and then bandaged onto the prepared limb or part.
- The cast will feel warm initially.
- POP will take 24–48h to dry and resin-based casts normally dry in 20–30min.
- Undertake regular observation of neurovascular status (see 📖 Neurovascular assessment, p. 490).
- Wearing gloves is mandatory for handling fibreglass material.
- Do not rest the freshly applied cast on a hard surface as it might distort or dent the plaster, which may interfere with its functional ability.
- Documentation and record keeping.
- The child or young person might be discharged after application in the emergency department or clinic.
- Parents/carers should be issued with clear written instructions regarding drying and checking for complications, and the use of aids or crutches as appropriate.

Removing the cast

- Casts can be removed with shears, but it is customary to use an oscillating saw. This may be frightening for the child as the saw emits a high frequency noise and can cause a vibrating sensation in the bone.
- Use play therapy or distraction techniques.
- May include 'splitting or bi-valving' the cast, which involves a single cut down the entire length of the cast (only appropriate for POP casts). Resin casts may require two-cuts down the length of the cast.
- A 'window' may be cut into the cast to facilitate inspection or wound dressing. The window should be replaced to protect the integrity of the cast.

Practice tips

- Keep the cast exposed to the air to facilitate drying and avoid using a hair dryer to dry the cast as this may cause burns.
- Keep the limb elevated when resting to reduce any swelling and rest on a towel as this will absorb moisture.
- Encourage exercise of fingers or toes.
- Features of a good cast include being light weight and well fitting, having a smooth interior and not causing constriction.

Pitfalls

The 5 'Ps' of ischaemia should be reported immediately and include:
- Pallor.
- Parathesia.
- Paralysis.
- Pain associated with passive movements.
- Pulselessness.

Compartment syndrome (see 📖 Recognition of compartment syndrome, p. 492), which constitutes an emergency when post-traumatic swelling may gradually compromise the circulation within a closed fascial compartment, causing ischaemia and death of the muscle, contributing to compartment syndrome.
- In hot weather a staphylococcal infection of the hair and sweat glands can lead to severe and painful dermatitis.
- The skin underneath the cast can become dry and scaly.
- Insertion of implements to scratch the skin underneath the cast can cause skin damage, risking infection or the implement can become lodged inside the cast risking further damage.

Associated reading

Chadburn L. (2006). Plaster care. In: Trigg E, Mohammed T. (eds). *Practices in Children's Nursing: Guidelines for Hospital and Community*, 2nd edn. Churchill Livingstone, Edinburgh.

Glasper A, McConochie J. (2010). Orthopaedic skills. In: Glasper A, Aylott M, Battrick C. (eds). *Developing Practical Skills for Nursing Children and Young People*. Hodder Arnold, London.

McDermott S, Nolan L. (2010). Musculo-skeletal system. In: Coyne I, Neill F, Timmins F. (eds). *Clinical Skills in Children's Nursing*. Oxford University Press, Oxford.

Royal College of Nursing (RCN) (2007). *Benchmarks for Children's Orthopaedic Nursing Care*. RCN, London.

Skin traction in children

Background

Skin traction is a non-invasive procedure performed on limbs (most often the lower limb) to produce traction on the underlying bone, muscle, or joint, via the skin and muscles. It involves applying adhesive or non-adhesive tape (extensions) to the skin, securing this, and applying counter traction that may be fixed or balanced. Adhesive tapes cannot be used if the child is allergic to Elastoplast. Examples of skin traction are simple skin traction (Pugh's), Gallows/Bryants traction, and Thomas splint traction (see 📖 Splints, p. 504). It is most commonly used to reduce, correct and maintain closed fractures.

Equipment

- *Adhesive or non-adhesive skin traction kits:* child or adult, depending on child size/age and allergy status. These contain the skin traction tapes with foam covered ends to protect the medial and lateral malleoli and a bandage.
- Tape to secure the bandage.
- *Balkan beams, pulleys and weights:* depending on type of traction required.
- *Thomas splint:* if required.
- Suitable distraction aids, e.g. story book, tape, etc.
- Appropriate and timed analgesia administered prior to the procedure.

❶ Ensure there is a competent practitioner to apply the traction.

Procedure

- Ensure this is the most appropriate method of treatment and competent practitioner to undertake the procedure.
- Gain informed verbal consent from person with parental responsibility and child (if old enough to consent).
- Check for allergies and reconsider tape, and other equipment if necessary.
- Prepare all equipment.
- Ensure child has adequate analgesia and it is working prior to the procedure.
- The child and parents may be shown photographs of how the traction may look if available, so that they can visualize what is going to be applied.
- Look for any breaks in skin integrity where skin tapes (extensions) or bandages may be applied.
- Apply the skin extensions to either side of the limb. In the lower limb, the extensions should be applied evenly to the medial and lateral sides of the leg, leaving the knee free. If the limb is held by the child in a particular position prior to the application, apply the extensions to the exposed side first. In lower limb fractures, the leg is usually held in external rotation. Therefore, the extensions should be applied to the medial side first.

- The extensions should be applied evenly, without creases and should follow the limb's natural contours. The foam areas should be evenly applied to protect the medial and lateral malleoli, and extend beyond the foot to allow for adequate plantar flexion of the foot.
- Once the extensions have been applied, the bandage should be applied evenly, starting at the distal area and securely taped. In the lower limb, the knee should be left exposed.
- The cord attached to the skin traction kit should be tied to produce a single cord if using simple skin traction or Gallows. The cord should be arranged as 2 even ends if applying to a Thomas splint.
- Attach to either the Thomas splint, or to weights via pulleys, ensuring that the limb is in the correct anatomical position, with the cords, pulleys, and weights in correct alignment and free hanging.
- The foot of the bed may be elevated to apply counter traction.
- Once applied, neurovascular assessment should be undertaken, to ensure that the application of skin traction (and the initial injury) has not resulted in neurovascular compromise.
- Complete nursing documentation.

Practice tips

- If non-adhesive extensions are required due to allergy, they require careful observation as they are much more likely to become dislodged.
- Wet areas on the skin extensions are an indication of blisters/sores under the extensions and should be investigated.

Pitfalls

- Young children on Gallows traction are at increased risk of choking, due to their position and should be observed at all times when eating.

Associated reading

Coyne I, Neill F, and Timmins F. (2010). *Clinical skills in children's nursing*. Oxford University Press: Oxford.

Hockenberry MJ and Wilson D. (eds). (2011). *Wong's nursing care of infants and children*, 9th ed. Elsevier Mosby: Missouri.

External fixation

Background

External fixators are devices used for the fixation of fractures, the correction of deformity or for bone lengthening.

There are several types of fixator:
- Monolateral external fixator.
- Circular frame fixators, e.g. Ilizarov frame and Taylor Spatial frame.

Monolateral fixator

This consists of pins inserted into the bone with a rail/bar connecting the pins and providing stability. It is commonly used to fix fractures or for lengthening of a bone.

Circular frame fixator

Ilizarov frame

This construct is made up of pins inserted into the bone and attached to circular rings. Larger strut pins may also be utilized to increase stability of the structure. Such fixators are useful in the management of fractures or for deformity correction as they allow for correction of multi-planar deformities. Limb lengthening can also be carried out simultaneously, if required, with these fixators. The bone is lengthened or corrected using clickers, spanners, and nuts or keys.

Taylor spatial frames

These frames consist of aluminium rings that are connected by six struts and the construct is attached by a series of pins inserted into the bone. The struts can be individually lengthened or shortened, and the bone manipulated in six axes. The programme for strut adjustment is created using specialized computer software and the struts are adjusted each day until correction has been achieved. The fixator then remains *in situ* until the bone has healed.

External fixators are used to treat:
- Fractures associated with severe soft tissue damage as wound management can still be carried out.
- Fractures associated with nerve or blood vessel damage.
- Severely comminuted and unstable fractures.
- Infected fractures where internal fixation is not appropriate.
- Some pelvic fractures.

Advantages

- Fracture stability is maintained as the fixator is a rigid structure.
- Associated wounds are easily accessible.
- Length of hospital stay will be reduced in comparison to alternative treatment options such as traction.

Disadvantages
- Pin site infection is a fairly inevitable complication of treatment with an external fixator.
- Long treatment times especially in lengthening and deformity correction.
- Schooling and family life will be affected by the fixator.
- Body image may be affected by the fixator. Clothing has to be adapted to accommodate the fixator.

Procedure and practice tips
- Where possible prepare the child and family fully for every aspect of treatment with an external fixator.
- Support the child psychologically, as well as physically throughout their treatment process.
- Monitor and record neurovascular status regularly.
- Encourage and support child and family in following any exercise regime ordered by physiotherapist.
- Carry out pin site care regularly according to local policy, observing and promptly documenting and reporting any signs of infection.
- Involve child and family in pin site care and provide appropriate teaching, encouragement, and support.
- Warn family that pin site infection is common. Teach and support them in recognizing the signs and symptoms of infection.
- An early return to school and normal family life should be facilitated wherever possible.

Pitfalls
- Osteomyelitis may develop as a result of pin site infection.
- If the frame is applied to the lower limb, but does not include the foot and ankle, plantar and dorsiflexion must be encouraged to prevent development of an equinus deformity.
- The child must be supported in accepting the frame, as treatment in an external fixator is often a lengthy process.
- Compliance with physiotherapy is paramount as there is potential for developing joint deformities, which may result in extension of the external fixator to span affected joints.

Pin site care

Background

Pin site care is an essential element of treatment with an external fixator. As the pins are inserted into the bone or pass through the bone, and communicate with the external environment, a route for infection to develop in the skin, soft tissues, or bone exists. Whilst localized infection is a fairly inevitable aspect of treatment, it must be prevented where possible and treated promptly if it does occur to prevent development of cellulitis, pin loosening, and osteomyelitis. Should this develop, frame removal may become necessary, which will inevitably lead to treatment failure.

Pin site reactionary changes can occur in the 72h following frame application. These are characterized by pin site erythema, localized soft tissue heat, and evidence of serous or haemo-serous fluid.

Symptoms of a pin site infection are localized redness, swelling, thick, yellow discharge, the presence of pus, and offensive odour. The child may also have increased pain in the infected pin site.

❶ The necessary regime or protocol for pin site care is an extremely contentious issue. There are many differing opinions on the correct method of cleaning pin sites with issues debated including whether pin sites should be massaged, if scabs or crusts should be removed from around the pin, and whether dressings should be applied.

❶ Due to the uncertainty regarding recommended practice and the high prevalence of consultant preference for localized pin site care protocols, it is therefore recommended that local policy be clarified and adhered to until national evidence-based guidance is published.

Practice tips

- Children and families must be fully prepared for pin site care before it is carried out for the first time.
- Children will be frightened when initially having their pin sites cleaned, and will need much reassurance and thorough age-appropriate explanations.
- Distraction is an essential part of pin site care in some children. Computer games, books, TV, or DVD's are all very useful resources.
- The child should be allowed to participate in pin site care if appropriate.
- Parents should be encouraged to undertake pin site care at their own pace.
- Parents, and the child where appropriate, must be taught recognition of the early signs of a developing pin site infection and action to be taken should infection be suspected.
- Infected pin sites should always be cleaned last.

Pitfalls

- Pin site infection must be treated promptly to avoid developing deep-seated infection, which may result in the need for frame removal and subsequent treatment failure.
- Children must be advised not to pick at their pin sites—the use of dressings may help to prevent this behaviour.
- Tenting of the skin will be painful and should be prevented where possible.

Associated reading

Lethaby A, Temple J, and Santy J (2008). *Pin site care for preventing infections associated with external bone fixators and pins*. Cochrane Database Systematic Review (4) CD 004551.

Moving and handling

Background

❶ During any handling task, if you need to lift more than 16kg and you are female, or 25kg if you are male, you should consider the child (or object if it's a box, etc.) to be fully dependent, conduct a risk assessment, and use manual handling assistance equipment.

Ensure that you have been fully trained and assessed as competent in the use of any manual handling equipment you use.

Procedure

- Always consider whether you need to undertake this activity:
  - Does the child *need* to be lifted or moved?
  - Could they move themselves with encouragement, information, clear guidance, or suitable aids?
- Prepare the equipment and environment:
  - Position furniture to best assist the task.
  - Move obstacles, and ensure area is clean and dry.
  - Gather appropriate moving and handling aids.
  - Ensure equipment is clean, safe, and the right size for the activity.

❶ Summon sufficient personnel to assist with the task—if there are not enough competent people available to undertake the activity safely do not do it!

- Prepare the child and family:
  - Provide appropriate explanation and gain consent.
  - Ensure child is fully aware of the procedure to be followed and what they should do, and that they are familiar with any handling aids which will be used.
  - Consider administration of analgesia in advance of procedure to achieve pain control if needed.
  - Involve child and family in activity, supporting with instruction and encouragement as appropriate.
  - Consider clothing and condition of child—will this hinder safe practice? Consider washing/changing, etc., before commencing process.
- Plan the moving and handling activity:
  - Review risk assessment and care plan.
  - Plan activity to minimize risk, i.e. consider what movement the child **is** able/allowed (in view of their condition) to achieve and plan with this in mind, with the use of moving aids to minimize the need for 'lifting'.
  - Ensure that all personnel involved, including child and family, are clear about procedure to be followed.
  - Determine and agree words to be used to prompt movement, e.g. '1,2,3 *move*'
  - Plan situation with the load to be moved, i.e. the child, as close to those who will move it as possible. If this will be difficult, use a slide sheet to bring the child closer before commencing main movement.
  - Adjust equipment/use of aids to provide the optimum working position for all personnel involved.

- Aim for:
  - Working at a comfortable height without the need to bend, twist, or stretch.
  - Stable base.
  - Back in neutral position.
  - Secure and stabilize equipment—utilize brakes, etc., as needed.
- When undertaking the movement:
  - Stay as close to the load to be moved as possible.
  - Position your hands to ensure optimum support for the child and adequate hold on any moving aids. Avoid gripping too tightly.
  - Spread feet and bend knees, maintaining your back in a neutral position.
  - Raise your head as the move begins and head into the direction of the lift/move.
  - Aim to use your own natural movement to assist the momentum of the movement of the load.
  - If you need to turn, try not to twist your torso, but turn by changing the direction of your feet.

Practice tips

- Using the power of your own weight and your posture will assist the success of any moving and handling task.
- *Remember*: children are often an 'in between' size, wriggly, and unpredictable. Make sure you consider all these things in your planning and execution.
- A child's cognitive level will influence their ability to comply with or follow guidance.
- Keep communicating with child, parent, and participating colleagues throughout manoeuvre.

Associated reading

Health and Safety Executive (HSE) (1995). *Reporting of injuries, diseases and dangerous occurences regulation (RIDDOR)*. HMSO: London.
Sales R and Jutting A. (2002). Manual handling and nursing children. *Paediatric Nursing* **14**(2), 36–42.

Assessing need for neck immobilization

Background

Due to the flexible nature of a child's cervical spine; unlike adult spines most paediatric spinal injuries occur either through the discs and ligaments, at the craniovertebral junction (C1, C2, and C3) or at C7/T1.

The relatively large mass of the head, moving on a flexible neck with poorly supportive muscles can lead to injury in the higher cervical vertebrae. Therefore, assessment of the cervical spine for a suspected injury is critical, poor management can lead to significant problems in later life and can be potentially fatal. See Box 17.2 for possible pitfalls.

Box 17.2 Possible pitfalls

▶When looking after a child or young person with a neck injury there are potentially many pitfalls related to assessment.
  These can include:
- Unclear mechanism.
- Non-accidental injury.
- Underlying medical/orthopaedic conditions.
- Communication issues due to age, stage of development, and anxiety/distress.
- A painful distracting injury.
- In the older child/adolescent check for intoxication.

Always have a high index of suspicion of neck injury with a unclear traumatic injury. If in doubt immobilize as able.

Any patient with a reduced Glasgow Coma Score (GCS)/paediatric GCS should be immobilized.

Indications for immobilization from history
- Clinical suspicion of a neck injury (GCS 15/15).
- Paraethesia in the extremities.
- Potentially dangerous mechanism of injury:
  - Fall from above 1m or five stairs.
  - Axial load to the head.
  - High speed road traffic accident (over 60mph).
- Roll over/ejection from vehicle.
- Bicycle collision or motorized recreational vehicle.
- Previous neck injuries/conditions.

▶In young children (below the age of 8yrs) mechanism of injury is a vital consideration when considering immobilization.

Step 1: initial clinical examination

▶Care should be taken not to move the cervical spine during initial assessment when suspicious of a neck injury. If able, gently remove clothing to visualize the cervical area, if necessary an assistant should maintain inline stabilization throughout.

- Look for bruising, swelling, lacerations.
- Palpate the cervical spine for midline tenderness, swelling, or deformity of spinous processes.

If any of these indications from step 1 are identified from the history or clinical examination, then a hard collar should be applied and the child/adolescent should ideally be immobilized unless there is significant distress. A distressed child moving uncontrollably may exacerbate a neck injury. Steps should be therefore taken to minimize distress (such as applying a hard collar and having parents hold the head, rather than using strapping to immobilize the child's neck).

If no indications for immobilization are identified from history or clinical examination then continue assessment to step 2.

Step 2: safe assessment features
- Simple rear end collision (establish whether child was secured in car seat).

▶▶Excludes:
- Pushed into oncoming traffic
- Hit by bus/large truck
- Rollover
- Hit by high-speed vehicle

- Low speed road traffic accident (RTA).
- Comfortable sitting position.
- Ambulatory since time of injury and no midline cervical spine (c-spine) tenderness.
- Delayed onset of neck pain.

If no safe assessment features are identified then apply hard collar and immobilization as able.

One or more safe assessment features
If one or more safe assessment features have been identified it is safe to go on to assess neck range of movement (Step 3).

Step 3: range of movement assessment
- Has the patient got left and right lateral rotation over 45 degrees?
- If the answer is yes then c-spine immobilization is not indicated.
- If there is limited or painful range of movement then c-spine immobilization should be applied.

▶▶If in doubt treat as a c-spine injury until proven otherwise, do not delay in applying immobilization.

Associated reading
Advanced Life Support Group (2005). *Advanced Paediatric Life Support: The Practical Approach*, 4th edn. Blackwell Publishing, London.
Bethel J. (2008). *Paediatric Minor Emergencies*. M&K Update Ltd, Keswick.

Kirschner (K) wire removal

Background

Kirschner wire (also known as a K-wire) is a rigid wire that can be used to hold bone ends in place following sustaining a displaced fracture. The wires are commonly inserted directly through the skin tissue thereby avoiding an open surgical incision.

K-wires are widely used to help maintain anatomical position of supracondylar elbow fractures and distal forearm/wrist fractures in children and young people following surgical correction of the fracture.

- Children who have undergone surgical correction for their fracture using K-wire fixation may have one or several K wires inserted.
- The K wire(s) is commonly left protruding through the skin surface and the arm then encased in a cast to help maintain position.
- The K-wires can be removed in out-patients once the fracture heals, usually between 3–4 weeks.
- The removal of K-wires is being evolved to nurses who have the skill and competency to undertake this practice.

Important considerations

- Local policies and procedures for the removal of K-wires should be in place.
- Parents and child should be given full verbal information supported by written information on the wire removal procedure so as to be able to give informed consent.
- Parents advised as appropriate to give analgesia, such as paracetamol an hour before their appointment time for K-wire removal.
- Assessment of the child is undertaken so as to ensure that wires can be effectively and safely removed without distressing the child. Children aged 5yrs or under may require admission to have their K-wires removed under anaesthetic/sedation.
- Play specialist providing distraction therapy.

❶ The practitioner undertaking the wire removal must have the experience and knowledge along with the appropriate level of skill to safely and effectively carry out this procedure.

Wire removal preparation

- Review the radiographs and patients clinical notes to ascertain the position, number of 'K' wires, and the surgical instruction for the wire(s) to be removed.
- Establish identity of patient.
- Establish rapport with child/young person and parent/carer.
- Introduce distraction therapy.
- The use of Entonox gas (NO) for the older child/young person in accordance with local policy should be considered.

Wire removal process
- Follow local policy for clean technique, expose the 'K' wire(s) by the removal or windowing of the cast as directed.
- If the wire has retracted under the skin tissue and is not visible it is advisable not to proceed and ask a surgeon for review.
- Remove each wire individually in the following manner:
  - Grip the wire firmly with the wire removers.
  - Turn the wire with 2–3 half turns to loosen.
  - Continue to rotate with half turns and gently maintain a steady pull in the line of the inserted wire until the wire has been completely removed.
- Place the removed wire in a sharps disposal box.
- Allow the wire tract to bleed momentarily and then apply a sterile swab. Maintain a steady pressure until haemostasis is achieved. Repeat this for each wire required to be removed.

Post wire removal care
- Using local protocols for dressing technique cleanse the K-wire tract site.
- Observe for any signs of infection.
- Observe for any over granulation of skin tissue around the wire site.
- Apply wound dressing.
- Wash and dry the remainder of the limb as appropriate.
- Re-apply cast as directed.
- Provide parent/carer information.

Practice tip
- Always keep the child as the focus and not the wire.

Associated reading
Loomes E and Parker K. (2005). Removing K wires: audit of practice. *Paediatric Nursing* **12**(1), 30–1.

Wound care

Wound assessment

Background

A wound is a breach in the skin surface that initiates a process of repair. Wounds in children most commonly result from injury, e.g. cuts, bites, puncture wounds, burns, lacerations, amputations. They may also be due to surgery or more rarely medical conditions such as meningococcal septicaemia. Initial accurate wound assessment is very important in order to instigate an individualized plan that will promote optimal wound healing conditions.

Equipment

- Disposable gloves/sterile gloves.
- Pain assessment tool.
- Plastic apron.
- Analgesia.
- Tape measure.
- Bowl of warm water/bath.
- Distraction aids/toys.
- Appropriate wound chart.

Procedure

History taking

Enquire about:

- Location, cause, timing, exact mechanism of injury.
- Estimated amount of blood lost.
- Any first aid treatment administered (what/when?).
- *Pain levels:* any pain relief administered (what/when?).
- The possibility of any foreign body left in the wound.
- When the child last ate/drank in cases likely to require surgery.
- *Child's general condition:* baseline observations including blood pressure (BP) should be taken.
- *Tetanus status:* refer to local policy and guidelines.
- *Any known allergies:* e.g. dressings, latex, plasters, etc.
- *Child's nutritional status:* can impact on wound healing.
- Any disorders that may affect healing.
- *Previous wound healing:* e.g. previous history of hypertrophic/keloid scarring.

Wound assessment

- *Minimize the risk of dust:* close windows, doors, switch off fans.
- Explain the procedure fully to the child and family, and gain consent.
- Assess the child's pain level using an age appropriate tool. If appropriate administer analgesia and allow sufficient time for it to take effect.
- Assess distress levels and the child's likelihood of compliance with the assessment.
- Enlist the help of the play specialist/parents to engage the child in age appropriate distraction in an attempt to reduce anxiety.
- If not contraindicated Entonox can be a useful aid.

- Put on plastic apron, wash hands, and apply gloves as per local policy.
- Remove any dressing from the wound–this can take time and patience especially with young children. It can be useful to soak off dried dressings in warm water. Toys can be placed into the water to encourage the child to put the affected area in. (Dressings can be soaked off in a bath depending on the extent of the wound).

Once uncovered inspect the general appearance of the wound:
- *Location:* an important consideration for dressing choice.
- *Size and depth:* measure length, width, document shape, and depth.
- *Colour and type of wound tissue:* granulation tissue, slough, necrosis.
- *Presence of exudate:* high, medium, low.
- *Odour:* may be indicative of infection. (Wound swab should be taken if infection is suspected and sent for culture and sensitivity.)
- *Periwound condition (skin surrounding the wound)*—observe for:
  - Redness, swelling, local heat, tracking—may indicate infection.
  - Signs of erythema, maceration—caused by leaking exudate.
  - Bruising—other potential injuries.
- *Wound margins:* are these distinct?
- Observe for exposed underlying structures, e.g. bones, tendons, nerves.
- *If the wound is situated on an extremity it may be necessary to assess neurovascular status:* temp, capillary refill, sensation, movement.
- Assess for any further injuries.
- Remove gloves, decontaminate hands as per policy, apply sterile gloves.
- Using aseptic non-touch technique (ANTT; see 📖 Aseptic non-touch technique, p. 174) cover the wound with an appropriate non-stick dressing and obtain an appropriate medical review if required.
- ❶ If there are any concerns regarding non accidental injury (NAI) local protocol, safeguarding policies must be adhered to. (📖 Safeguarding children, p. 24.)
- Wash hands, dispose of all equipment, and document episode of care.

Practice tips

- Some children may be extremely distressed by the procedure; think about who needs to review the wound–If medical review is required and it is safe to do so it may be beneficial to delay the initial review until all personnel are available.
- Children can be encouraged to assist with the removal of dressings. This affords them an element of control and can improve participation and compliance.
- Use of digital photography can assist with the initial and future wound assessment/s.

Pitfalls
- Failure to undertake accurate pain assessment.
- Failure to provide appropriate pain relief.
- Failure to provide appropriate preparation.
- Mistaking erythema limited to the wound edges as a sign of infection when it may in fact be a normal response to the inflammatory phase of wound healing.
- ❶ Failure to identify NAIs. It is important to ensure that the wound is consistent with the mechanism of injury and to be observant for other potential clues, e.g. delayed presentation, wounds in unusual places, injury, or history not consistent with age, and/or developmental level.

Associated reading
Trigg E. Mohammed T. (eds) (2010). *Practices in Children's Nursing: Guidelines for Hospital and Community.* Churchill Livingstone, Edinburgh.

Cleaning a wound

Background

Equipment

Procedure

Cleaning a wound

Background

An external wound is damage that has occurred to the skin. The mechanism of injury often affects the way a wound is treated. Wound types commonly seen in children include lacerations, abrasions, and punctures. Regardless of the cause all wounds must be kept clean to reduce the risk of infection and promote healing. (Please note there is variation in local policy as to how often wounds should be cleaned.) It is argued that wounds which are free from debris and appear healthy do not require cleaning. If, however, debris or necrotic tissue is present then cleaning is necessary to prevent infection.

Equipment

- Dressing trolley.
- Disinfectant wipes as per local policy (for cleaning trolley).
- Alcohol gel.
- Disposable gloves and apron.
- Sterile dressing pack including (dressing towel, sterile gloves, gauze, gallipot, and waste bag). Contents of dressing packs vary from Trust to Trust—ensure all items listed are available.
- 0.9% NaCl (normal saline) warmed.
- Syringe 20–30mL.
- Plastic needle.
- Sterile forceps.
- *Documentation:* including appropriate wound chart.
- Distraction aids/play specialist.

Procedure

- Ensure privacy and dignity is maintained and the environment is appropriate: minimize risk of dust. Close windows, doors, switch off fans.
- Explain the procedure to the child, and parent/carer, and gain consent.
- Administer analgesia and allow at least 30min to take effect.
- Assess the child's level of understanding. If the child is able to understand and follow instructions, consider using Entonox–provides effective short acting pain relief which is ideal for painful procedures and can be used in conjunction with paracetamol or ibuprofen–this is often determined by the local policy or pain team.[1,2]
- Position the child so they are comfortable and the wound is exposed.
- Enlist the help of a play specialist for distraction. Parents/carers can be involved in distraction. (Refer to Chapter 6.)
- Decontaminate hands as per policy (📖 Hand hygiene, p. 168).
- Wipe the dressing trolley clean using appropriate disinfectant wipes and allow time for the surface to dry.
- Put on apron and decontaminate hands according to local policy.
- ANTT should be used throughout this procedure (see 📖 Aseptic non-touch technique, p. 174).
- Open the dressing pack onto a clean trolley and pour warmed normal saline into a gallipot.
- Decontaminate hands as per policy and put on sterile gloves.

- Position the sterile dressing field around the wound.
- Take a wound swab if infection is suspected and send for culture and sensitivity.
- Remove any large visible debris from the wound using sterile forceps.
- Draw warm saline into the syringe and irrigate the wound.
  ❶ Mechanical cleansing is not recommended as it can damage the fragile granulation/epithelializing tissue formed when a wound heals via secondary intention. It also increases the potential for infection as fibres can be left in the wound.
- Repeat the previous step until the wound is clean.
- If irrigation has caused the wound to bleed, apply pressure using a sterile dressing towel or dressing until the bleeding subsides.
- See 📖 Dressing a wound, p. 534.
- Dispose of waste according to local policy and decontaminate hands as appropriate.

Practice tips

- Irrigating the wound with saline helps prevent damage to new tissue. The optimum pressure required to clean a wound is 8–12psi. Pressures higher than 15psi can cause trauma to the wound and result in bacteria being driven into the tissue. Pressures lower than 6psi may result in inadequate cleansing of the wound.
- Chronic wounds can be cleaned using warm tap water. Sterile normal saline is not necessary to clean this type of wound unless the child is severely immunocompromised.
- Regardless of the solution used it should be warmed to body temperature to avoid cooling the wound and slowing down cellular repair.

Pitfalls

- ❶ Cotton wool should never be used for wound cleaning as fibres can be left in the wound and become a focus for infection.
- If bleeding continues seek medical advice.
- ❶ Needles should not be used for irrigation in children due to the risk of needle stick injury and causing unnecessary fear for the child. A smaller syringe can be used to create a greater pressure or, alternatively, plastic needles equivalent to an 18G needle can be used. Some hospitals stock irrigation devices specific for this purpose.

Associated reading

Dougherty L, Lister S. (2008). *The Royal Marsden Hospital Manual of Clinical Nursing Procedures*, 7th edn. Wiley-Blackwell, Oxford.
Willcox M. (2004). Cleaning simple wounds: healing by secondary intention. *Nursing Times* **100**(46), 57.

[1] Vater M, Hessell D. (2000). Nitrous oxide and oxygen mixture (Entonox) and acute procedural pain. *Paediat Perinatal Drug Ther* **4**(2), 35–44.

[2] Glover H, Finley C. (2009). *Guidelines for Entonox Administration to Children by Demand System*. East Cheshire NHS Trust, Macclesfield.

Dressing a wound

Background

The majority of wounds in children will be acute traumatic or surgical wounds. Dressings are applied to wounds in order to promote healing, but also to protect them from contamination. Many wound care products can be left in place for up to 7 days, but may require changing if there is excessive exudate, which causes strike-through (leakage of exudate through the dressing that can lead to infection entering the wound).

An ideal dressing should

- Be easy to apply and remove even to difficult wounds.
- Be atraumatic on removal. Causing minimal damage to the wound bed and rounding skin.
- Reduce pain in the wound.
- Protect the wound and surrounding tissue.
- Promote moist wound healing.
- Be comfortable and well tolerated by the child.
- Manage exudate and odour.

Equipment

- Dressing trolley.
- Disinfectant wipes as per local policy (for cleaning trolley).
- Sterile dressing pack including (dressing towel, sterile gloves, gauze, gallipot, and waste bag). Contents of dressing packs vary from Trust to Trust–Ensure all items listed are available.
- Alcohol hand rub.
- Disposable apron and gloves.
- 0.9% NaCl (normal saline) warmed.
- Sterile scissors (in case dressing needs to be cut to size).
- Chosen wound care product.
- Documentation including wound chart if appropriate.

Procedure

- Ensure privacy and dignity is maintained, and an appropriate environment is provided.
- Undertake an accurate and ongoing assessment of the wound and surrounding skin in order to select the appropriate dressing. (📖 Wound assessment, p. 528.)
- Ensure appropriate analgesia has been administered prior to the procedure (at least 30min).
- Check that the patient has no known allergies.
- Check there are no potential contraindications to the proposed dressing/wound care product.
- Explain the procedure to the child and parent's/carer's and gain consent.
- Employ distraction techniques as appropriate for the age of the child, i.e. books, DVD's, and music (see 📖 Distraction, p. 150).
- Decontaminate hands as per policy.
- Wipe the dressing trolley clean using appropriate disinfectant wipes and allow time for the surface to dry.
- Put on apron and decontaminate hands as per policy.

- Principles of ANTT should be employed throughout this procedure (📖 Hand hygiene, p. 168 and 📖 Aseptic non-touch technique, p.174).
- Open the dressing pack onto a clean trolley and pour warmed normal saline into a gallipot.
- Decontaminate hands and apply gloves as per policy.
- If a dressing is in situ carefully remove it (see 📖 Practice tips, p. 535).
- Decontaminate hands as per policy and apply sterile gloves.
- Clean the wound, in accordance with local policy.
- Apply the selected wound care product as per manufacturer's instructions.
- If the dressing needs to be cut to size use sterile scissors.
- If the dressing is not adhesive secure with tape applying a secondary dressing if required.
- Discard all equipment as per local policy.
- Decontaminate hands as per policy and clean the trolley.
- Document the care given in the patients records.

Practice tips

- Successful wound healing requires effective ongoing wound assessment and constant re-evaluation of the wound.
- Encouraging the child to participate during the dressing procedure, e.g. removing bandages can help the child assume a sense of control over their experience, and can help to reduce their anxiety.
- Dressings are sometimes difficult to remove due to dried blood/ exudate. In these cases it can be helpful to soak the dressing off in warm soapy water. (Dressings can be soaked off in a bath depending on the extent, position of the wound.)
- Putting small toys into the water, e.g. rubber ducks can encourage the child to place their hands in the water.
- The use of one of the available adhesive removers may also help.
- Where wounds are in difficult areas to dress such as on the face or scalp they should be left 'exposed' as attempting to dress them will often cause children more distress than the actual wound.

Pitfalls

- Children can be non-compliant with wound care and may not tolerate dressing removal particularly if it is traumatic; choosing the correct dressing in the first instance is very important.

Associated reading

Dressings.org. (2009). *Alphabetical list of dressings data cards*. Available at: 🕸 http://www. dressings.org/dressings-datacards-by-alpha.html.

DressingsOnline.com. *Dressings, Wound Dressings, Surgical Dressings and Wound Care Products.* Available at: 🕸 http://www.dressingsonline.com/ (accessed 20 September 2010).

Trigg E, Mohammed T. (eds) (2010). *Practices in Children's Nursing: Guidelines for Hospital and Community.* Churchill Livingstone, Edinburgh.

Applying steristrips

Background

Steristrips are strips of adhesive tape; they vary in width and are used for the closure of small wounds in order to aid healing.[1] They can be used on lacerations, closed surgical wounds, and skin tears but are unsuitable for open surgical wounds, burns, or abrasions as there are no clear edges to be brought together. Steristrips can also be used following the removal of sutures or staples to provide further reinforcement. They are often used in preference to sutures as they result in less scarring and are easier to apply and remove. Steristrips are ideal for children as they cause less pain and anxiety and can be left to fall off by themselves in 5–10 days. This reduces the disruption and further anxiety that can be caused by having stitches removed.

A wound should be carefully assessed and cleaned prior to its closure. (see 📖 Dressing a wound, p. 534).

Equipment

- Dressing trolley.
- Sterile disposable forceps.
- Disposable apron.
- Sterile breathable dressing.
- Disinfectant wipes (as per policy).
- 0.9% NaCl (normal saline) warmed.
- Dressing pack (including sterile gloves, gauze, dressing towel, waste bag): Contents of dressing packs vary—ensure all items listed are available. Distraction aids/play specialist.
- Steristrips

Procedure

- Ensure privacy and dignity is maintained, and an appropriate environment is provided.
- Explain the procedure to the child and parent/carer and gain consent.
- Utilize play specialists/parents to help distract the child throughout the procedure (see Chapter 6).
- Ensure adequate pain relief has been administered in good time.
- Decontaminate hands as per policy and wipe the dressing trolley clean using disinfectant wipes and allow time for the surface to dry.
- Put on apron, and decontaminate hands as per policy.
- Principles of ANTT should be employed throughout this procedure (📖 Hand hygiene, p. 168 and 📖 Aseptic non-touch technique, p. 174).
- Open the dressing pack onto a clean trolley and pour warmed normal saline into a gallipot, decontaminate hands, and apply sterile gloves.
- Irrigate the wound (see 📖 Cleaning a wound, p. 532).
- Assess the wound to determine whether steristrips are the most appropriate method for closure. If the wound is deep, bleeding excessively, or covers a joint, or area that excretes moisture alternative methods should be used.
- Remove each steristrip from the pack using gloved fingers.
- Oppose the edges of the wound together as closely as possible using gloved fingers.

- To apply the first steristrip, start at the middle of the wound attach half of the strip to one side, then gently press across the wound ensuring the strip is securely attached, and effectively holding the wound edges together.
- Continue applying each strip, approximately 3mm apart, working outwards from the middle of the wound. This gap allows any discharge to drain out of the wound preventing it from forming a collection which can lead to infection.
- Cover the wound with a sterile breathable dressing such as a gauze or film dressing to prevent the child from picking at the strips and avoid infection. Decontaminate hands and discard all equipment correctly.
- Observe the child for signs of infection around the wound site (redness, swelling, increased tenderness).
- Monitor the child's temperature.

If the child is to be discharged provide discharge advice on:
- *Potential signs of infection:* parents should be provided with a contact number in case of concern.
- *Medication:* prophylactic antibiotics may be prescribed (what, when, how).
- Make an outpatient appointment for the child to return for removal of steristrips, refer the child to the paediatric community team for removal.

Practice tips

- You may find it useful to have an assistant (also wearing sterile gloves) to close the edges of the wound together as you apply the steristrips.
- Additional steristrips can be applied parallel to the wound to prevent the edges from curling up.
- Film dressings may be applied over the wound to provide extra protection. These are breathable but waterproof and provide further protection against infection or re-opening of the wound. They also allow the wound to be observed without removing the dressing.

Pitfalls

- ❶ Wounds must be clean prior to their closure in order to prevent infection. If thorough cleansing is not possible due to the child's distress or the complexity of the wound, consideration should be given to sedation or surgery.
- Wounds that have exposed bones or evident tendon damage are not suitable for steristrip closure. Surgical intervention should be sought.
- Steristrips should be kept dry to prevent them from falling off and reduce the risk of the wound re-opening.
- Avoid the use of steristrips on joints as the wound is likely to re-open.
- Avoid use on areas that will sweat, areas that are covered in hair as the strips will be less likely to adhere effectively.

Associated reading

Dougherty L, Lister S. (2008). *The Royal Marsden Hospital Manual of Clinical Nursing Procedures*. 7th edn. Wiley-Blackwell, Oxford.

[1] Autio L, Orson KK. (2002). The Four S's of Wound Management, Staples, Sutures, Steristrips and Sticky Stuff. *Holistic Nurs Pract* **16**(2), 80–8.

The use of glue in wound closure

Background

Glue or medical adhesive can be used to adhere the edges of a wound together. It may be used on sites such as the head, face, and body, but its success is reliant on the ability to keep the wound clean and dry, as well as ensuring the closure is not completed under tension.

Equipment

- Dressing trolley, disinfectant wipes as per policy (for cleaning trolley).
- Disposable apron.
- Dressing pack (including sterile gloves, gauze, dressing towel, waste bag). Contents of dressing packs vary from Trust to Trust—ensure all items listed are available.
- 0.9% NaCl (normal saline) warmed.
- Glue and applicator as required.
- Steristrips (may be useful for difficult closures).
- Dry dressing dependent on the site of the wound.
- An assistant if distraction or a second pair of hands is required.

Procedure

- Ensure privacy and dignity is maintained, an appropriate environment is provided.
- The wound should be assessed and a decision made on the appropriateness of the closure technique.
- The likely hood of any foreign body in the wound should be established and excluded prior to the application of glue.
- Explain procedure to the child and family in terms they understand. Gain consent.
- Position the child comfortably. Sitting on a parents lap may provide good positioning as well as reassurance to the child.
- Decontaminate hands as per policy and wipe the dressing trolley clean using disinfectant wipes and allow time for the surface to dry.
- Put on apron and decontaminate hands as per policy.
- Principles of ANTT should be employed throughout this procedure (□ Hand hygiene, p. 168 and □ Aseptic non-touch technique, p. 174). Open the dressing pack onto a clean trolley, and pour warmed normal saline into a gallipot.
- Decontaminate hands as per policy and apply sterile gloves.
- Thoroughly clean the wound using warmed sterile 0.9% saline.
- Dry the skin around the wound using sterile gauze swabs.
- Bleeding may occur following cleaning. Apply direct pressure to site.
- Bring the two edges of the wound together using your gloved fingers.
- Ensure gloved fingers are close enough to the wound to enable the edges to be brought together without any puckering of the skin. Ensure the wound is not under tension.
- Once the two edges are together if bleeding continues the wound can be gently dabbed dry using sterile gauze swabs.
- A thin line of glue should be applied over the top of the two edges.
  ❶ Glue should never be placed inside the wound.

- Hold the two edges of the wound together until the glue begins to set. (Refer to manufacture's guidelines for the specific timings of product.)
- A dry dressing may be placed over the wound site if necessary.
- Decontaminate hands; discard all equipment as per policy and document the procedure in the child's notes.

Practice tips

- Distraction of the child during procedure may enhance co-operation.
- Steristrips may be a useful aide in bringing the two edges of a wound together in some instances. Even difficult Y- or V-shaped lacerations may be brought together using a combination of glue and steristrips. If this technique is used, do not use steristrips to pull the edges together.
- In some instances, subcutaneous (SC) fat may protrude from the wound. This should be gently re-inserted into the wound using sterile forceps prior to the two edges being brought together.
- If the wound continues to ooze once the two edges have been brought together; a 'spot welding' technique may be used before the glue is applied:
  - Bring the two edges of the wound together using your gloved fingers as before.
  - Apply glue over the top of the two edges in small spots. Use sterile gauze swabs to dab the wound between each application.
  - Continue until there is a thin layer of glue covering the complete length of the wound.
  - Hold both edges of the wound together until the glue begins to set.
- For scalp lacerations the hair should be gently parted to reveal the wound and ensure no hair is trapped in the wound during the closure.
- Extra care should be taken when closing wounds around the delicate eye area to ensure the glue does not stick the child's eyelids together. ❶ Always ensure flow control applicators are used in this area. The eye can also be covered using gauze to help prevent this occurring.
- Appropriate advice should be given to the child and family regarding the care of the closed wound, the need to keep the area clean and dry, signs that may indicate the wound requires further review.
- Information should also be given regarding instances where the wound may need a further consultation such as redness or swelling.

Pitfalls

- The wound may reopen if it is knocked or the glue is picked off. If this occurs within the first 24h following closure glue may be re-applied successfully.
- In areas where an abrasion is close to the wound site stinging may occur when the glue is applied.
- Glue cannot be used for lacerations where bleeding persists as the glue is unable to set.
- Glue should not be used in areas that are damp, moist, e.g. lips, mouth.
- Areas of the body that experience pressure or movement, e.g. the sole of a foot, joints are not suitable for the use of glue for wound closure.

Sutures

Background

Sutures are widely used for the repair of wounds and lacerations. They work well in areas of high tension, areas of oily or hairy skin, and areas which require frequent washing. Sutures come in absorbent and non-absorbent form. The non-absorbent suture retains strength, whereas the absorbent suture loses strength as it remains in place.[1] With children where possible it is advisable to use absorbable sutures as this avoids the need for removal. Where this is not possible sutures should generally be removed as follows:

- From the face in 3–5 days.
- From the scalp extremities in 7–8 days.
- From mobile joints, chest, palms, feet in 10–14 days.
  - (NB. Please refer to local policy and individual patient requirements).

Equipment

- Dressing trolley.
- Disinfectant wipes as per policy (for cleaning trolley).
- Sterile suture removal pack (containing sterile field, sterile forceps, sterile stitch cutters, scissors). Contents of dressing packs vary from Trust to Trust—ensure all items listed are available.
- Sterile gloves.
- Disposable apron and gloves if applicable.
- Alcohol gel.
- Sharps box to dispose of stitch cutter.

Procedure

- Ensure privacy and dignity is maintained/an appropriate environment is provided.
- Explain procedure to the child and family and gain consent.
- If appropriate ensure adequate analgesia is administered at least 30min prior to the procedure.
- Employ age appropriate distraction techniques (see Chapter 6).
- Decontaminate hands as per policy and wipe the dressing trolley clean using appropriate disinfectant wipes and allow time for the surface to dry.
- Put on apron and decontaminate hands as per policy.
- Principles of ANTT should be employed throughout this procedure (☐ Hand hygiene, p. 168 and ☐ Aseptic non-touch technique, p. 174).
- Open the dressing pack onto a clean trolley and pour warmed normal saline into a gallipot.
- Decontaminate hands and apply gloves as per policy.
- Remove any dressing that is *in situ* and dispose of as per local policy.
- Review the wound to ensure it is fully healed.
- Seek medical review prior to removal if there is a likelihood of wound dehiscence following suture removal or signs of infection. (Wound swab should be taken if infection is suspected and sent for culture and sensitivity.)
- Decontaminate hands and apply gloves as per local policy.

- If necessary clean the wound to ensure a clear view of the sutures (⬚ Cleaning a wound, p. 532).
- Decide which suture to remove first (see ⬚ Practice tips, p. 541).
- Using sterile forceps gently pull the knot of the suture upwards away from the skin (see ⬚ Pitfalls, p. 541).
- Using the sterile stitch cutter insert the blade convex side down underneath the suture and cut on one side.
- Cut as close to the skin as possible to reduce the amount of suture pulled back through the deeper layers of the wound.
- Using forceps, while still holding the knot gently pull to release the suture from the skin.
- Place the removed suture on some gauze.
- Continue until all sutures are removed.
- If bleeding occurs apply pressure using sterile gauze until the bleeding stops.
- Steristrips may be applied post suture removal to further strengthen the wound if required.
- Dispose of all equipment as per local policy.
- Decontaminate hands as per policy.
- Clean the trolley.
- Document all appropriate information.

Practice tips

- If children have a number of sutures *in situ*, it is often best to start with those likely to be the most easily removed.
- It can be useful to allow the child a choice regarding which order to remove the sutures.
- Stitch cutters are extremely sharp. An assessment should be made in relation to the child's potential tolerance to the procedure. If there are concerns it may be safer to use sterile scissors.

Pitfalls

- Care must be taken not to cut off the knot as this could result in part of the suture remaining in the wound.
- ❶ Raising the knot too far away from the skin is likely to cause the child significant pain, trauma, and upset.

Associated reading

Dougherty L, Lister S. (eds) (2008). *The Royal Marsden Hospital Manual of Clinical Nursing Procedures.*, 7th edn. Blackwell Publishing Ltd, Oxford.

[1] Autio L. Olson K. (2002). The four S's of wound management: staples, sutures, steri-strips, and sticky stuff. *Holistic Nurs Pract* **16**(2), 80–8.

Removing clips/staples

Background
Surgical clips/staples are frequently used to close the skin portion of an incision, they are made from surgical steel and do not dissolve. The typical surgical wound takes about 7–14 days to heal sufficiently to remove clips/staples. A few exceptions will be wounds on the face and scalp. In these cases clips/staples should be removed earlier to reduce the potential for unsightly scar formation.

Equipment
- Dressing trolley.
- Disinfectant wipes as per policy—for cleaning trolley.
- Dressing pack (including sterile gloves, gauze, dressing towel, waste bag). Contents of dressing packs vary from Trust to Trust—ensure all items listed are available.
- Sterile single use clip/staple remover.
- Sterile forceps.
- 0.9% NaCl (normal saline) warmed.
- CSSD bag for used instruments.
- Sharps bin for clips/staples that have been removed.
- Adhesive skin strips.

Procedure
- Ensure Privacy and dignity is maintained, and an appropriate environment is provided.
- Explain the procedure to the child/family and gain consent.
- Employ distraction techniques as appropriate for the age of the child, e.g. books, DVD's, and music. (See Chapter 6.).
- Ensure appropriate analgesia has been administered prior to the procedure (at least 30min before).
- Decontaminate hands as per policy and wipe the dressing trolley clean using appropriate disinfectant wipes and allow time for the surface to dry.
- Put on apron, and decontaminate hands as per policy.
- Open the dressing pack onto a clean trolley and pour warmed normal saline into a gallipot.
- Principles of ANTT should be employed throughout this procedure (📖 Hand washing, p. 168 and 📖 Aseptic non-touch technique, p. 174).
- Decontaminate hands and put on gloves as per policy.
- Remove any dressing from the wound.
- Decontaminate hands as per policy and put on sterile gloves.
- Cleanse the wound thoroughly, according to local policy, before removing the clips/staples.
- Clear away any dried blood or other material that may have adhered to the clips/staples as this will make it harder to grasp and hold them.
- Begin at one end of the wound and not in the middle as this ensures that no clips are missed, and that they do not get caught in the clip/staple remover.

- Ensure that the middle of the clip/staple is positioned correctly in the lower jaw of the remover (there is a small groove in the lower jaw of the remover that the clip/staple should be aligned with before the upper jaw is engaged).
- Squeeze the handles of the clip/staple remover completely to close the remover, this bends the clip/staple in the middle and pulls the edges out of the skin.
- Gently move the clip/staple away from the wound when both ends are visible.
- Place the removed staples/clips into a gallipot.
- Repeat the procedure until all clips are removed.
- After removal of clips/staples apply adhesive skin strips to prevent dehiscence and a simple dressing to protect the wound from rubbing on clothing, bedding.
- Discard equipment as per local policy.
- Decontaminate hands as per policy.
- Clean trolley.
- Document all relevant information.

Practice tips

- Remove alternate clips/staples to check for any dehiscence of the wound, if none occurs, remove the remaining clips/staples.
- Reassess the wound following staple/clip removal for any signs of dehiscence.

Pitfalls

- Don't lift the clip/staple remover, while squeezing the handle, as this can tear the skin and put pressure on the newly-healed suture line.
- Don't remove any remaining clips/staples if dehiscence occurs; seek appropriate review if dehiscence is evident.

Associated reading

Dougherty L, Lister SE. (2008). *The Royal Marsden Hospital Manual of Clinical Procedures*,. 7th edn. Blackwell Publishing, Oxford.

Richardson M. (2004). Procedures for cleansing, closing and covering acute wounds. *Nursing Times. net* 100(4), 54. Available at: ℘ http://www.nursingtimes.net/nursing-practice-clinical-research/procedures-for-cleansing-closing-and-covering-acute-wounds/205033.article (accessed 20 September 2010).

Care and removal of a wound drain

Background

Wound drains are used to remove fluid such as blood and exudate from a wound site in order to promote healing and reduce the risk of infection. There are various types of drain which can be separated into the two categories of closed–draining into a sterile vacuum container, or open–draining without suction into a dressing.[1] Closed drains aid healing as the vacuum produced actively drains the wound, enhancing blood flow, and stimulating cell growth. Open drains consist of one or more soft rubber tubes which are placed into the wound and aid healing by facilitating drainage of the wound.

Equipment

- Dressing trolley.
- Disinfectant wipes as per policy (for cleaning trolley).
- Disposable apron and gloves.
- Dressing pack (including dressing towel, sterile gloves, gauze, and waste bag). Contents of dressing packs vary from Trust to Trust–ensure all items listed are available.
- Sterile forceps.
- Sterile stitch cutter.
- 0.9% NaCl (normal saline) warmed.
- Sterile dressing.
- Sharps box–to dispose of stitch cutter.
- CSSD bag for used instruments.
- Distraction aids/play specialist.

Procedure

Please note: The output from a drain should be monitored as per local policy and the drain should be removed once drainage is minimal. The surgical team should be consulted prior to removal. Drains may need to be removed if they become blocked.

- Ensure privacy and dignity is maintained, and an appropriate environment is provided.
- Explain the procedure to child and carer and gain consent. Role play can help younger children understand, and books or computer aids can be useful for older children.
- Utilize play specialists to provide distraction and if appropriate, involve parents/carers (see Chapter 6).
- Administer analgesia and allow time for it to take effect. The child's level of understanding and co-operation should be assessed as Entonox provides effective, short acting analgesia for painful procedures if the child can co-operate.[2] This could be used in conjunction with morphine, paracetamol or ibuprofen to provide longer lasting pain relief (this is often determined by the pain team or local policy).
- Decontaminate hands as per policy and wipe the dressing trolley clean using disinfectant wipes and allow time for the surface to dry.
- Put on apron and decontaminate hands as per policy.

- Open the dressing pack onto a clean trolley and pour warmed normal saline into a gallipot.
- Principles of ANTT should be employed throughout this procedure (📖 Hand hygiene, p. 168 and 📖 Aseptic non-touch technique, p. 174).
- Decontaminate hands and put on gloves as per policy.
- Remove any dressing from the wound.
- Decontaminate hands as per policy and put on sterile gloves.
- Clean the drain site with warmed normal saline if required to allow a clear view of the sutures.
- Clamp the wound drain or release the suction prior to its removal.
- Using sterile forceps lift the knot of the suture and cut as close to the skin as possible using a sterile stitch cutter, then gently pull free.
- Remove the drain by steadily pulling the tubing. (If resistance is felt, stop pulling, reassure patient, secure the drain, and seek assistance).
- Following removal apply pressure to the wound site using a sterile towel/dressing until bleeding has subsided. If bleeding does not cease, continue to apply pressure, and seek medical assistance.
- Once bleeding has subsided cover the drain site with a sterile breathable gauze dressing to prevent infection.
- Measure any fluid in the drain and then discard according to local policy, documenting all output on the patients fluid balance chart.
- Decontaminate hands as per policy.
- Observe the wound site for further bleeding or discharge.
- Continue to monitor the patient for any signs of deterioration such as, pain or bleeding.

Practice tips

- Clamping drain prior to removal prevents suction during removal. This reduces discomfort for the patient and helps to prevent tissue damage.
- If the drain site shows signs of infection, a swab should be taken and sent with the tip of the drain for culture and sensitivity.
- Parents/carers can be an invaluable source of distraction and comfort for a child, aiding co-operation and alleviating fear. However, they may be as distressed as the child and therefore involving them in the procedure may not always be appropriate. Parents/carers should be given the option of being involved, but should not feel obligated.

Pitfalls

- Losses from a wound site greater than 3mL/kg/h would require intravenous replacement. If losses of this volume are evident post-drain removal, consideration should be made as to whether the drain should be reinserted.

Associated reading

Walker J. (2007). Patient preparation for safe removal of surgical drains. *Nursing Standard* **21**(49), 39–41.

[1] Walsh M. (2002). *Watson's Clinical Nursing and Related Sciences*, 6th edn. Bailliere Tindall, London.

[2] Bruce EA, Howard RF, Franck LS. (2006). Chest drain removal pain and it's management: a literature review. *J Clin Nurs* **15**(2), 145–54.

Ear, nose, and throat system

Assessment of the ear

Background

Although the ears can give rise to symptoms all through life, in children the most debilitating conditions are acute otitis media and serous otitis media, which often occur in early childhood. Hearing or lack of hearing can affect speech development in the early years, which in turn can lead to slow educational development.

Equipment

- Adequate light source.
- Otoscope.
- Aural speculae: variety of sizes.

Procedure

History taking: the ear

- How long have the symptoms been present?
- Ascertain level of hearing. Ask the child whether they hear well or ever struggle to hear in specific situations. How are they doing at school? Do the teachers have any concerns?
- Is there any discharge from the ear? Does the discharge affect both ears? What is its quantity? What colour is the discharge? Is it mucoid?
- Is it painful or painless? Is it wax?
- Has there been an infection noted?
- Is there any pain? Where is the pain? Is it bilateral or unilateral? Is there any itching? Was the pain relieved by the discharge? Is there pain and/or swelling behind the pinna?
- Is there any history of foreign body (FB) insertion?
- Is there any family history of ear problems or deafness in the family?
- Is there a past history of any infectious diseases, such as measles, mumps, or meningitis, which can lead to deafness.
- Is there a history of previous ear surgery, e.g. insertion of grommets?

Examination of the ear

Explain the procedure and gain verbal consent.

Examination of the external ear

- Examine the pinna, behind the pinna, and the outer meatus.
- Is the pinna normal in size?
- Are there any previous surgical scars either behind or in front of the ear, which could indicate that there has been previous surgery?
- Is the pinna unusually low down on the face? (This may indicate other problems such as craniofacial anomalies).
- Is the pinna red or inflamed?

Examination of the auditory meatus and tympanic membrane
- Check that the otoscope is working and that the light source is bright.
- Holding the otoscope as you would a pen, with your little finger resting against the patient's face insert the specula gently into the meatus. Using the largest size specula that will fit comfortably into the ear, carefully check the ear canal and the eardrum.
- Observe for signs of infection, FB, abnormal anatomy, discharge, grimacing, or pain.
- Can you see the ear drum?
- Is it obscured by wax?
- Does the ear drum look normal? The normal appearance of the ear drum varies and can only be learned by practice. Practice will lead to recognition of abnormalities.
- Document your findings.
- Refer any concerns to appropriate personnel.

Practice tips
- Use a disposable speculum and the largest one that is comfortable for the child. A speculum which is 4.25mm in diameter is commonly used in children.
- Hold the otoscope like a pen. Extend the little finger and use it as an anchor on the child's face. The right hand should hold the otoscope to the right ear and the left hand to the left ear.
- Make sure that you, the patient, and the parent/carer are comfortable.
- If the child is young, encourage the parent/carer to participate in the examination and show them how to hold the child, so the child feels reassured.

Pitfalls
- Use an otoscope that has a bright white light. If the light is yellow, you will not see the structures well.

Associated reading
Graham J, Scadding G, Bull P. (eds). (2007). *Pediatric ENT*. Springer, Berlin.
Wormald P, Browning G. (1996). *Otoscopy—a structured approach*. Arnold, London.

Examination of the nose

Background

Before any physical ear, nose, and throat (ENT) assessment, listen to the patient, elicit symptoms, and take a careful history. The questions that need to be asked depend on what the child has presented with. Explain all aspects of the examination, and ensure that the patient and parent/carer understand and give consent. Once you have taken a detailed history a careful physical examination can be performed.

Equipment

- Metal tongue depressor (to examine misting from the nostrils, alternatively you could use a mirror or spoon).
- Otoscope and disposable speculum.
- Nasal speculum (usually only older children will tolerate use of a nasal speculum).

Procedure

History taking

- How long have the symptoms been present?
- Take a general health history, particularly any bleeding disorders or systemic disease that may be applicable.
- Is there any bleeding? If so from which side? How frequently?
- Is there any history of trauma?
- Is there any pain?
- Is there any history of FB insertion?
- Is there any blockage? If so are both nostrils blocked? Is the blockage present constantly or is it intermittent?
- Is there any running? If yes is it bilateral or unilateral? What colour is it? Does it smell offensive?
- Is there any sneezing? Does the sneezing occur at any particular time of day?
- Is there any history of atopy?

Examination of the nose

- Explain the procedure to the child and family and gain consent.
- Look at the face. Is there any asymmetry?
- Look at the position of the nose. The tip of the nose can be lifted gently and the vestibule can be inspected showing the front of the nasal septum.
- Assess airflow through the nose. Hold something metal, e.g. a tongue depressor, mirror, or spoon just below the vestibule, and observe the misting pattern.
- A baby's nose can be assessed by holding a small piece of cotton wool under the nostril to observe whether it moves as the air is expelled through the nostril.
- A nasal speculum can be used to examine the anterior nasal cavities, although in practice, children are not keen!

- An alternative option is an otoscope, which can be placed gently into each nostril. Children will usually tolerate this method of examination.
- The normal nasal mucosa is moist and pink and some secretions may be present.
- In children, a FB may be observed that would need to be removed (see 📖 Removal of foreign body from nose, p. 556).
- Prominent blood vessels may be observed, which can often be the site of epistaxis (see 📖 Epistaxis control, p. 554).
- Document your findings.

Practice tips

- If the child is anxious, they could sit on the parent/carers knee facing you. Encourage the parent/carer to place one hand on the child's forehead and the other around the chest. This allows you to examine the child, but is also reassuring for the child.

Associated reading

Bluestone C, Stool S, Cuneyt A, et al. (2003). *Pediatric Otolaryngology*, 4th edn. Saunders, London.
Drake-Lee A. (1996). *Clinical Otorhinolaryngology*. Churchill Livingstone, London.

Examination of the throat

Background
- The throat is comprised of the oral cavity, the pharynx and the larynx.
- A fibre optic nasendoscope is required to examine the larynx and pharynx.
- This is only tolerated by a minority of children and often an examination under general anaesthetic is required. It is however possible to examine the oral cavity.
- The most prevalent problem seen in paediatric ENT departments is a sore throat.

Equipment
- Adequate light source.
- Tongue depressor.

History taking
When assessing the child's throat, it is important to elicit the symptoms of the sore throat to ascertain what the problem is. The questions to ask are:
- How long has the child had a sore throat?
- Where is the pain?
- How often does the child have this pain?
- Is it associated with pyrexia?
- Are they able to tolerate diet and fluids when the pain is present?

Examination of the throat
- Explain the procedure to the child and family and gain verbal consent.
- Look in the child's mouth using an appropriate light source.
- If necessary use a tongue depressor to obtain a satisfactory view.
- The lips should be examined first, then the buccal mucosa and teeth, and then the floor of the mouth.
- Using the tongue depressor if necessary the tongue can be lowered, so the palate and tonsils can be examined.
- Check for any signs of enlargement of the tonsils, a bifid uvula (see 📖 Practice tips, p. 553), and any white patches or ulceration.
- If the child's sore throat is associated with general malaise and pyrexia, the indications are that it is infectious in origin.
- Most children with a sore throat can be managed in primary care. However, if they have the following symptoms they should be referred to a specialist service:
  - Peri-tonsillar abscess (quinsy).
  - Unilateral swelling of the tonsil.
  - Swelling of the tonsils that is causing an upper airway obstruction.
  - A history of sleep apnoea.

Practice tips

- If the child is anxious, they could sit on the parent/carers knee facing you. Encourage the parent/carer to place one hand on the child's forehead and the other around the chest. This allows you to examine the child and also is reassuring for the child.
- The presence of a bifid uvula could indicate that the child has a sub-mucous cleft. If you see a bifid uvula, a medical opinion should be sought.

Pitfalls

❶ Removal of tonsils has an associated morbidity and mortality. It is essential that the child is assessed by an experienced practitioner before a tonsillectomy is performed.

Associated reading

Bluestone C, Stool S. Cuneyt A, et al. (2003). *Pediatric Otolaryngology*, 4th edn. Saunders, London.
Graham J, Scadding G, Bull P, (2007). *Pediatric ENT*. Springer, Berlin.
🖑 http://www.prodigy.nhs.uk.

Epistaxis control

Background

Epistaxis in children is common and most children will suffer a bleed from the nose at some time. In children, the site of bleeding is usually just inside the nostril, on the nasal septum (the middle harder part of the nostril). Here, the blood vessels are fragile and the reason for the bleed is often due to a break in a blood vessel within the nose. Bleeding can be unilateral or bilateral.

Equipment

- Disposable apron and gloves.
- Otoscope and speculum.
- Nasal speculum (often only able to use these in an older child).
- Tissues/gauze swabs (to clean the rest of the face).
- Crushed ice.
- Vomit bowl for the patient to hold under their chin.

Procedure

Epistaxis may occur due to:
- An injury to the nose.
- Blowing the nose too hard or too frequently.
- A child picking his/her nose.
- Putting a FB into the nose.
- Local disease within the nasal cavity.
- Systemic disease, such as leukaemia.
- As a result of anticoagulant therapy.

Questions to ask

- How long have symptoms been present?
- Which side does the bleeding come from?
- How frequently does the child have nose bleeds?
- Is there any past medical history?

Treatment

- Reassure both the child and the parent/carer.
- Explain the procedure to the child and family and gain consent.
- Wash hands as per policy.
- Apply gloves and apron.
- Sit the child down either on their own or on the parents/carers knee. Make sure the child sits upright, with their head tilted forwards so that the blood does not run back into the throat.
- Pinch the soft part of the nose (below the bridge) between the thumb and finger for at least 10min. Squeeze firmly and do not let go until the 10min has elapsed.
- Apply crushed ice or a bag of frozen peas wrapped in a towel to the bridge of the nose. This will cause the blood vessels in the nose to constrict and help slow the bleeding.

- If bleeding is severe or does not stop after 10min reapply pressure and obtain baseline observations of pulse and blood pressure (BP). A medical assessment should be sought and it may be advisable to take bloods for full blood count (FBC) and clotting.
- Sometimes it may be necessary to pack the nose to stop bleeding. This must been done by an experienced practitioner.
- Once bleeding has stopped dispose of all equipment, wash hands and document the episode of care.

Practice tips

- Advise child/parent/carer that the child should not have any hot drinks for the next 24h.
- Advise child/parent/carer that the child should wipe the nose, rather than blow it for the next 24h.
- Once bleeding has ceased yellow/white soft paraffin can be applied just inside each nostril to keep the skin inside the nose moist and prevent the formation of scabs.
- A child who has regular nosebleeds should see an ENT specialist so investigations can be undertaken. It may be necessary to cauterize some of the blood vessels at the front of the nose that give rise to bleeding. This can be done by an ENT specialist either in clinic (if the child is compliant and willing) or under a general anaesthetic (GA).

Pitfalls

- Do not tilt the child's head backwards as they are likely to swallow blood.
- Do not put cotton wool up into the nostrils. The cotton wool can adhere to the bleeding point and when removed the bleeding often recommences.
- A child who returns recurrently with what appear to be simple nosebleeds should undergo a blood screen to ascertain whether they have an underlying bleeding disorder.

Associated reading

Barnes K. (2003). *Paediatrics—A Clinical Guide for Nurse Practitioners*. Elsevier Science Ltd, London.
Graham J, Scadding G, Bull P. (eds)(2007). *Pediatric ENT*. Springer, Berlin.
Patient UK (2010). *Nosebleeds (Epistaxis)*. Available at: http://www.patient.co.uk/health/Nosebleeds-(Epistaxis).htm.

Removal of foreign body from the nose

Background

Nasal FBs are a common occurrence in young children presenting to emergency departments or primary care services. Generally diagnosis will follow either a witnessed incident or a history from the child that they have inserted something into their nose. Possible diagnosis should also be considered when a child presents with unilateral discharge, often with an offensive odour. Additional symptoms could include: bleeding, nasal pain or snoring. Diagnosis will be confirmed with direct visualization of the FB following examination using a suitable light source.

Equipment

If the 'kissing technique' described here (☐ Steps of the 'kissing technique', p. 556) is not effective and alternative techniques are necessary the following equipment may be required:

- Auroscope.
- Appropriate light source.
- A right-angle hooked probe.
- Fine forceps.
- Suction device and appropriately-sized suction catheter.

Procedure

Only a suitably qualified practitioner such as a doctor, or nurse practitioner should undertake removal of any FB; therefore, the role of the qualified or student nurse will be to assist in this procedure.

There are a number of techniques available to remove nasal foreign bodies; however, nowadays the non-invasive 'kissing' technique is generally the first method of choice. The 'kissing' technique or 'parent kiss' requires co-operation from the child's parent, but it is recommended because it is non-invasive, and therefore safer and less distressing for young children.

Steps of the 'kissing technique'

- Explain the procedure to the parent, gain consent, and ensure they are happy to try the technique.
- Explain to the child that mummy/daddy is going to give them a 'big' or 'magic kiss'.
- The child then sits sideways on their parents lap, with the affected nostril against the parent's body.
- The parent occludes the unaffected nostril with their finger.
- The parent then needs to cover the child's mouth with his or her own and give a short, sharp puff.
- The FB will then either pass out of the nostril fully, caught hopefully in a gauze/tissue, or reach the tip, where it can then be stroked out gently by running pinched fingers from the bridge of the nose downwards.
- If the 'kissing' technique is unsuccessful then alternative techniques may be required.

Alternative techniques
- Using direct visualization provided by a good light source, the doctor or nurse practitioner will either hook or suck out the FB.
- Re-examine the nostrils to ensure no further FB or signs of trauma.
- Reassure the child and family.
- Usually no further treatment or follow-up is required and assuming sedation has not been used the child and family can usually be discharged immediately.
- Document removal of FB and procedure used.
- ❶ In order to prevent further damage or aspiration, the practitioner should have a low threshold for considering referral to ENT if the FB is difficult to remove/causing the child pain or distress.
- ❶ It is vital to remember that the safety and patency of the child's airway must be maintained at all times.

Practice tips
- If a parent feels unable to attempt the 'kiss', or cannot understand this instruction the same manoeuvre can be attempted using a bag valve mask. However, this is often a little more distressing for the child.
- In order to prevent unnecessary distress to the child during attempts to remove the FB, it is essential to utilize distraction techniques with the support of a play specialist if available (see Chapter 6).
- Safe, therapeutic holding techniques, such as 'blanket wrapping' for younger children, may be helpful.
- Sedation should be considered for a child who is very distressed and uncooperative.

Pitfalls
- ❶ Although very rare, there is the potential risk of aspiration if a FB is pushed into the nasopharynx and inhaled. Thus, caution must be exercised when managing a FB in a child's airway.

Associated reading
Davies FCW (2003) *Minor Trauma in Children.* Arnold, London.
Purohit N, Ray S, Wilson T, Chawla OP. (2008). The 'parent's kiss': an effective way to remove paediatric nasal foreign bodies. *Ann R Coll Surg Engl* **90**(5), 420–2.
Royal College of Nursing (2010). *Restrictive Physical Intervention and Therapeutic Holding for Children and Young People.* RCN, London.

Ear toilet

Ear toilet is the removal of debris, wax, FBs, and excess discharge from the external auditory meatus. It allows for examination of the external auditory meatus and the tympanic membrane.

❶ Aural toilet of ears should only be performed by staff that have received appropriate training, and are confident in their knowledge and skills to assume responsibility as registered practitioners.

Equipment
- Otoscope.
- Disposable speculum.
- Jobson–Horne probe.
- Cotton wool.

Procedure
- Explain the procedure in age appropriate terms to the child and family, and gain consent.
- Check for any history of ear disease or previous surgery.
- Conduct a comprehensive examination of the ear (see 📖 Assessment of the ear, p. 548).
- Explain the findings and subsequent plan of treatment to the child and parent/carer.
- Reassure the child and parent/carer throughout the treatment.

Aural toilet
- Secure a good light with head mirror and lamp.
- Insert a speculum into external auditory meatus.
- If assessment of the external auditory meatus indicates infection, take a swab for culture and sensitivity, and send to the laboratory.
- If discharge is present utilize a dry mop technique:
  - Secure cotton wool to Jobson–Horne probe.
  - Dry mop the discharge using a rotating action.
  - Change the cotton wool as necessary.
- Re-examine the ear intermittently.
- If there is debris, wax, or a FB present, refer to an appropriately trained member of staff, e.g. ENT nurse specialist/medical staff for advice as to the best method for removal (see 📖 Removal of foreign body from the ear, p. 560).

Following the procedure
- Explain all findings to child and parent/carer.
- Dispose of instruments and waste according to infection control and local policy, and decontaminate hands appropriately.
- Document the procedure and all findings.
- If any abnormality is observed, refer promptly to appropriate medical personnel.

Practice tips

- If you have confirmed that there is a FB present, think carefully about the treatment plan. In children there is often only one chance to remove the FB. If it is deep, awkward, or the child is very distressed refer straight to an experienced ENT practitioner. (See 📖 Removal of foreign body from the ear, p. 560.)

Pitfalls

- ❶ Do not attempt to insert anything into a child's ear or undertake any task for which you have not received training.
- ❶ Water irrigation can be used as tolerated, although this practice is now rarely used in children. If the child only has one hearing ear, or is known to have a perforation or a cochlear implant it is not advisable to use water irrigation.

Associated reading

Graham J, Scadding G, Bull P. (2007). *Pediatric ENT*. Springer, Berlin.
Thurgood K, Thurgood G. (1995). Ear syringing a clinical skill. *Br J Nurs* **4**(12), 682–7.
Wormald P, Browning G. (1996). *Otoscopy: a Structured Approach*. Arnold, London.

Removal of foreign body from the ear

Background

As with nasal FBs, children commonly present to both emergency care and primary care settings with foreign objects in their ears.

A witnessed event or the child's own history is usually the first indicator that a child has a FB in their ear. Occasionally, small insects can also find their way into the ear; the child will usually describe hearing or feeling them buzzing or tickling, or complain of acute (often severe) ear pain. A delayed diagnosis of FB may be discovered if a child presents with pain, deafness, or a discharge from the ear. As with nasal FB, diagnosis is confirmed following direct visualization using an auroscope/otoscope.

Equipment

The equipment to be prepared will depend on the object requiring removal, but the information given here can be used as a guide:

- Light source.
- Auroscope/otoscope.
- *Small right-angled forceps (such as Tilley's forceps):* useful for soft material, such as paper, cotton wool, or some foodstuffs, e.g. sweetcorn!
- *Syringe and warmed water:* if needing to irrigate light objects (such as insects). ❶ Contraindicated in any object that could swell, such as paper and vegetable matter.
- *Suction:* helpful for light solid objects, such as beads.
- *Small angled hook or probe:* used to pass behind and hook forward a heavier solid object (such as a small stone).

Procedure

❶ Only a suitably qualified practitioner such as a doctor, or nurse practitioner should undertake removal of any FB. The role of the qualified or student nurse will be to assist in this procedure.

A number of factors must be considered before attempting to remove a FB from a young child's ear:

- Consider the age and potential compliance of the child. This will affect the decision as to which technique will be most suitable.
- Consider distraction techniques, if possible with the help of a play specialist.
- Consider use of suitable therapeutic holding techniques.
- Ensure a good light source is available.
- Consider the need for sedation if the child is very young or very distressed.
- If attempting removal, the choice of instrument will usually depend on the object to be removed and its location.

Once all considerations have been made:

- Ensure procedure is explained to the child and family, and that consent has been gained.
- Position the child, to ensure that the affected ear is easily accessible.

- Depending on the FB and technique being used, the practitioner will then lift the pinna upwards and outwards, and under direct visualization remove the FB.
- After removal, re-examine the ear using an auroscope/otoscope, to ensure there is not an additional FB and to exclude trauma.
- Reassure child and family.
- Usually no further treatment or follow-up is required, and assuming sedation has not been used, the child can be discharged immediately.
- Document removal of FB and the procedure used.

Practice tips

- *Positioning:* sit a younger child, toddler, or infant on the parents/carers lap with the unaffected ear resting against their chest. The parent/carer can then support and cuddle the child with one arm, and use their other hand to gently support the child's head. If using therapeutic holding techniques it may be helpful to gently wrap a younger child in a blanket, but the procedure should not be undertaken if the child is distressed and moving.
- Always remember to re-examine the ear after FB removal in case of additional FB.

Pitfalls

- Consider referral to a specialist ENT team if FB is located deeply, i.e. within the medial two-thirds of the auditory canal.
- ❶ Foreign body removal in a young child should not be attempted unless the child is co-operative, and the practitioner competent and confident in the procedure, if in doubt discuss with specialist team.

Associated reading

Davies FCW. (2003). *Minor Trauma in Children*. Arnold, London.
Royal College of Nursing (2010). *Restrictive Physical Intervention and Therapeutic Holding for Children and Young People*. RCN, London.

Cleft lip and palate: pre-operative care

Background

A cleft of the lip and or palate is one of the most common congenital abnormalities affecting approximately 1000 children within the UK each year. It is often considered rather low on the list of disabling deformities despite the fact that it can affect appearance, feeding, speech, hearing, maxillary growth, and dentition. Cleft lip can be defined as a gap through the soft tissue of the mid-face usually extending from the top lip upwards towards the nose. A cleft palate can be defined as a gap through the roof of the mouth usually extending into the nasal cavity. There are varying categories of both cleft lip and palate, which differ in terms of severity. Isolated cleft palate is now being viewed as a separate condition to cleft lip and palate. The majority of care required pre-operatively by children with a cleft is routine, but there are a number of specific issues that need attention prior to surgery.

Procedure

Preoperative care: lip and palate repair

Routine pre-operative care plus:

- *Clinical photographs:* national protocol dictates that views of the face and palate are taken for every child undergoing cleft surgery.
- *Some children are fitted for arm splints preoperatively:* arm splints are optional and parents are offered the choice of using them in order to prevent their children from placing fingers, toys, etc., into their mouth and damaging their surgery. If used, arm splints are recommended for the first 48h post-operatively (local Policy differs between cleft centres as arm splints are not used in all centres).
- *Advice is given against the use of dummies/comforters post-operatively:* the child's sucking pattern is different when using a dummy than when feeding. Increased risk of infection and potential damage to the palate repair are the main reasons for discouraging the use of dummies post-operatively. If, however, the child is extremely upset, allowing them to suck on a clean dummy for a few minutes in order to help them to settle is unlikely to do any harm.
- Emotional support for the parents and family is essential:
  - Parents have often been aware that their child is going to need surgery from 16 weeks gestation onwards. This can lead to the pregnancy being medicalized and cause increased stress. Thus, effective antenatal support is essential.
  - Children who require lip surgery will look very different following their surgery. This can be traumatic for the parents who may need emotional support and time to adjust.
  - The child's feeding pattern post-operatively is also likely to have been altered. It may take 2–3 days for this to become fully re-established. This is worth discussing pre-operatively.
- Nose and throat swabs should be taken pre-operatively (refer to local policy).

- Methicillin-resistant *Staphylococcus aureus* (MRSA) and beta haemolytic Streptococci pose the greatest risk to cleft surgery.
- If MRSA is present on swabs inform the surgeons who will make a decision as to whether to proceed with surgery.
- Follow local policy guidelines in relation to the management of MRSA.
- *Bloods*: routine/specialist bloods, if required, are usually taken in theatre once the child is anaesthetized (check local policy).

Pre-operative care: issues specific to palate repair
- Due to the difficulty in obtaining clear clinical photographs of the palate these will usually be taken in theatre once the child is asleep.
- Special anaesthetic review pre-operatively is not usually necessary unless there are concerns regarding the patency/stability of the child's airway (see 📖 Practice tips, p. 563).

Practice tips

- If swabs are positive for beta haemolytic Streptococci, 24h worth of antibiotics will be needed pre-operatively. In addition, the child will need to complete a 10-day course following surgery. Surgery may be cancelled otherwise (check local policy).
- Cleft children with potential airway management difficulties, e.g. those with Pierre Robin sequence will need to be seen by an anaesthetist pre-operatively. The purpose is to assess the child's suitability for/ readiness for surgery. In some cases, surgery may need to be delayed.
- A paediatric intensive care unit (PICU)/paediatric high dependency unit (PHDU) bed should be booked for any child who is considered at risk for post-operative difficulties. (Local policy does vary; in some hospitals all cleft children go to PHDU routinely during the immediate post-operative period).
- Occasionally, some cleft children with underlying medical conditions require admission pre-operatively under the care of the lead paediatrician for further investigation prior to surgery.

Pitfalls

- A significant number of children who have a cleft also suffer from cardiac problems (isolated cleft palate children especially). Thus, it is important to check that all cardiac reports and test results are present.

Associated reading

Martin V, Bannister P. (eds). (2004). *Cleft Care: a practical guide for health professionals on cleft lip and/or palate*. APS Publishing, Salisbury.
Moller KT, Glaze LE. (eds) (2009). *Interdisciplinary issues and treatment*. 2nd edn.: Pro Ed, Austin.
Watson ACH, Sell DA, Grunwell P. (eds) (2001). *Management of Cleft Lip and Palate*. Whurr, London.

Cleft lip repair: post-operative care

Background
Cleft lip is one of the most common congenital facial deformities with approximately 1:6–700 births in the UK each year (for definition see 🕮 Cleft lip and palate: pre-operative care, p. 562).

Equipment
- A spare nasopharyngeal airway (NPA).
- Correct size suction catheters for airway size.
- Oxygen saturation monitor.
- Apnoea alarm (check local policy).
- Gloves.
- NaCl 0.9%.
- Soft white/yellow paraffin.

Procedure
Airway management
Babies are obligate nose breathers until 6 months of age. Therefore, they have difficulty in compensating when their airway has become smaller. A cleft child's airway is reduced in size post-surgery due to closure of the lip and nose, and normal post-operative swelling:
- Ensure working oxygen and suction is available.
- Elevate head of cot to help reduce swelling.
- Lie baby on their side to assist in the drainage of secretions from the oro/nasal cavity.
- An apnoea alarm may be required for 24h post-operatively (check local policy).
- Continuous O_2 saturation monitoring for first 24h. Aim to maintain saturations >94% (reduces the risk of increased respiratory effort).
- Observe for signs of respiratory distress including:
  - *Lip sucking*—1° sign that the baby is getting tired (see 🕮 Practice tips, p. 565).
  - Nasal flaring (can be difficult to see due to swelling from surgery).

Nasal pharyngeal airways
If *in situ*
- Ensure airways are secure.
- Suction airways at least every 2h for the full duration the airways remain *in situ* (more often if required).
- Document the length of the NPA.
- Suction up to 3mm beyond the end of the NPA to ensure the airway remains clear. Suctioning beyond this can cause bleeding and damage to the nasal passages.

If NPA becomes blocked
- Apply 1–2 drops of normal saline into the NPA then repeat suction.
- If this is not effective and there are signs of increased respiratory effort seek prompt medical advice.

Feeding
- Offer feed (breast or bottle) as soon as the baby appears ready.
- Feed little and often at the baby's own pace until normal feeding is re-established.
- Parents may need to adjust their normal feeding technique (assisted feeding method is common for children with a cleft). ❶ Assisted feeding is a specialist feeding technique. *Do not* use this technique unless assessed as competent to do so.
- Ensure there is an adequate intake of fluids (75% of total requirement) in each 24h period post-operatively. Ensure this is tolerated without increased signs of respiratory effort.
- Apply soft white paraffin to the lips and corners of the mouth.
- *Pain relief:* give regular analgesia as prescribed (paracetamol and ibuprofen)
- Regular analgesia should be continued for a minimum of 1 week following discharge home.

Emotional support
The baby's face will have changed, often dramatically; parents/carers need a lot of emotional support at this time.

Lip/suture care
- *Dissolvable sutures:* clean with NaCl 0.9% or cooled boiled water.
- Use dressed applicators (cotton buds).
- Roll moistened applicator down over the suture line once. Remove any blood or scabs (if they come off easily).
- Repeat using a fresh applicator each time, until clean.
- When clean roll a dry applicator once along the suture line.
- Apply soft white paraffin to the suture line and lips.
- This should be repeated 2–3 times a day for the first week.
- *Second week:* leave the suture line to settle and clean as normal.
- *Glue:* if glue has been used, leave this in place to come off in its own time. Ensure the area around the glue is kept clean.
- Arrange for removal of sutures if appropriate (local policy).

Practice tips
- Lip sucking ≈ one of the 1° signs of respiratory distress. This sign is peculiar to cleft lip children. They suck in their lower lip on inspiration. If lip sucking is observed reposition the child and commence gentle suction of the nasal passages/NPA's. Give O_2 if required and as prescribed. ❶ Persistent lip sucking requires prompt medical review.
- A cleft nurse specialist will usually do a post-operative home visit within 2 weeks of discharge (check local policy).

Pitfalls
- Babies tire very quickly. If concerned, take appropriate action.
- Poor lip care and infection can lead to scarring and have a long-term psychological impact on the child and family.
- A good post-operative scar care regime should be implemented (check local policy).

Cleft palate repair: post-operative care

Background
Cleft palate occurs in approximately 1–600 births in the UK (for definition see ☐ Cleft lip and palate: pre-operative care, p. 562). The cause is thought to be multifactorial with both genetic and environmental factors playing a role. It is estimated that 30% of children with a cleft palate may have additional complications.

Repairs can be done in stages. The age at which surgery takes place ranges from 8 to 13 months. Second stage repairs take place at an older age (local practice varies with regard to this please refer to local policy).

Equipment
- Oxygen saturation monitor.
- Nasogastric tube (NGT), FG Ch 6, pH paper, syringes -min 20mL enteral feed.
- Sterilizing unit and solution.
- Bottles, teats, teacher beakers.

Procedure
Post-operative care: airway
- Reduced in size due to closure of the cleft and post-operative swelling.
- Elevate the head of cot to aid breathing and help reduce swelling.
- Monitor oxygen saturations >94% for 24h post-operatively (longer if required).
- Observe for signs of increased respiratory effort (↑ respirations, nasal flaring, ↑ intercostal recession).
- Lay the child on their side to assist in drainage of oral secretions.
- There may be some pooling of secretions in the back of the oral cavity (this may necessitate very gentle oral suction).

Circulation
It is usual to have some oozing following surgery. Blood-stained secretions may come from the nose, these should become darker over the next few days. ❶ Excessive oozing requires surgical review.

Eating and drinking
- Many children find drinking difficult initially following a palate repair.
- When the child is able, start with yogurt/ice-cream type foods.
- Encourage small frequent amounts of soft/pureed diet (4 weeks).
- Allow the child to take the lead with feeding.
- ❶ Do not force feed.
- No hard or sharp foods to be given for 4 weeks post-surgery.
- Rinse the child's mouth with water after all foods, except bio/natural yogurt.
- Observe the palate at least 2–3 times/24h for signs of infection, breakdown, and sloughy areas.

Nasogastric tube

Use of NGT post-operatively is variable. If used:

- Aspirate old blood on return to the ward (blood is often swallowed during surgery).
- 1st night post-operatively give milk/liquids, pain relief/antibiotics via NGT if refused orally.
- Remove NGT the morning after surgery.
- ❶ Do not re-pass an NGT if it comes out. (Unless the child is supported by nasogastric feeds pre-operatively. If this is the case refer to the surgical team.)

Pain relief

- Follow local protocol.
- Give analgesia frequently and pro-actively.
- Advise parents to continue giving regular pain relief at home for as long as needed.

Emotional support

- The child will feed differently post-operatively. It may take several days for the child to re-establish their normal feeding.
- Support, reassure, and encourage the parents and child through this time.

Practice tips

- Children have to relearn how to swallow following surgery; therefore, they may not swallow secretions as normal initially.
- If excessive bleeding is evident, give ice cold water or ice-cream to help stop the bleeding and seek prompt medical/surgical help.
- Regular analgesia is essential.
- Avoid foods with skins, flakes, and pips for 3–4 weeks following surgery, as these can get caught in the repair and cause infection.
- Use fizzy water or soda water if the palate appears to get 'sloughy' 2–3 days post-operatively. The bubbles help to remove debris and keep the mouth clean.
- Oral hygiene is paramount, encourage parents to continue cleaning their child's teeth (age appropriate).

Pitfalls

- Children post-palate repair will often tolerate diet better than fluids, it is better to add extra fluid to the child's food, rather than persisting with fluids if the child is becoming distressed.
- Patience is required with feeding post-operatively. Each child is different and some may take longer to return to their normal routine than others.
- ❶ Inadequate pain relief leads to potential delays in feeding and discharge.

Associated reading

Martin V, Bannister P. (eds) (2004). *Cleft Care: a practical guide for health professionals on cleft lip and/or palate.* APS Publishing, Salisbury.

🔗 http://www.clapa.com.

🔗 http://www.nurses4cleft.org.uk.

Ophthalmology

History taking and assessment

Background

Assessing vision and examination of the eye are essential in order to detect conditions in a child that can be a sign of serious systemic illness or result in blindness. Undetected eye problems, such as strabismus, glaucoma, cataracts, and neurological disorders can lead to poor school performance. Early detection can save a child's vision and detecting conditions, such as retinoblastoma can save a child's life.

- Examination of the eyes should be performed in all newborns and at subsequent routine health assessments.
- Visual acuity measurements can be performed from about the age of 3yrs and upwards.
- Infants and children with a high risk of eye problems include prematurity, genetic, or metabolic disorders, developmental delay, neurological problems, and eye abnormalities, family histories of cataracts, or retinoblastoma, or systemic disease associated with eye problems.

History taking

Parents' observations are valuable. Ask:

- Does your child usually seem to see well?
- Do they hold objects close to their face when trying to focus?
- Do they appear to have eyes that cross over or appear lazy?
- Do their eyelids droop or their eyes appear unusual?

Ask about:

- Trauma.
- Previous similar episodes.
- Systemic illness and family history of eye disease or vision problems.
- Preschool or early childhood use of glasses in parents or siblings.
- If there is visual disturbance then ask for how long.
- Distinguish any blurred vision as opposed to double vision.
- Is there any pain, redness, watering, or discharge in the eyes?
- Is the problem unilateral or bilateral, and have they noticed any changes in the appearance of the eye.

Examination procedure

Use a systematic approach.

- Explain procedure as appropriate to child and parent/carer and gain consent.
- Use age/cognitive level appropriate distraction/play, involving other personnel as needed.
- Start with the outer eye and work inwards using a pen torch.
- Look at the outer eye for redness and swelling, such as peri-orbital oedema.
- Are their eyelids symmetrical? Observe for any drooping that may indicate ptosis or nerve damage.
- Check the skin around the eye lids for inflammation and swelling, or crusting of the lashes.
- The surface of the eye should be bright and shiny, look for any redness.

- If there is any suggestion of injury to the cornea then the eye should be stained with fluorescein and then examined with a blue light. Any problems on the surface of the cornea will show up green.
- Pupils should be central, round of equal size, and respond equally to light and accommodation. Small differences can occur normally, but should be noted for reference in case of subsequent head injury.
- Ensuring the eyes are in alignment is of considerable importance in pre-school and early school aged children. Development of strabismus (squint/crossed eye) can occur at any age and can be a sign of serious disease in the orbit, eye, or brain. The corneal reflex test and cover test are used for diagnosis.

Practice tips

- Redness around the periphery of the eye or lid linings indicates conjunctivitis. The most common cause is lacrimal duct obstruction which usually occurs during the first 3 months of age as persistent purulent discharge from one or both eyes.
- The presence of cloudy or asymmetrically enlarged corneas could indicate glaucoma and should be promptly referred to ophthalmology.
- Slow or poorly reactive pupils may indicate retinal or optic nerve dysfunction. Asymmetry of pupil size can indicate 3rd cranial (oculomotor) nerve palsy or damage to the sympathetic nervous syndrome (Horner syndrome). Pupil asymmetries greater than 1mm needs investigating as can be attributable to serious neurological disorders.
- Use a toy or a puppet to focus the child's eyes.
- Minimize distractions that may interfere with eye examination.
- If possible avoid performing eye examination when the infant or child is tired, anxious, or hungry.
- Eye examination is best performed prior to other procedures that may upset the child.

Associated reading

Denniston A, Murray P. (2009). *Oxford Handbook of Ophthalmology*. Oxford University Press, Oxford.
Shaw M, Lee A, Stollery R. (2010). *Ophthalmic Nursing*, 4th edn. Wiley-Blackwell, Oxford.

Visual acuity measurement

Background

In general children do not complain of visual difficulties and so visual acuity measurement should begin at the earliest possible age practical which is about 3yrs. The most sophisticated test that the child is capable of should be used in order to obtain the most accurate results. In general, the tumbling E test or HOTV should be used in children age 3–5yrs and the Snellen letters or numbers in children 6yrs and older. If a child is unable to perform a test after 2 attempts or you suspect an abnormality they should be referred to an ophthalmologist for further assessment.

Procedure

0–3yrs

Vision assessment in children 0–3yrs of age or any non-verbal child is achieved by assessing the child's ability to fix and follow objects.

- Ensure that the child is fully awake and alert before performing the test as poor attention can mimic a poor vision response.
- Determine if each eye can fix on an object, maintain fixation, and follow the object into various gaze positions.
- Perform the test on both eyes to start with, then each eye separately by covering the other. Poor fixation and following with both eyes after age 3mnths indicates bilateral eye or brain abnormality and should be referred for further assessment.

3yrs and older

Various tests are available including picture tests such as Allen cards, suitable for children aged 2–4yrs of age. Test for children older than 4yrs include wall charts containing Snellen letters or numbers. For children unable to perform visual acuity testing by letters and numbers the tumbling E test and the HOTV test (a letter matching test involving just the letters H O T, and V) may be used.

Snellen chart

The Snellen chart is used to test distant visual acuity and consist of lines of different letters stacked one on top of the other. The letters are large at the top decreasing in size from top to bottom.

- The chart is placed on a wall at eye level in a well lighted area.
- The child stands 6m from the chart and covers on eye with an occluder.
- A child who has corrective eye glasses should be screened wearing them.
- Tell the child to keep both eyes open during the testing.

- The child reads each line of letters until he or she can no longer distinguish them. Under each line on the chart there is a number that is used to record the results. A common acuity test score is 6/6 and represents the average eye. The top number 6 represents the distance from the child to the chart. The bottom number represents the distance the average eye can see the letters on a certain line of the eye chart.
- If a child sees 6/9, at 6m from the chart the child can see what an average eye could see at 9m. If any letters on a line are missed encourage the child to keep reading until he can't distinguish any more letters, but record the number of letters missed using a minus sign. If the child missed two letters on the 9 line record the score as 6/9–2.

HOTV matching test

This test is designed for children unable to verbally identify letters and numbers on a Snellen eye chart. The test consists of a wall chart which contains only the letters H, O, T, and V. The child is provided with a small board containing a large letter H, O, T, and V. The examiner points to a letter on the wall chart and the child matches the correct letter on the testing board.

Allen cards

Allen cards consist of flash cards containing 7 schematic figures; tree, bear, telephone, horse, truck, house, and birthday cake. When viewed at 6m these figures represent 6/9 vision. It is important that testing is only performed with the figures that the child can readily identify.

- The child should first be shown the cards from about 50cm distance with both eyes open.
- Ensure the child understands the testing procedure then begin to move backward 1m at a time, continuing until the child misses the figures.
- To calculate the acuity score the furthest distance the child is able to identify the figures accurately is the numerator. 9 is used as the denominator. Therefore, if a child were able to identify the figures accurately at 6m the visual acuity would be recorded as 6/9.

Opthalmoscopy

Opthalmoscopy may be possible in some very co-operative 3- or 4-yr-olds who are able to fixate on a toy while the opthalmoscope is used to evaluate the retinal vessels and optic nerve.

Eye care

See 📖 Eye care, p. 110.

Eversion of the eyelid

Background
Everting the upper eyelid may be necessary in order to examine the palpebral conjunctiva for foreign bodies, inflammation, infection, or trauma.

Equipment
• Gloves.
• Cotton applicator(s).
• Distraction aids.

Procedure
This procedure will only be possible if the child is very co-operative and able to keep still.
• Provide a full explanation of the procedure to the child and parent, and gain consent.
• Wash hands and wear gloves.
• Ask the child to look down with the eyes slightly open.
• Gently grasp the upper eyelashes and pull the lid downward.
• Place a cotton applicator above the lid edge and push down gently with the applicator while still holding the eyelashes to turn the lid over.
• Hold the eyelashes against the upper ridge of the bony orbit below the eyebrow to maintain the everted position of the lid.
• Inspect the palpebral conjunctiva for foreign bodies, swelling, or trauma.
• Gently remove any foreign bodies by using the tip of the applicator.
• Return the eyelid to normal by asking the child to look up and blink.
• The eyelid should return to normal.
• Visual impairment support for children with visual disability.

Background
Severe visual impairment can affect all areas of a child's development:
• Emotional and social.
• Communication.
• Psychomotor.
• Knowledge and understanding of the world (spacial awareness, self-awareness).
• Self-help skills.

Health professionals involved with the child and their family will need active listening skills, empathy, effective communication, and good knowledge of the relevant support services available in the community for children with a visual impairment and complex needs.

Procedure: general principles of care

- Provide informal advice, to explain the impact visual impairment may have on a baby's general development.
- Reassure the parents that though their child/baby will have a different way of learning every day skills, compared with fully seeing babies and children. Though it may take longer, those skills will be acquired.
- Local child development centre and the local visual impairment services will provide assessment and recommendations on coping strategies.
- Signpost appropriate statutory and voluntary services for further support.
- Offer advice on certificate of visual impairment (CVI) registration and benefit entitlements, if appropriate. If the child is eligible for registration, the ophthalmologist arranges CVI. Both the specialist and the child's main carer then sign the certificate.
- Liaise with the health visitor or school nurse.
- Liaise with the visually impaired teacher for the visually impaired child, and acting as a point of contact.
- Liaise with special educational needs co-ordinators teams (SENCO) and with child development centres.
- With the parents consent, refer the child/baby to the visual impairment service.
- On an occasional basis, make contact with the sensory team at the local social services.

Associated reading

℘ http://www.cafamily.org.uk.
℘ http://www.nbcs.org.uk.
℘ jhttp://www.rnib.org.uk.

Dermatology

Assessing skin integrity and topical treatment

Background

Skin conditions in children (<14yrs of age) comprise approximately 21% of all persons consulting with skin disease. This age group represents 19% of the population and data from NHS Direct for 2008 showed that 4% of all calls related to skin rashes; the commonest age group was children aged 1–4yrs (31.8%) with a further 15.3% for children <1yr and 15.1% in the 5–14-yr-old age group.[1]

Equipment

- A warm and well lit room, preferably natural lighting or artificial lighting that will not change the natural colour of the skin.
- A magnifying lamp or light.
- A gown or sheet to maintain dignity as each area of the skin is exposed for examination.
- Sampling equipment for laboratory examinations:
  - Microbiological samples of scales, crusts, exudate, and tissue (including hair and nails) for microscopy and culture testing for yeast and fungus, bacteria, virus, parasites.
  - Examination of blood for diagnosis and monitoring of drug therapies, sent for clinical chemistry, haematology, immunology.
  - Diagnostic biopsies—immunofluorescence (IMF) looks at immune complexes, also sent for histological examination.

Procedure

Assessment of the child with a skin condition should include the following.

History of the skin condition
- Duration.
- Episodes of flare and remission.
- Does it occur at different times of the year?
- Family history of skin disease.
- School and hobbies–do they have an impact?
- Medications: applied to the skin, taken by mouth, prescribed, or purchased by the parents.
- Allergies.
- Previous and present treatments, and their effectiveness.
- Are there any treatments, actions, or life style changes, which have influenced the condition, such as diet, homeopathy, illness, or stressful events?

A general assessment

- A great deal can be observed in the child's face, which may give insight to how they feel and are coping with the skin condition. They may be withdrawn, not sleeping, and be very conscious about their appearance and the reactions of others.
- There are psychological and disease specific scores, which can measure the impact of skin disease on the individual.

Physical skin assessment

- Make a point of touching your patient:
  - This will give you clinical information about skin texture and temperature.
  - Breaks down physical barriers, as many dermatology patients experience stigma and isolation because of their visible condition.
- Consider religious and cultural preferences before the physical examination.
- The skin tells a story and can give many clues, so it needs to be examined thoroughly (from the scalp to toes including hair, nails and flexures), looking at the following.

Distribution

Is it acral (hands, feet), extremities of ears and nose, in light exposed areas, or mainly confined to the trunk

Character

- Is there redness (erythema), scaling, crusting, exudate.
- Are there excoriations, blisters, erosions, pustules, papules.
- Are the lesions all the same (monomorphic), e.g. drug rash, or variable (polymorphic), e.g. chickenpox.

Shape

Are the lesions small, large, annular (ring-shaped), linear.

Consideration of the skin as a sensory organ

- Assess pain, itching, and soreness associated with the skin condition.
- Itching (pruritus) is the principal symptom of primary skin disease.
- Systemic causes of itch, includes pregnancy, chronic renal failure, cholestasis, thyroid dysfunction, haematological disorders, iron deficiency, and internal malignancy.

Patient's knowledge about his or her skin condition

- As many skin conditions may be life-long, and involve flare up's and remissions, children/young people and their families need to have an understanding of their condition, the management, and long-term implications.

Documentation

- Findings, such as birth marks, scars, bruising, wounds, and loss of digits should be documented and dated.
- Findings should be documented using appropriate terminology or descriptions on a body map.

Primary lesions

Primary lesions are those present at the initial onset of the disease:

- *Macule:* a flat mark, circumscribed area of colour change—brown, red, white, or tan.
- *Papule:* elevated 'spot', palpable, firm, circumscribed lesion generally <5mm in diameter.

- *Nodule:* elevated, firm, circumscribed, palpable, can involve all layers of the skin, >5mm in diameter.
- *Plaque:* elevated, flat topped, firm, rough, superficial papule >2cm in diameter. Papules can coalesce to form plaques.
- *Wheal:* elevated, irregular-shaped area of cutaneous oedema, solid, transient, changing, variable diameter, red, pale pink or white in colour.
- *Vesicle:* elevated, circumscribed, superficial fluid filled blister <5mm in diameter.
- *Bulla:* vesicle >5mm in diameter.
- *Pustule:* elevated, superficial, similar to vesicle, but filled with pus.

Secondary lesions
Secondary lesions are the result of changes over time caused by disease progression, manipulation (scratching, rubbing, picking), or treatments.
- *Scale:* heaped-up keratinized cells, flaky exfoliation, irregular, thick or thin, dry or oily, variable size, silver, white or tan in colour.
- *Crust:* dried serum, blood or purulent exudate, slightly elevated, size variable.
- *Excoriation:* loss of epidermis, linear area usually due to scratching.
- *Lichenification:* rough, thickened epidermis, accentuated skin markings caused by rubbing or scratching.

Topical treatment application
- Drugs used on the skin must be dissolved or suspended in bases such as lotions, creams, ointments, sprays, gels, tapes.
- The choice of product will depend on the diagnosis and condition of the skin.
- Penetration of the drug through the skin depends on a number of factors:
  - The concentration of the drug.
  - The base.
  - The diffusion of the drug through the stratum corneum.
  - The thickness of the stratum corneum (this will vary at different sites).
  - Hydration of the skin.
  - Temperature.
  - Occlusion with dressings, nappies, etc.

Practice tips
- In practice there are a significant range of skin colours and hair types:
  - Lesions, which in white skin appear red or brown, appear black or purple in pigmented skin.
  - Mild degrees of redness (erythema) may be masked completely.
  - Inflammation commonly leads to pigmentary changes—both lighter (post-inflammatory hypopigmentation) and darker (post-inflammatory hyperpigmentation), which may persist for a long time after the initial skin condition has settled.
- When treatment is commenced, ensure there is a clear care plan/documentation guiding administration.

Pitfalls

- It is easy just to look at lesions in isolation.
- Many skin conditions present in specific sites and with a classic distribution. These may be missed if the skin is not examined as a whole.
- Listen to the child or parents descriptions as their observations also provide very useful information and clues.
- Having a sound understanding of the anatomy and function of the skin will also inform clinical decisions.

Associated reading

British Dermatological Nursing Group. Available at: ℜ http://www.bdng.org.uk.

Lawton S (2005). Assessing the patient with a skin condition. *Pract Nurse*. **30**(5), 43–8.

New Zealand Dermatological Society. Available at: ℜ http//www.dermnetnz.org.

Office for National Statistics (2001), *KS02 Age structure: Census 2001, Key Statistics for Local Authorities*. Available at: ℜ http://www.statistics.gov.uk/StatBase/ssdataset.asp?vlnk=6556&Pos (accessed 24 February 2011).

Quality of Life Scores, Available at: ℜ http://www.dermatology.org.uk/quality/quality-life.html.

[1] Schofield J, Grindlay D, Williams H. (2009). *Skin Conditions in the UK. A Health Care Needs Assessment*. Centre of Evidence Based Dermatology, University of Nottingham. Available at: ℜ http://www.nottingham.ac.uk/SCS/Divisions/EvidenceBasedDermatology/index.aspx (accessed 24 February 2011).

Endocrinology

Diabetes care

Background

Diabetes mellitus (DM) is a chronic lifelong endocrine condition. Environmental factors trigger an autoimmune response to destroy insulin producing cells in the pancreas, resulting in Type 1 diabetes (Insulin dependent). Subsequently patients lose their ability to control blood glucose (BG) levels and are reliant on insulin therapy for survival. Long term poor BG control leads to multiple complications, with life expectancy on average reduced by 15yrs. Causes are mainly environmental (viral). 90% of people have no relative with diabetes. Genetic elements can be traced to Human leucocyte antigen markers predisposing individuals. DM typically affects <25-yr-olds, with a peak incidence in age of 10–14-yr-olds; although there is a rising incidence in under 5-yr-olds.[1]

Other forms of diabetes are much less common in children, but include Type 2 diabetes and maturity onset diabetes mellitus of the young (MODY), and secondary diabetes, e.g. cystic fibrosis-related diabetes. This chapter focuses on care of type 1 diabetes.

Presentation

Presentation can be variable in length of onset, featuring a range of symptoms that can also range in severity:

- Hyperglycaemia.
- Polydipsia.
- Polyuria (excessive urine production, especially at night).
- Fatigue/tiredness.
- Weight loss.
- Glycosuria.
- Ketones detected in blood/urine.
- Diabetic ketoacidosis (DKA; severe symptom, 100% mortality if untreated with insulin).

Investigations

- Laboratory BG, Blood/urine ketone, venous blood gas for acid base status, U & E, thyroid function test (TFT), Coeliac serology, HbA1c.
- Consider Islet cell antibodies if no ketonuria and autosomal dominant family history diabetes (consider diagnosis of MODY or type 2 diabetes).

Aims of management

- Optimal glycaemic control.
  - Target BG 4–7mmols/L pre-meal, without significant disabling hypoglycaemia.
  - Individual targets may be set for younger children, or if hypoglycaemia warning symptoms are lost.
- Frequent self BG monitoring (see 📖 Blood glucose monitoring, p. 98).
- Appropriate hypoglycaemic management.

- Aim for HBA1c <7.5% (59mmol/mol). Clinical marker for long-term prognosis.
- Suitable insulin regimen.
- Healthy eating regime and regular exercise.
- Concordance with treatment.
- Empowering and motivating to self-care.
- Good quality of life.
- Reduce risk of long-term severe complications:
  - Cardiovascular, macrovascular, and microvascular damage.
  - Retinopathy (eventually blindness).
  - Nephropathy (eventually renal failure).
  - Neuropathy.
- Psychological support/access to Child and Adolescent Mental Health Services (CAMHS).
- 3–4-monthly clinical reviews.
- Annual reviews.
  - <12yrs urinary albumin, creatinine screening, thyroid function.
  - >12yrs in addition; retinal screening, screening for lipid profiles, blood pressure (BP) checks.
- Bi-annual screening for other autoimmune conditions.
- In adolescence, include education to manage alcohol safely, risks of smoking, and recreational drugs, basic pre-conceptual awareness.
- Effective transition to adult services.

Practice tips

- If newly diagnosed treat DKA if present. Other presentations require immediate initiation of subcutaneous insulin therapy.

Pitfalls

- Careful consideration of family history could indicate differential diagnosis.

Associated reading

British Society for Paediatric Endocrinology and Diabetes (2009). *Recommended DKA Guidelines*. Available at: http://www.bsped.org.uk/professional/guidelines/docs/DKAGuideline.pdf (accessed 20 February 2011).

National Institute for Clinical Excellence. (2004). *Clinical Guideline 15 Type 1 Diabetes: Diagnosis and Management of Type 1 Diabetes in Children, Young People and Adults*. Available at: http://www.nice.org.uk/nicemedia/pdf/CG015childrenfullguideline.pdf (accessed 20 February 2011).

Diabetes UK. Available at: http://www.diabetes.org.uk.

Juvenile Diabetes Research Foundation. Available at: http://www.jdrf.org.uk.

MODY— http://projects.exeter.ac.uk/diabetesgenes.

[1] Royal College of Paediatrics and Child Health. (2009). *Growing up with Diabetes: Children and Young People with Diabetes in England* Research report. Available at: http://www.diabetes.org.uk/Documents/Reports/CYP_Diabetes_Survey_Report.pdf (accessed 20 February 2011).

Insulin administration

Background

Insulin needs to absorb at a steady rate, to evenly regulate BG levels. It is administered based upon close BG monitoring (see 📖 Blood glucose monitoring, p. 98), as well as part of diabetes care for Type 1 diabetes (see 📖 Diabetes care, p. 584). The regime most appropriate to the individual will determine the type of insulin used.[1] Insulin cannot be ingested in tablet form, as it is inactivated by gastro-intestinal (GI) enzymes, therefore it must be injected. It is administered into subcutaneous (SC) fatty tissue (Fig. 22.1) and can be administered by:

- Insulin syringes (less commonly used by children).
- Insulin pen devices.
  - Disposable 3-mL pre-filled insulin pens, containing insulin of choice.
  - Pens with ½- or 1-unit increments.
- Insulin pumps (see 📖 Continuous subcutaneous insulin infusion, p. 589).

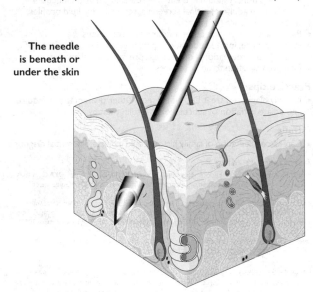

The needle is beneath or under the skin

Fig. 22.1 Subcutaneous injection.
Reproduced from www.gosh.nhs.uk, © GOSH Trust September 2007 with kind permission from Great Ormond Street Hospital NHS Trust.

Equipment

- Prescription.
- Insulin.
- Insulin syringe and needle, *or* insulin pen (pre-filled/insulin cartridge in pen device) and needle.
- Sharps bin.

Procedure

- Prepare insulin. In a hospital setting, adhere to local medicine protocol and general drug administration principles (see 📖 Drug administration, p. 196).

Pen device

- Ensure a new needle is *in situ*.
- Prime the needle with an air shot.
- Check correct dosage and dial this on the pen.

Syringe

- Draw up insulin into insulin syringe to the required amount.
- Select appropriate site (see Fig 22.2).
  - Speed of insulin absorption varies from site to site.
  - With pre-exercise, avoid injecting the limb about to be used.
  - Develop a pattern of using different sites during the day.
  - Injecting in the same site causes lipohypertrophy (lipo's).
- Consider skin 'pinch up'.
- Insert needle into skin, at a 90° angle.
- Administer insulin and keep needle *in situ* for 10s.
- Remove needle.
- Dispose of needle/syringe safely in sharps container.
- Document.

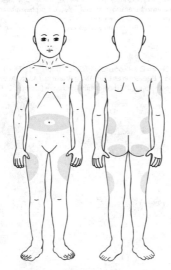

Fig. 22.2 Subcutaneous injection sites.
Reproduced from www.gosh.nhs.uk, © GOSH Trust September 2007 with kind permission from Great Ormond Street Hospital NHS Trust.

Practice tips

- Make a suitable choice of needle length.
  - Pen needle lengths: 4, 5, or 6mm.
  - 8mm needed for very obese patients and 8mm is recommended for children and young people with pinch up technique.
- Syringes have a max. dose of 30units (0.3mL), 50units (0.5mL), 100units (1mL).
- Ensure appropriate use of a skin fold 'pinch up' technique.
- Consider the use of distraction/play specialist (see 📖 Distraction, p. 150).
- Consider issues of privacy and dignity, especially with young people.

Pitfalls

- Avoid intramuscular (IM) injections—increases hypoglycemia risk.
- Ensure correct insulin is administered at the correct time, such as before meals or long-acting insulin to be given before bed.
  - Patients will have their own individual routines and insulins, which should be adhered to.

Associated reading

National Institute for Health and Clinical Excellence. (2010). *Insulin Therapy in Type 1 Diabetes—Management.* Available at: ⅋ http://www.cks.nhs.uk/insulin_therapy_in_type_1_diabetes/management/scenario_managing_injection_problems/advice_on_insulin_administration#-479184 (accessed 20 February 2011).

RCPCH Publications Ltd. (2011). *British National Formulary (BNF) for Children.* BMJ Publishing Group Ltd, London.

⅋ http://www.diabetes.org.uk.

---

[1] National Institute for Clinical Excellence. (2004). *Clinical Guideline 15 Type 1 Diabetes: Diagnosis and Management of Type 1 Diabetes in Children, Young People and Adults.* Available at: ⅋ http://www.nice.org.uk/nicemedia/pdf/CG015childrenfullguideline.pdf (accessed 20 February 2011).

Continuous subcutaneous insulin infusion

Background

Continuous subcutaneous insulin infusion (CSII) (also known as insulin pump therapy) is the continuous infusion of a variable dose of rapid-acting insulin into the subcutaneous tissue at a rate that is set according to the child's requirements (*basal rate*). When the child eats, a *bolus* dose of insulin can be given by pressing buttons on the pump. CSII is an alternative treatment method for type 1 diabetes mellitus. In comparison with insulin injections, CSII more closely mimics the action of the non-diabetic pancreas. The child/family must learn with the help of their diabetes specialist team to adjust the insulin doses (basal and bolus) according to the child's requirements.

The pump contains a reservoir that holds the insulin. Attached to this is a thin catheter with a small needle/indwelling cannula at the other end. The needle/cannula is inserted into the subcutaneous tissue and can usually be left *in situ* for 2–3 days, after which a new infusion set should be inserted. As with insulin injections it is important to rotate sites to avoid lipohypertrophy.

Equipment

- Insulin pump. The equipment required depends upon the type of pump and cannula in use. For detailed information consult the local diabetes team/user manuals.
- Insulin reservoir and giving set.
- Rapid acting insulin.
- Cannula and insertion device.
- Clean paper tape.

Procedure

For changing the giving set and reservoir

- Check the insulin and prescription as per local policy.
- Using a clean technique, avoid touching the key parts.
- Fill the reservoir with the prescribed insulin (each manufacturer has a different reservoir and therefore different method of filling).
- Remove any air bubbles.
- Use the pump menu to rewind the piston.
- Attach the catheter giving set to the reservoir, following the manufacturers' instructions.
- Load and/or prime the set as described by each company manual.
- Explain the procedure to the child/family.
- Clean the insertion area if it is visibly dirty.
- Position the child according to the child's preference and cannula location. For infants and toddlers it may be easier if they are lying down.

- Cannulae can be inserted into the same places that insulin injections can be given:
  - The abdomen avoiding the umbilical region.
  - Lateral aspects of the upper arms.
  - Lateral aspect of thighs.
  - Upper-outer quadrant of buttocks.
  - The abdomen and buttocks are the preferred sites owing to the greater amount of subcutaneous tissue, therefore less risk of IM insertion.
- Follow the manufacturer's instructions to insert the cannula (the angle of insertion depends upon the cannula/device used).
- Once inserted, if using a cannula, remove the needle and dispose according to local guidelines.
- Fill the cannula as instructed by the pump.

Practice tips

- Remove insulin from the fridge approximately one hour before set change to allow it to reach room temperature, as cold insulin is more difficult to draw up without bubbles.
- For young children it is advisable to tape the catheter in loops to the body to prevent pulling or playing with the tubing.
- In infants a dressing such as duoderm can be used to prevent IM insertion as infants may have less subcutaneous tissue.
- It is recommended that people using an insulin pump test their BG level a minimum of four times a day (see 📖 Blood glucose monitoring, p. 98).
- If the BG is elevated (>14mmol/L or 252mg/L) check blood ketone levels, give a correction bolus and recheck the BG after 2h. If it hasn't decreased, change the reservoir, giving set and cannula and give a further bolus. Continue to monitor 2-hourly. If the BG remains elevated give a bolus using a rapid acting insulin pen and contact the pump manufacturer for further advice.

Pitfalls

- No long-acting insulin is used; therefore, the child will only have a small insulin depot. Any interruption to the supply of insulin (e.g. occlusion, leaking equipment, broken pump) puts them at increased risk of diabetic ketoacidosis. However, the child can be disconnected from their pump for a period of up to 1h before needing to be reconnected.
- If hypoglycaemic; give fast acting glucose (e.g. Lucozade, or glucose tablets), slower-acting carbohydrate is not required following this due to the smaller insulin depot compared to treatment by injection. This could cause the child to become hyperglycaemic.

Associated reading

Hanas R. (2007). *Type 1 Diabetes in Children, Adolescents and Young Adults*, 3rd edn. Class Publishing, London.

Haematology and immune system

Transfusion of blood and blood products

Background

Types of blood products

- Red cells.
- Platelets.
- Fresh frozen plasma (FFP).
- Cryoprecipitate.

Indications for transfusion

Red cells

- To replace acute blood loss due to haemorrhage, trauma, or surgery.
- Red cells are also transfused to children when they have significant anaemia* to increase the oxygen carrying capacity of the blood.
- To provide supportive care and treatment for certain types of chronic or malignant diseases, e.g. thalassaemia and leukaemia.

*The decision to transfuse in anaemia will usually be dependent on the clinical status of the child.

Platelets

For the prevention and treatment of haemorrhage in patients with thrombocytopaenia (reduced platelet count).

Fresh frozen plasma and cryoprecipitate

Transfused when there are coagulation factor deficiencies associated with severe bleeding.

Key concepts

❶ When transfusing blood and/or blood products ensure you have:
- The right patient.
- At the right time.
- The right product.

All members of staff involved in the collection, checking, and administration of blood and blood products should complete appropriate training as per local guidelines.

Red cell ABO compatibility

A child's blood group is determined by whether their red cells carry the anti-A, anti-B antigen, neither, or both (see Table 23.1) Healthy individuals make antibodies against the antigens that are not present in their own cells.

Table 23.1 Red cell ABO compatibility

Patient's ABO blood group	Patient's red cell antigen	Compatible red cells
A	Anti-B	A, O
B	Anti-A	B, O
AB	Anti-A and anti-B	A, B, AB, O
O	Neither	O

Calculating volumes for transfusion and recommended transfusion rates
Red cells
- Typical dose: volume (mL) = desired Hb rise (g/dL) × weight (kg) × 3.
- All red cells should be transfused within 4h of being removed from designated storage fridge.
- Typical administration rate 5mL/kg/h (max. 150mL/h).
- Faster infusion rates may be required in severe haemorrhage as per medical staff direction.

Platelets
- Typical dose:
  - Child <15kg: 10–20mL/kg.
  - Child >15kg single adult pack (typically 180–300mL).
- Typical administration rate 10–20mL/kg/h (usually 30–60min).

FFP and cryoprecipitate
- FFP typical dose: 10–20mL/kg.
- Cryoprecipitate typical dose: 5–10mL/kg.
- Typical administration rate 10–20mL/kg/h (usually 30–60min).

Equipment
- Working oxygen and suction near patient.
- Patient identification band.
- Patient information booklet.
- Blood prescription chart.
- Alcohol hand rub dispenser.
- Thermometer.
- Blood pressure (BP) monitor and appropriate sized cuff.
- Oxygen saturation monitor and probe.
- Observation chart.
- Patent and suitable venous access (access large enough to tolerate flow and rate of blood product).
- Blood transfusion compatibility form.
- Syringe and 0.9% saline solution (to check patency of venous access).
- Sterile chlorhexidine/alcohol swab.
- Blood administration giving set (with a 200µ filter).
- Electronic infusion device (only if manufacturers state suitable for blood transfusion).
- Well-fitting gloves (as per local policy).

Procedure

Pre-transfusion

- Provide the child and parents with appropriate information and explain procedure:
  - Use local blood transfusion information booklets.
  - Medical staff prescribing the blood product should discuss potential risks and benefits of the blood transfusion with the child and family.
  - Ensure child and family are aware of signs of an adverse reaction, and that they know to inform someone as soon as possible.
  - Obtain appropriate blood transfusion prescription ensuring it is prescribed correctly, with any special blood requirements documented, e.g. cytomegalovirus (CMV) negative, irradiated, etc.
  - Ensure correct volumes are prescribed utilizing equations given in 📖 Calculating volumes for transfusion and recommended ransfusion rates, p, 593. If volumes prescribed differ from those advised, discuss with medical staff to establish reasoning.
- Check that the child has appropriate and patent venous access (flush with 0.9% NaCl bolus) utilizing aseptic non-touch technique (ANTT).
- Ensure the child is wearing a correct and fully completed ID band.
- Obtain and record the child's baseline observations, to include: temperature, pulse, respiratory rate, BP, oxygen saturations, and conscious level (Alert, Voice, Pain, Unresponsive (AVPU) or Glasgow Coma Score (GCS)).
- Take blood transfusion prescription to the designated blood storage fridge/blood bank to collect the product required.
- Check the details on the prescription against the blood product label, and the compatibility form. To include: patient identification details, expiry date of unit, the donation number (matches on unit and compatibility form), special requirements, blood group compatibility.
  - If there is any discrepancy *do not* take the blood product, check details with blood bank staff.
  - Follow local policy for the collection of blood products from the designated storage area/blood bank.
- Once taken to clinical area, the blood product should be used as soon as possible. If there is no fluid warmer, it should be left for a short period (used within 30min) to prevent the cold fluid causing shock.
- Check all details with qualified second checker.
- When all details checked and confirmed, utilize appropriate blood product administration set and prime this with blood product.
- Positively identify child prior to commencing transfusion, with second checker. Where possible ask the child to verbally identify themselves (full name and date of birth), or check with parents. Ensure all details match on name band and prescription.
- Once all details are confirmed with exact matches, connect blood product to intravenous access using ANTT (first, check patency again with bolus of 0.9% saline).
- Programme electronic infusion device with correct rate (mL/h) as per prescription. If child is not receiving a full unit, then ensure a 'volume to be infused' has been programmed into pump, as prescribed, to prevent over transfusion.
- Commence transfusion.

- Both qualified staff should sign for the transfusion and document the start time and date.

During transfusion
- A qualified member of staff should remain with the patient for the first 5min of the transfusion.
- Observations should be repeated 15min from the start of the transfusion: temperature, pulse, respirations, BP, and oxygen saturations. Check local guidelines for observation frequency—protocols may vary.
- If any signs of a transfusion reaction are evident, then the transfusion should be stopped and medical staff contacted (see 📖 Managing transfusion reactions, p. 598).
- If required, administer diuretic at prescribed dose and time.
- Maintain fluid balance record.

Post-transfusion
- Obtain and record a full set of observations (as 📖 During transfusion, p. 595).
- Disconnect blood product and flush venous access device 0.9% saline using ANTT (do not flush giving set through with 0.9% saline as this will dislodge debris from the filter).
- Dispose of blood/blood product bag, as per local policy.
- Document end time and date of transfusion.
- Ensure that all fluid administered is recorded on fluid balance chart including cannula patency flushes if child is having their fluid balance strictly monitored.

Practice tips
- Some children do not like looking at the blood product whilst it is being transfused. Use a pillow case to cover the bag.
- When the giving set has been primed with the blood product, be aware that it may splash when removing the cap. Holding the end of the line with an alcohol wipe may prevent this.
- Do not administer blood products overnight, unless it is an emergency or directed by medical personnel, as it is difficult to observe the child closely and their sleep will be disturbed with frequent observations.
- Observe venous access site hourly throughout transfusion to monitor for signs of extravasation—stop transfusion if this occurs and inform medical staff immediately.
- Sometimes, it may be necessary to remove a connector or bung from the end of the intravenous (IV) access device to enable adequate flow of blood or platelets.
- Platelet transfusions should never be given using an electronic infusion device as this destroys the platelets.
- If administering platelets via a cannula, they may not flow if the cannula is positional, or stiff. In an emergency, you may need to use a 50-mL syringe to administer the platelet transfusion.
- If the child is receiving IV fluids, parenteral nutrition (PN) or IV drugs via another lumen of central venous line (CVL) or another IV access point, check with medical staff if these should continue during transfusion, especially if there is a risk the child may become fluid overloaded.

- Do not let the child leave the clinical area without supervision from a qualified member of staff with the equipment to manage an adverse reaction.
- Remember that for followers of the Jehovah's Witness faith, the administration of blood and blood products is prohibited. Medical staff should discuss this with the child and family. Alternatives will be used where possible. However, in life-threatening situations, two consultants can make the decision to administer blood and blood products. Legal advice should be sought.

Associated reading

Watson D and Hearnshaw K. (2010). Understanding blood group and transfusion in nursing practice. *Nursing Standard* **24**(30), 41–8.

Managing transfusion reactions

Managing transfusion reactions

Background

Transfusion of blood and blood products carries the risk of a transfusion-related reaction. These adverse reactions vary from mild allergic reactions to anaphylaxis or multi-organ failure.

Signs or symptoms of acute transfusion reaction

- Urticaria (raised red rash).
- Pruritus (itching).
- Flushing.
- Fever.
- Rigors.
- Tachycardia.
- Hyper or hypotension.
- Chest pain.
- Abdominal pain.
- Shortness of breath.
- Respiratory distress.
- Nausea.
- Feeling unwell.
- Feelings of 'impending doom'.

Mild allergic reaction

These reactions usually result in urticaria and pruritus shortly after the transfusion has started. This mild reaction is more often seen in platelet and FFP transfusions due to the high plasma content.

Equipment

- IV chlorphenamine (dose as prescribed).
- Syringes ×2.
- Needle ×2.
- NaCl 0.9% solution.
- Thermometer.
- BP monitor and appropriate sized cuff.
- Oxygen saturation monitor and probe.

Procedure

- Slow transfusion or stop if symptoms severe (do not disconnect transfusion from IV access).
- Obtain repeat observations of temperature, pulse, respiratory rate, blood pressure, oxygen saturations.
- Contact medical team and ask for prompt review.
- Consider the administration of IV chlorphenamine.
- Continue with transfusion after 30min if symptoms subside (transfusion may need to be slowed down).
- Increase frequency of observations.
- If recurrent problem child may need premedication with IV chlorphenamine for subsequent transfusions.

Febrile non-haemolytic transfusion reaction

The child will experience a rise in temperature (>1.5°C above baseline), and may also have a rigor. This is most commonly seen with red cell and platelet transfusions.

It is important to note that the fever and rigors associated with these reactions could be the first sign of a severe haemolytic reaction.

Equipment
- Paracetamol (oral or IV dependent on patient status and IV access).
- Thermometer.
- BP monitor and appropriate sized cuff.
- Oxygen saturation monitor and probe.

Procedure
- Slow the transfusion (stop if symptoms severe and seek medical assistance—do not disconnect transfusion from IV access).
- Obtain repeat observation of temperature, pulse, respiration rate, BP, oxygen saturations.
- Give paracetamol (if prescribed) if temperature rise <1.5°C above baseline and patient otherwise well (otherwise seek prompt medical review).
- Restart transfusion at slower rate.
- Increase frequency of observations.

Anaphylaxis (severe allergic reaction)

This can result in life-threatening cardiovascular collapse, bronchospasm and airway compromise.

Equipment
- High flow oxygen (15L via non-rebreathe mask).
- IV chlorphenamine.
- Salbutamol nebulizer.
- Intramuscular (IM) adrenaline.
- 0.9% saline solution.
- Arrest trolley.
- Thermometer.
- BP machine and appropriate sized cuff.
- Oxygen saturation monitor and probe.

Procedure
- ❶ Stop transfusion.
- ❶ Call for help (activate paediatric arrest call if required or seek urgent senior medical assistance).
- Maintain airway and administer high flow oxygen.
- Obtain observations of temperature, pulse, respiration rate, BP, and connect to continuous oxygen saturation monitoring.
- Disconnect transfusion product from IV access (keep for returning blood product and giving set to blood bank once patient stabilized).
- Follow anaphylaxis protocol once medical assistance on ward.
- Inform blood bank and obtain blood samples from the patient as directed.
- The child will usually need to be transferred to the intensive care unit.
- Follow local trust protocol for documenting and reporting serious adverse drug reactions.

ABO incompatibility/acute haemolytic reaction

Incompatible transfused red cells will react with the patient's anti-A or anti-B antibodies leading to an acute severe reaction. These reactions occur soon after commencing the transfusion with symptoms including: restlessness, fever, feelings of 'impending doom', chest pain, abdominal pain, shortness of breath, hypotension, and shock. The child may later have haemoglobinuria (high haemoglobin levels in urine) and renal failure can follow.

These reactions more commonly occur as a result of errors in the checking procedure at one or more stages of the transfusion process.

Equipment
- High flow oxygen (15L via non-rebreathe mask).
- 0.9% saline solution.
- Thermometer.
- BP machine and appropriate sized cuff.
- Oxygen saturation monitor and probe.
- Empty unused sharps bin.
- Bedpans/urine bottles (for monitoring urine output).
- Catheter (may be required).
- Urine testing strips.
- Blood bottles (for urea & electrolytes (U&E) and liver function tests (LFTs), repeat cross-match).

Procedure
- ❶ Stop the transfusion.
- ❶ Call for help (activate paediatric arrest call if required or seek urgent senior medical assistance).
- Maintain airway and administer high flow oxygen.
- Obtain frequent observations of temperature, pulse, respiration rate, BP and connect child to continuous oxygen saturation monitoring.
- Check patient ID band, compatibility label on unit being transfused and compatibility form from blood bank.
- Disconnect unit and giving set.
- Urgently inform blood bank and return unit intact to blood bank in unused sharps bin.
- Maintain IV access with 0.9% saline.
- Monitor urine output and catheterize child if necessary. Test urine for presence of haemoglobin.
- Maintain urine output 1–2mL/kg/h (furosemide may be required).
- Send baseline U&Es and LFTs, obtain a fresh cross-match sample and send to blood bank urgently.
- The child will often need to be transferred to the intensive care unit (ICU).
- Follow local trust protocol for reporting and documenting serious adverse events.

Transfusion transmitted infection

Bacterial contamination of blood products is rare, but is still a potential complication of transfusions. More commonly seen in platelet transfusions than red cells, the symptoms of this reaction mimic those of an acute haemolytic reaction or severe allergic reaction, including rapid onset of hyper- or hypotension, rigors, and collapse.

Equipment
- As for acute haemolytic reaction.
- Broad spectrum IV antibiotics.

Procedure
- As per acute haemolytic reaction.
- In addition take repeat full blood count (FBC), blood cultures, coagulation screen, biochemistry.
- Commence broad spectrum IV antibiotics.
- Discuss with haematologist.

Transfusion related acute lung injury (TRALI)

The plasma of one of the donors contains antibodies that react strongly with the child's leucocytes, which can lead to symptoms of breathlessness, non-productive cough and fever. There are typical appearances evident on chest X-ray.

Equipment
- High flow oxygen (15L via non-rebreathe mask).
- Thermometer.
- BP machine and appropriate sized cuff.
- Oxygen saturation monitor and probe.
- Empty unused sharps bin.
- Arrest trolley (may be required).

Procedure
- ❶ Stop the transfusion.
- ❶ Call for help (activate paediatric arrest call if required or seek urgent senior medical assistance).
- Maintain airway and administer high flow oxygen.
- Obtain frequent observations of temperature, pulse, respiration rate, BP and connect child to continuous oxygen saturation monitoring.
- Disconnect unit and giving set.
- Urgently inform blood bank and return unit intact to blood bank in unused sharps bin.
- The child will usually need to be transferred to intensive care as mechanical ventilation is often required.
- Follow local trust protocol for reporting and documenting serious adverse reactions.

Practice tips

- Children who are unconscious, have reduced conscious levels, or those who cannot talk are more difficult to assess for signs of a transfusion reaction, and therefore more frequent observations will be necessary.
- Obtain a transfusion history prior to any transfusion, so that you are aware of any previous reactions.
- Children who have previously experienced a transfusion reaction may have a pre-medication of IV steroid and IV antihistamine prior to commencing the transfusion.
- Liaise with the parents or family to ensure someone remains with the child during the transfusion (particularly for the first 30min).
- Communicate with the child and family so that they are aware to inform a member of staff if the child feels unwell, they are concerned, or if they are showing signs of a transfusion reaction.
- Ensure that all members of staff on the ward are aware that a transfusion is in progress and who is receiving it.
- If the child experiences an adverse reaction it is important to keep the child and parents informed of their condition and the care required.
- Keep calm and focused on the child.
- In any emergency situation always ensure you have easy access to the child and surroundings.
- If the child is distressed, encourage one parent to stay with the child and reassure them (but always ensure you have easy access to the child and equipment).

Associated reading

Gray A et al. (2007). Safe transfusion of blood and blood components. *Nursing Standard* **21**(51), 40–7.

Care of the immunocompromised child or young person

Background

Children and young people may be immunocompromised for a variety of reasons these include:

- Chronic disease processes, such as severe combined immune deficiency syndrome (SCIDS).
- Administration of medications, such as chemotherapy and corticoid steroids, which affect the body's ability to provide immunity.

Children who are immunocompromised need to be protected from contracting bacterial, viral, and fungal infections, usually dealt with by a functioning immune system. It is important to remember that children with health problems may have many portals for the entry of infection into their bodies such as CVL, gastrostomy, and wounds amongst others. Local policy should always be adhered to and practice may vary particularly in specialist treatment areas, such as bone marrow and organ transplantation.

Vaccinations may be offered to some immune-compromised children.

Equipment

In hospital

- A single room suitable for reverse barrier nursing, preferably with a double door and air lock facility. Air lock is vital for severely immunocompromised children, such as those receiving bone marrow transplants, or post-organ transplant.
- Protective outer wear in accordance with local policy, e.g. gloves, aprons, face masks.
- Hand-washing facilities inside and outside the room.
- Single use equipment or specific equipment for that child/young person for example multi-parameter monitor.
- Consider nurse allocation and ward area in which the child shall be nursed to help avoid cross-contamination.
- In some circumstances provision of sterile water and avoidance of certain foods is recommended.
- Use of ANTT where appropriate.

Procedure

In hospital

- Careful observe the child/young person for signs and symptoms of infection.
- Provide appropriate treatment for existing infection, in accordance with local policy.
- Maintenance of hand hygiene.
- Limit visitor numbers when deemed necessary.
- Adhere to local infection control policy.
- Prepare and educate with regard to reverse barrier nursing and hand hygiene for the child/young person and their family.
- Arrange play therapy and access to age appropriate communication tools, such as email to help alleviate boredom and feelings of isolation.

At home/school/college/work

- Maintenance of usual activities and social interaction as is safe and desirable for the child/young person.
- Education for the child/young person and any others involved in their care, including teachers, child minders, etc., should be provided in verbal and written form on areas such as:
  - Avoidance of any building works as brick dust may contain aspergillus.
  - Avoidance of some pets that may carry disease.
  - Avoidance of individuals known to have contagious infections.
  - Maintenance of good personal hygiene.
  - Notification for the child/young person and their family if someone in their nursery/school/college has a known contagious disease, such as chickenpox.
  - Monitoring and acting upon pyrexia, pain, or symptoms of sepsis.
- Ensure a pathway for self and immediate referral to specialist health care is provided in case of suspected onset of sepsis.
- Ensure appropriate community support is available for the child/young person and their family.

Practice tips

- Be aware of local policy with regard to initiation of treatment in immunocompromised children.
- Be aware of local septic screening protocol for immunocompromised children.
- Some children may receive treatments to help improve their immunity.

Pitfalls

- Temperature measurement equipment may vary, ensure continuity of assessment.
- Encourage children/young people to observe CVL site/gastrostomy site, etc., for signs of infection and to maintain hygiene.

Associated reading

Abbas A, Lichtman A. (2010). *Basic Immunology: Functions and Disorders of the Immune System*, 3rd edn. Saunders Elsevier, Philadelphia.

Hemsworth P. (2006). Pet ownership in immunocompromised children: a review of the literature and survey of existing guidelines. *Eur J Oncol Nurs* **10**(2), 117–27.

Royal College of Paediatrics and Child Health (2002). *Immunisation of the Immunocompromised Child: Best Practice Statement*. RCPCH, London.

Index